Motor Unit Number Estimation (MUNE)

Proceedings of the First International Symposium on MUNE, Snowbird, Utah, USA, 13–15 July 2001

EDITED BY

M.B. BROMBERG

Department of Neurology, Neuromuscular Program and EMG Laboratory, University of Utah, 50 N. Medical Drive, Room 3R152, Salt Lake City, UT 84132, USA

SUPPLEMENTS TO CLINICAL NEUROPHYSIOLOGY
VOLUME 55
2003

ELSEVIER

AMSTERDAM – BOSTON – LONDON – NEW YORK – OXFORD – PARIS – SAN DIEGO
SAN FRANCISCO – SINGAPORE – SYDNEY – TOKYO

ELSEVIER SCIENCE B.V.
Sara Burgerhartstraat 25
P.O. Box 211, 1000 AE Amsterdam, The Netherlands

First edition 2003

Library of Congress Cataloging in Publication Data
Symposium on Motor Unit Number Estimation (1st : 2001 : Snowbird, Utah)
Motor unit number estimation (MUNE) : proceedings of the First International Symposium on MUNE, Snowbird, Utah, USA, 13-15 July 2001 / edited by M.B. Bromberg.
p. cm. -- (Supplements to Clinical neurophysiology ; .v.55)
Includes bibliographical references and index.
ISBN 0-444-50723-X (hb : alk. paper)
1. Motor neurons--Congresses. 2. Electromyography--Congresses. 3. Electrodiagnosis--Congresses. I. Title: MUNE. II. Bromberg, M. B. (Mark B.) III. Title. IV. Series.

QP369.S945 2003
616.7'407547--dc21 2003044055

British Library Cataloguing in Publication Data
International Symposium on MUNE (1st : 2001 : Snowbird, Utah)
Motor unit number estimation (MUNE) : proceedings of the First International Symposium on MUNE, Snowbird, Utah, USA, 13-15 July 2001. - (Supplements to Clinical neurophysiology ; v. 55, 2003)
1. Motor neurons - Congresses 2.Neurophysiology - Congresses
I.Title II.Bromberg, M. B. III. Clinical neurophysiolgy
612.8'252

ISBN 044450723X

ISBN: 0-444-50723-X
ISSN (series): 1567-424X

∞ The paper used in this publication meets the requirements of ANSI/NISO Z39.48-1992 (Permanence of Paper).
Printed in The Netherlands.

Preface

My personal interest in motor unit number estimation (MUNE) arose after reading a description of the spike triggered averaging technique in 1988. Shortly thereafter, I tried the technique on a patient with ALS and found large motor units and a low motor unit count. With the addition of fiber density and macro-EMG information, I was impressed that I was seeing first hand some of the underlying lower motor neuron changes in ALS. I quickly became acquainted with other MUNE techniques and the history of the technique. The original incremental stimulation technique described by Alan McComas in 1971 seemed particularly elegant in its simplicity and its grounding in basic neurophysiology. Shortly thereafter, the principles and issues of MUNE were explored in a series of papers by William Brown and colleagues that brought home the complexities of MUNE. William Brown's exploration resulted in several modifications to the incremental technique as well as the development of the F-wave and multiple point stimulation techniques. Interest in MUNE was rekindled in the late 1980s, and the statistical MUNE technique developed by Jasper Daube represented a new way to estimate motor unit size. Over the past 10 years there have been many informal discussions about MUNE during national and international meetings, but the brief time available and the limited number of participants hindered a full discussion. Three years ago I thought it timely to attempt to organize a full meeting on MUNE. An international meeting was a bold proposal, but all of my colleagues were supportive, and the symposium became a reality.

Mark B. Bromberg
Salt Lake City, UT, USA

Dedication

I dedicate the proceedings to my father, Walter Bromberg, MD, who influenced me more than he knew.

Introduction

The First International Symposium on MUNE represents for me a long-term desire to bring together investigators interested in MUNE to hear and discuss the issues. The field of MUNE arose from the original publication by Alan McComas and coworkers in 1971 on a noninvasive electrophysiologic method to estimate the number of motor units innervating a human muscle. Prior to this symposium there had been no previous meeting that focused on MUNE. As interest in MUNE grew, the American Association of Electrodiagnostic Medicine supported a special interest group (SIG) in MUNE at their annual meeting. It was during one of the SIG meetings that the term "Motor Unit Number Estimation" was agreed upon. A one-day satellite workshop was held in conjunction with international meetings on single fiber EMG and computerized and quantitative EMG in 1993 in which several MUNE techniques were demonstrated.

The First International Symposium was successful in bringing together physiologists, clinical electromyographers, EMG industry representatives and a representative from the Food and Drug Administration. Prior to the publication of these Proceedings there has been no monograph devoted to MUNE, and it is hoped that these Proceedings represent an accurate report for those who could not attend.

The Proceedings are organized to follow the Symposium's agenda. Speakers were asked to submit a manuscript of their talk. Open discussions were held after each series of talks. The discussions were recorded and have been edited to make them flow smoothly. This format should provide the reader with a good understanding of the symposium, and the ability to find information about specific topics.

Acknowledgements

For me, MUNE represents basic neurophysiology in a clinical setting. Since my research career started in basic neurophysiology, I first acknowledge Arnold Towe, my mentor during my postdoctural fellowship at the University of Washington, for giving me a solid base for viewing the nervous system and critical ways of reviewing data. Several years later I decided to shift my career from basic to clinical science, and Sid Gilman was a role model of a clinical scientist. I could not have been made the career change without the support and help of Judith Abrams, and I acknowledge her pivotal role in successfully making this change. She also gave me an appreciation for the role of statistics and was an immeasurable help with my early research efforts, particularly in MUNE. When I changed to clinical neurophysiology, my clinical mentor, James Albers, give me a similar solid base for viewing the peripheral nervous system and critical ways of gathering and reviewing data. I also acknowledge Erik Stålberg for his support and for giving me my foundation in quantitative EMG. In the area of MUNE, William Brown helped with my early efforts with the spike triggered averaging technique. Jasper Daube has provided a continuous stream of provocative discussions about MUNE and has been a major advisor for my efforts for this symposium. It has been my great pleasure to know and work with Alan McComas, the father of MUNE, who has been a most enthusiastic supporter of my efforts.

I have had many colleagues helping me in my MUNE research efforts. Shortly after becoming acquainted with MUNE, we participated in a small multicenter drug trial for ALS that used the spike triggered averaging MUNE technique as a secondary endpoint measure. This perhaps represented the first use of MUNE in a drug trial, and I acknowledge Walter Bradley and Rup Tandan for their foresight in considering MUNE as an endpoint measure, and Timothy Fries for collecting MUNE data at the second site. This trial was academically productive for me, and I acknowledge the support and assistance of Dallas Forshew in gathering data.

The symposium truly represented a joint effort by many people. My steering committee, Jasper Daube, Catherine Lowmen-Hoerth, and Jeremy Shefner, was most helpful in organizing and giving shape to the program. My local colleagues, Gordon Smith, Victoria Lawson and Kathy Swoboda have been supportive. Elly Tjoa, from Elsevier Science, has been supportive in putting together the Proceedings.

The Symposium would not have been possible without the financial support of the Harris and Amanda Simmons Foundation, and the Symposium is in memory of Margaret Pahnke, Amanda Simmons' mother. John Edwards from the University of Utah Development Office has been helpful and wrote the biographical sketch of Margaret Pahnke. Aventis Pharmaceuticals has continued their longstanding support for ALS with generous financial for the symposium, along with Elan Pharmaceuticals. MUNE represents a unique relationship between clinicians and EMG equipment manufacturers, and Nicolet Biomedical, Neuroscan Medical Systems, Medtronic and Oxford Instruments were supportive not only financially but also with demonstration equipment and active participation in the symposium.

My heartfelt thanks goes to Rosalie Lammle from the Continuing Medical Education Office. Rosalie was there from the beginning to the end, and literally made everything happen!

On a personal side, I acknowledge the support of my wife, Diane Banks-Bromberg, who always listened and whose excellent suggestions smoothed out the kinks along the way. I also acknowledge my daugher, Katherine Sarah Bromberg, who has kept me young and on my toes.

Remembrance

This Symposium is in memory of Margaret Pahnke.

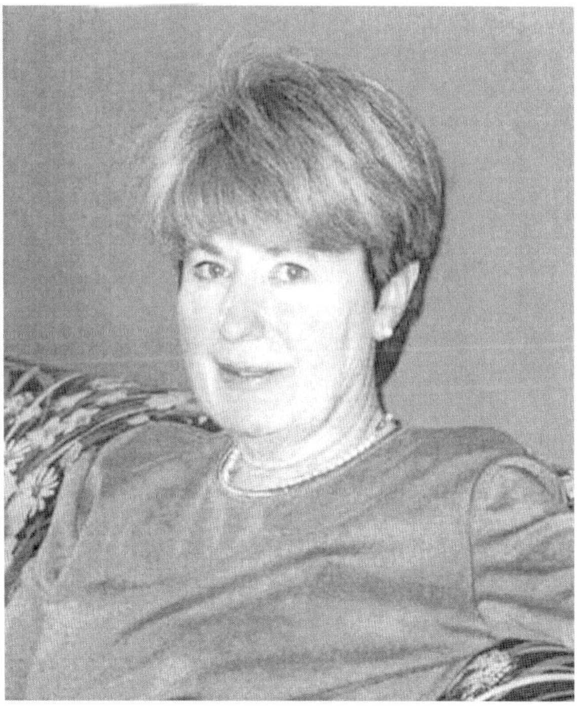

Margaret Pahnke
June 12, 1940 to February 14, 2001

Margaret Pahnke died from ALS.

In dealing with her fate she taught her family lessons they would never have learned otherwise. Lessons about acceptance without capitulation, lessons about the lasting impact a mother has on her children, and lessons about living life.

In a way Margaret had it her way, both ways. As a stay-at-home mother she raised five daughters and a son.

But before marriage and kids and after raising the children she packed in a lot of living of another kind. As a single woman she worked in San Francisco and began a life long love affair with the city.

After the kids were raised she worked in the sometimes frenzied world of the Utah Legislature, then for the Utah arts Council, and finally as an administrative assistant in the University of Utah Government Relations office.

She always found time for another true passion – travel. Like reading and learning it was something she could not get enough of. She traveled for pleasure, she traveled to help educate her children and she traveled on behalf of yet another passion, the Children's Dance Theater.

However, the one destination that always eluded her was Paris. Getting there became an obsession, but somehow it did not happen until 1999. It was to be a very personal trip, just Margaret and her husband, Ralph. But when they arrived the city was in the throes of a massive strike. Places were closed down and public transportation barely existed. The couple ended up walking around the "City of Lights". It was not convenient, but walking has always been the best way to experience a great city. It was during these Parisian strolls that Margaret began feeling something was not quite right.

Upon her return to Salt Lake, she resumed work and playing tennis but in December she realized her left leg was not working. After a frustrating month of tests, came the crushing news... Amyotrophic Lateral Sclerosis.

She was referred to Dr. Mark Bromberg in the University of Utah's Neurology Department. There, one day, gathered the entire family. In a 3-h session Margaret's limited and horrifying future was laid out. Daughter, Amanda Simmons, remembers "everyone cried except Mom".

Margaret accepted the description of her short future with a heroic stoicism. Amanda remembers her attitude as very much, "why not me? Why should it be someone else?"

Life's cruel curveballs did not stop there. During Margaret's final year lightning struck and heavily damaged the Pahnke home. Amanda Simmons says during the 4 months it took to rebuild the home all of Margaret's children "got to take care of her. It gave us a whole new perspective on how she raised us".

Margaret died in February of 2001, 7 weeks after moving back into her home and 53 weeks after being diagnosed.

It is in her honor that the Harris and Amanda Simmons Foundation has contributed the funds to help support this conference.

It would have been Margaret's hope that some of the people attending will make a significant contribution in the management and treatment of ALS.

After all, to paraphrase her attitude.

Why Not You?

Why should it be someone else?

Written by John Edwards

List of Contributors

Arasaki, K., EMG/EEG Laboratory, Department of Neurology, NTT East Kanto Medical Center, 5-9-22 Higashi-Gotanda, Shinagawa-ku, Tokyo 141-0022, Japan.
Armon, C., Department of Neurology, Loma Linda University School of Medicine, Loma Linda, CA 92354, USA.
Barkhaus, P.E., Medical College of Wisconsin and Milwaukee, VA Medical Center, Milwaukee, WI, USA.
Bouquiaux, O., Department of Physical Medicine and Rehabilitation, CHU Sart Tilman, B35, B-4000 Liège, Belgium.
Bromberg, M.B., Department of Neurology, University of Utah School of Medicine, Room 3R152, 50 North Medical Drive, Salt Lake City, UT 84132, USA.
Brown, W.F., Department of Neurology, Tuft's University, Boston, MA, USA.
Bryan, W.W., Division of Clinical Trial Design and Analysis, Office of Therapeutics Research and Review, Center for Biologics Evaluation and Research, Food and Drug Administration, 1401 Rockville Pike, Rockville, MD 20852, USA.
Butler, J., Department of Medicine, Division of Neurology (4U1), McMaster University Medical Centre, 1200 Main Street West, Hamilton, ON L8N 3Z5, Canada.
Chan, K.M., Division of Physical Medicine and Rehabilitation, 513 Heritage Medical Research Center, University of Alberta, Edmonton, AB T6G 2S2, Canada.
Conwit, R.A., Department of Neurology, Johns Hopkins Bayview Medical Center, 4940 Eastern Avenue, Baltimore, MD 21224, USA.
Daube, J.R., Department of Neurology – E8B, Mayo Clinic, Rochester, MN 55905, USA.
Delwaide, P.J., University Department of Neurology, B-4000 Liège, Belgium.
De Pasqua, V., Department of Physical Medicine and Rehabilitation, CHU Sart Tilman, B35, B-4000 Liège, Belgium.
Doherty, T.J., Department of Physical Medicine and Rehabilitation, University of Western Ontario, London, ON N6A 1Y6, Canada.
Fehlings, D., Bloorview MacMillan Centre, Toronto, ON, Canada.
Galea, V., School of Rehabilitation Science, McMaster University Medical Centre, Hamilton, ON L8N 3Z5, Canada.
Gooch, C.L., Department of Neurology, Columbia Presbyterian Medical Center, 710 West 168th Street, New York, NY 10032, USA.
Griggs, R., University of Rochester, New York, NY, USA.
Kaufmann, P., Department of Neurology, Columbia Presbyterian Medical Center, 710 West 168th Street, New York, NY 10032, USA.
Kirsch, S., Bloorview MacMillan Centre, Toronto, ON, Canada.
Krajewski, K., Department of Neurology and Center for Molecular Medicine and Genetics, Wayne State University School of Medicine, UHC 8D, 4201 St. Antoine, Detroit, MI 48201, USA.
Lawson, V.H., Department of Neurology, University of Utah, 50 North Medical Drive, Room 3R210, Salt Lake City, UT 84132, USA.
Leedham, J., Neuroscan, 18713 Potomac Station Drive, Leesburg, VA 20176, USA.
Lewis, R.A., Department of Neurology, Wayne State University School of Medicine, UHC 8D, 4201 St. Antoine, Detroit, MI 48201, USA.
Li, J., Department of Neurology, Wayne State University School of Medicine, UHC 8D, 4201 St. Antoine, Detroit, MI 48201, USA.
Lomen-Hoerth, C., Department of Neurology, Box 0114, University of California, San Francisco, School of Medicine, 505 Parnassus Avenue, M348, San Francisco, CA 94143-0114, USA.
Maertens de Noordhout, A., University Department of Neurology, B-4000 Liège, Belgium.

Martin, J., Department of Medicine, Division of Neurology (4U1), McMaster University Medical Centre, 1200 Main Street West, Hamilton, ON L8N 3Z5, Canada.
McComas, A., Department of Medicine, Division of Neurology (4U1), McMaster University Medical Centre, 1200 Main Street West, Hamilton, ON L8N 3Z5, Canada.
Metter, E.J., National Institute on Aging, Gerontology Research Center, Baltimore, MD, USA.
Nandedkar, D.S., Rensselaer Polytechnic Institute, Troy, NY, USA.
Nandedkar, S.D., Oxford Instruments Medical Systems, 12 Skyline Drive, Hawthorne, NY 10532, USA.
Olney, R.K., Department of Neurology, Box 0114, University of California, San Francisco, School of Medicine, 505 Parnassus Avenue, San Francisco, CA 94143-0114, USA.
Petajan, J.H., Department of Neurology, University of Utah, 50 North Medical Drive, Salt Lake City, UT 84132, USA.
Quartly, C., Faculty of Health Sciences, McMaster University, Hamilton, ON L8N 3Z5, Canada.
Shefner, J.M., Department of Neurology, Upstate Medical University, 750 E. Adams Street, HSC Syracuse, Syracuse, NY 13210, USA.
Shy, M.E., Department of Neurology and Center for Molecular Medicine and Genetics, Wayne State University School of Medicine, UHC 8D, 4201 St. Antoine, Detroit, MI 48201, USA.
Sica, R., Division of Neurology, Hospital Ramos Mejía, Urquiza 609, 1221 Buenos Aires, Argentina.
Slawnych, M.P., Faculty of Medicine, Health Sciences Centre, University of Calgary, 3330 Hospital Drive N.W., Calgary, AB T2N 4N1, Canada.
Smith, A.G., Department of Neurology, University of Utah, 50 North Medical Drive, Room 3R152, Salt Lake City, UT 84132, USA.
Smith, B.E., Department of Neurology, Mayo Clinic Scottsdale, 13400 East Shea Boulevard, Scottsdale, AZ 85259, USA.
Sorenson, E.J., Department of Neurology – E8B, Mayo Clinic, Rochester, MN 55905, USA.
Stålberg, E.V., Department of Clinical Neurophysiology, Uppsala University Hospital, S-751 85 Uppsala, Sweden.
Stashuk, D.W., Department of Systems Design Engineering, University of Waterloo, Waterloo, ON N2L 3G1, Canada.
Swoboda, K.J., Department of Neurology, University of Utah School of Medicine, 3R210, 50 North Medical Drive, Salt Lake City, UT 84132, USA.
Trojaborg, W., Department of Neurology, Columbia Presbyterian Medical Center, 710 West 168th Street, New York, NY 10032, USA.
Turnbull, J., Department of Medicine, Division of Neurology (4U1), McMaster University Medical Centre, 1200 Main Street West, Hamilton, ON L8N 3Z5, Canada.
Upton, A.R.M., Department of Medicine (Neurology), McMaster University, Hamilton, ON L8N 3Z5, Canada.
Wang, F.C., Department of Physical Medicine and Rehabilitation, CHU Sart Tilman, B35, B-4000 Liège, Belgium.
Windebank, A.J., Department of Neurology – E8B, Mayo Clinic, Rochester, MN 55905, USA.

Contents

Section VII. MUNE Correlations with Other Metrics

Section VIII. MUNE in Clinical Practice

Section IX. MUNE in Clinical Trials

Section X. MUNE in Animal Studies

Section XI. MUNE Relationship with Industry and Regulatory Agencies

Section XII. Consensus

Section I

Special Lecture

Motor Unit Number Estimation (Supplements to Clinical Neurophysiology Vol. 55)
Editor: M.B. Bromberg

Chapter 1

Review of MUNE over 30 years

Roberto Sica[a] and Alan McComas[b,*]

[a]*Division of Neurology, Hospital Ramos Mejía, Urguiza 609, 1221 Buenos Aires, Argentina*
[b]*Department of Medicine, Division of Neurology (4U1), McMaster University Medical Centre, 1200 Main Street West, Hamilton, ON L8N 3Z5, Canada*

The importance of studying motor units

There are several good reasons why motor unit number estimation (MUNE) deserves attention. First, such studies supply information about the structure and organization of the human brainstem and spinal cord, and about the innervation of muscles, which would otherwise not be available. Further, these electrophysiological determinations can be obtained in living human beings, a fact which is quite remarkable given that the only other cells, for which total estimates can be made during life, are the different types of blood cell. Second, MUNE offers the possibility of studying age effects on motoneuron populations. Third, the natural history of muscle denervating disorders, such as amyotrophic lateral sclerosis (ALS), spinal muscular atrophy (SMA), poliomyelitis and different types of peripheral neuropathy, can be established. Related to this, is the opportunity to look at the results of therapeutic interventions by means of serial MUNEs. Another reason for MUNE research is to look at the power of collateral reinnervation as a compensatory phenomenon in denervating disorders. MUNE may also draw attention to hitherto unsuspected pathophysiological aspects of diseases. Finally, MUNE offers the electromyographer a powerful new diagnostic tool. Some of these applications are considered below, while others are dealt with more fully elsewhere in the symposium proceedings.

In addition to providing a historical review of MUNE, the present chapter provides an answer to a puzzling question, namely, why it was that a methodology with such important and obvious applications was not widely adopted after the initial reports appeared. Why, indeed, were 30 years to elapse before this, the first international symposium on MUNE?

Anatomical studies of motor unit numbers

Sir Charles Sherrington appears to have been the first to recognize that a single motor nerve fiber and the colony of muscle fibers which it supplies constitute a unit of contraction. In a paper, written with Liddell (Liddell and Sherrington, 1925) on recruitment and reflex inhibition, he referred fleetingly to the motor unit as "the motoneuron-axon and its adjunct muscle fibers", and he drew attention to its all-or-nothing responsiveness. Four years later, in delivering the Ferrier Lecture to the Royal Society of London, Sherrington (1929) defined the motor

**Correspondence to*: Dr. Alan J. McComas, Division of Neurology (4U1), McMaster University Medical Centre, 1200 Main Street West, Hamilton, ON L8N 3Z5, Canada. Tel.: (905)-525-9140x22519; fax: (905)-521-2656; e-mail: mccomas@fhs.mcmaster.ca

doi: 10.1016/S1567-424X(03)00001-1

unit as "an individual motor nerve-fiber together with the bunch of muscle-fibers it activates. Each such 'motor unit' has centrally, of course, a nerve-cell of which a group or 'pool' represents the muscle in the spinal cord". Sherrington went on to interpret the excitatory and inhibitory reflexes of the spinal cord in terms of the numbers of motor units involved and, by extension, on the central excitatory and inhibitory states impinging on the motoneurons. At the time of these pioneering studies, Sherrington was Regius Professor of Physiology at Oxford and was in the last years of a remarkably successful career, a career which had culminated in the study of the reflex activity of the mammalian spinal cord. It is intriguing to speculate what might have happened if Sherrington had continued his work a little longer and if his research team had not dispersed. With his optical recording system he had equipment which was sensitive enough to detect the reflex twitches of individual motor units in the cat hindlimb (Eccles and Sherrington, 1930), and he had taught himself to dissect motor axons from a nerve trunk, so that a study of single motor units, and even the first physiological MUNEs, would have been quite feasible. Instead, Sherrington retired, and his two most talented students, Denny-Brown and Eccles, left Oxford; not long after the second world war broke out.

Before the diaspora occurred, Eccles and Sherrington (1930) did collaborate in one investigation of motor units, namely, the numbers which were present in different cat muscles. To obtain these values, the dorsal nerve root ganglia were excised and, after sufficient time had elapsed for the sensory fibers to degenerate, the surviving myelinated fibers in the muscle nerve were counted and assumed to be motor. The values which Eccles and Sherrington obtained were about 640 for the semitendinosus, 430 for the medial gastrocnemius and 250 for the soleus. However, although the authors had noted that the myelinated nerve fibers tended to fall into two groups, in terms of their diameters, they assumed that both populations innervated skeletal muscle fibers and that the total count reflected the number of motor units. It was left to Leksell (1945), in Sweden, to show that the thinner (γ) axons supplied the small muscle fibers within the muscle spindles, and that only the thicker (α) axons innervated the skeletal fibers.

The first anatomical estimates of human motor unit numbers appeared well after the war had ended, by Feinstein et al. (1955) in Wohlfart's laboratory in Lund. While it was a simple, albeit, tedious task to count the large myelinated fibers in stained cross-sections of muscle nerves that had been taken from cadavers, the major uncertainty which these authors faced was the proportion of these axons which were α-motor, as opposed to sensory axons from the muscle spindles and tendon organs. However, the Lund group had previously examined the muscle nerve of a patient who had died after having had severe poliomyelitis and it was then possible to compare the counts of the larger fibers with those of the corresponding nerves from non-neurological cadavers. By subtraction, it appeared that the α-motor fibers made up approximately 60% of the large-diameter population and this was the percentage which Feinstein et al. (1955) adopted for their calculations.

The motor unit numbers of Feinstein et al. are given in Table 1, which also contains the results of other anatomical studies of human muscles, all of them made using Feinstein et al.'s ratio of 60 : 40 for motor and sensory axons, respectively. It can be seen that the extraocular muscles and the muscles of the jaw and neck all have large numbers of units. In contrast the small muscles of the hand each have about 100 units, while the larger muscles of the limbs have more units, in proportion to their sizes. Two of the values in Table 1 appear anomalous in the light of other data; these are the extremely high estimates for the opponens pollicis and the biceps brachii obtained by Christensen (1959). Other than axon branching, one possible reason is that the normal programmed death of motoneurons had yet to occur in some of the fetuses. However, the results of animal studies make it unlikely that this could account for a difference of an order of magnitude from the values in adults or, for that matter, in newborn children (cf. Fig. 1 in Campbell et al., 1973). In Table 1, the values of most interest to current MUNE practitioners are those for the hand muscles. Of these,

TABLE 1

ANATOMICAL ESTIMATION OF NUMBERS AND SIZES OF MOTOR UNITS IN VARIOUS HUMAN MUSCLES

Muscle	Reference	No. of motor units	Muscle fibers/unit
External rectus	Feinstein et al. (1955)	2970	9
Superior rectus (2)	Christensen (1959)	1779	23
Temporalis	Carlsöö (1958)	1331	936
Masseter (2)	Carlsöö (1958)	1425	2373
Platysma	Feinstein et al. (1955)	1096	25
Biceps brachii	Christensen (1959)	3552	163
Brachioradialis (2)	Feinstein et al. (1955)	333	>410
Opponens pollicis (6)	Christensen (1959)	6047	13
Thenar (median n.)	Lee et al. (1975)	203	–
First dorsal interosseous	Feinstein et al. (1955)	119	340
First lumbrical	Feinstein et al. (1955)	96	108
Abductor digiti minimi (10)	Santo Neto et al. (1985)	380	190
Opponens digiti minimi (4)	Carvalho et al. (1988)	158	100
Flexor digiti minimi (10)	Santo Neto et al. (1998)	130	108
Sartorius (2)	Christensen (1959)	740	300
Rectus femoris (2)	Christensen (1959)	609	305
Gracilis	Christensen (1959)	275	527
Semitendinosus	Christensen (1959)	712	713
Med. + lat. gastrocnemii	Christensen (1959)	778	2037
Med. gastrocnemius	Feinstein et al. (1955)	579	1934
Tibialis anterior	Feinstein et al. (1955)	445	562
Plantaris (5)	Carvalho (1976)	204	372

Note: Unless otherwise indicated, values derived from single muscles.

the estimate for the median-innervated thenar muscles obtained by Lee et al. (1975) is especially noteworthy, in that the range of the α-motor fiber diameters was determined from impulse conduction velocity measurements.

Although it is tempting to accept anatomical values, such as those in Table 1, as the true numbers of units, they are no more than estimates and, in certain respects, the values are at least as fallible as the physiological results (see below). In the first place each estimate is usually derived from only one muscle nerve, so no account is taken of the variability between subjects. Second, in some muscle nerves the frequency histograms of nerve fiber diameters are not bimodal, so that it is impossible to know the sizes of the axons that should be counted. Third, some motor axons begin to branch before they reach the muscle belly and sometimes, as in the case of the extensor digitorum brevis (EDB), a proportion of the axons will run through the muscle belly to supply other muscles. Finally, it is now clear, from the exhaustive anatomical study by Boyd and Davey (1968) of muscle nerves in the cat hindlimb, that the ratio of motor to sensory axons varies considerably from one muscle to another. For this reason, the choice of 60.40 by Feinstein et al. (1955), and then by others also studying human muscles, carries some uncertainty. Nevertheless, the estimated numbers of motor units provide the best basis presently available for comparison with the physiological values.

The first physiological motor unit estimates: a personal account by AJM

In 1967, I took the opportunity to spend part of the summer at Johns Hopkins Hospital with Dr. Richard Johns and, on occasion, acted as subject for some experiments that he and Dr. Colin Brown were carrying out on the relative excitabilities of motor and sensory axons. One day, being alone in the laboratory, it occurred to me to see if the recording system would be capable of detecting single motor unit potentials, using surface electrodes over the hypothenar eminence. The intensities of the stimuli to the ulnar nerve at the wrist were reduced until the responses became "all or nothing" in nature. This critical condition was, of course, evidence that a unitary event was involved, in this case, the stimulation of a single motor axon. It took but an moment to compare the peak-to-peak amplitude of the lowest threshold hypothenar motor unit potential with that of a maximum response, and to derive a rough estimate of the numbers of functioning motor units. It is interesting to ask why such a simple method had not been employed earlier. The explanation may lie in the EMG culture of the time for, largely due to the painstaking work of the Buchthal school in Copenhagen, it was felt that detailed study of muscle could only be undertaken with needle electrodes.

Although MUNE was thought to be feasible on the basis of the very first trial, it took 2 years to bring a satisfactory methodology to fruition. Roberto Sica, Peter Fawcett and Malcolm Campbell were also involved in this work, which was undertaken in the muscular dystrophy laboratories in Newcastle upon Tyne (UK). It was Malcolm who would disappear down the hospital corridor and, like a faithful retriever, return half an hour later with a subject for testing, while Roberto could always be counted upon to obtain a perfect oscilloscope photograph when one was needed.

An important step in those early days was to choose the EDB as the most suitable muscle for this kind of study. This choice was based partly on the anatomical isolation of this muscle on the dorsum of the foot, for it was thought that an active recording electrode positioned over the muscle belly would pick up little evoked activity from the only other muscles supplied by the deep peroneal nerve in the foot, the dorsal interossei. As was shown in the first publication of the methodology in 1971 (McComas et al., 1971b), this supposition was true. The relatively thin, flat muscle belly also made EDB attractive, for the deeper motor units would still be sufficiently close to the active electrode for their action potentials to be detected. What we did not know, was that the EDB muscle, even in healthy subjects, often shows histological and histochemical evidence of chronic denervation, as was shown later by Jennekens et al. (1972) in Newcastle and attributed by them to the wearing of tight-fitting shoes. I still wonder if this explanation is correct. However, it is certainly true that the EDB, of all the muscles tested to date, is the one most sensitive to any generalized denervating process. Indeed, this characteristic makes the muscle especially valuable in the search for evidence of a peripheral neuropathy.

The development of incremental MUNE

In the quest for an active electrode to record from all the motor units in EDB, it was thought that the ideal one should be able to cover the entire muscle belly. Accordingly a shallow silver cup was fashioned, with curved edges to fit snugly on to the skin, and this was packed with cotton wool soaked in saline. Unfortunately this electrode proved totally unsatisfactory, for not only did saline trickle out from under the edges of the cup, but the recorded motor unit potentials often had bizarre shapes. This last problem was attributed to the complexities of volume conduction from motor units with fibers extending to the edges of the cup; also, the motor unit potentials were obviously being degraded by an electrode that covered the "sources" as well as the "sinks" of the action currents. Regretfully, the expensive silver cup was discarded, and probably still lies in a laboratory cupboard, either completely forgotten or a continuing cause of puzzlement to a later generation of neuroscientists. It was supplanted by a strip electrode placed over the endplate zone of the muscle, this zone having been found by systematically exploring the muscle belly with a probing electrode and noting the sites at which the evoked M-waves had the largest and steepest initial negative deflections. Since all the motor units in

EDB appeared to have their endplates in the same part of the muscle, synchronous activation caused their evoked responses to summate. The first strips were made out of thin silver foil, 6 mm in width, and were held in place with adhesive tape. It was many years before self-adhesive EKG electrodes became available and we were able to use these instead, having first cut them in half.

At the outset, we were very much aware of the studies of Henneman and his colleagues in the cat (McPhedran et al., 1965; Wuerker et al., 1965), which had been published two years earlier and were the most significant advance in motor unit research since the time of Sherrington. By dissecting ventral root fibers, they were able to record the contractions of single motor units. They showed that not only did the motor units differ in their contractile speeds but, even within the same muscle, there were large variations in the twitch and tetanic tensions, reflecting differences in the sizes of the units themselves. Therefore, in order to obtain meaningful MUNEs, it would be necessary for us to base the calculation not on the motor unit potential generated by the axon with the lowest threshold to electrical stimulation, but on as large a population of motor unit potentials as possible. We anticipated that, as the stimulus intensity to the peroneal nerve was gradually increased above threshold value, other motor axons would be activated in an orderly sequence, with each new motor unit potential appearing as a discrete step in the evoked response. Such, indeed, appeared to be the case, as is evident from Fig. 1. The approximate number of motor units in the EDB muscle was then found by dividing the mean amplitude of the increments into the amplitude of the maximum M-wave. The voltage–time integrals (areas) of the action potentials would have been a superior type of measurement to amplitude, since it would have been less influenced by temporal dispersion of the response. Not having a computer, we could have performed such analyses graphically, but it would have been laborious and hardly suited for online investigations. A few years later, however, Ballantyne and Hansen (1974) overcame this problem with their semi-automated version of MUNE.

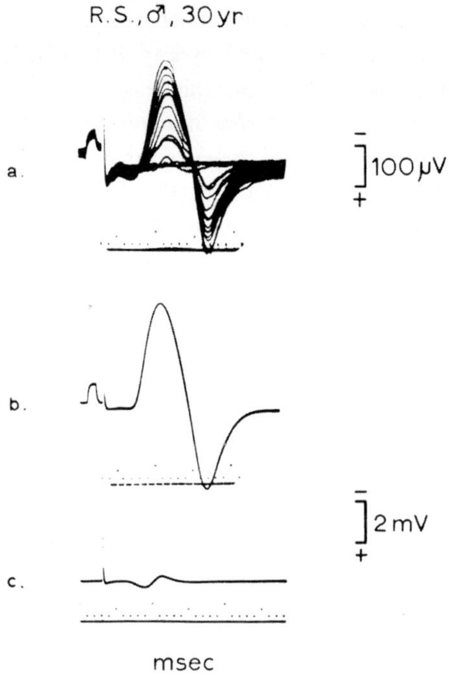

Fig. 1. The first published MUNE, obtained on the EDB muscle of one of the authors (McComas et al., 1971b). The incremental and maximal responses were captured on a variable persistence storage oscilloscope and then on a Polaroid film. Note the voltage calibration pulse before the shock artifacts. In this recording there were 11 response increments and the estimated number of units was approximately 200. Reproduced with permission from McComas et al. (1971b).

Assumptions and limitations of incremental MUNE

Most of the assumptions and limitations of the method were set out in the first full paper (McComas et al., 1971b), published one year after two initial reports (Campbell and McComas, 1970; Campbell et al., 1970). Among the potential problems was the reliability of the sample of motor unit potentials employed in the estimate. Thus, we usually relied on 10 increments for the sample, since a greater number involved the use of lower amplification and consequently there was more difficulty in detecting small motor unit potentials. The possibility that the electrical stimuli were preferentially exciting the largest motor axons, themselves innervating the greatest numbers of muscle fibers, was also a concern, since this might have been predicted from the classic studies on isolated peripheral nerves by Gasser and Erlanger (1924). We were able to show that this bias was not present in our own studies, by use of a collision technique. These negative results suggested that, when nerves are excited through the skin, the thresholds of the fibers are determined more by the resistance of the tissue pathway between the skin and the nodes of Ranvier, than by the dimensions of the fibers themselves, at least within a certain range.

The greatest problem with MUNE, however, was that of "alternation". We observed that, even when the stimulus intensity was held constant, the responses often fluctuated. We attributed this phenomenon to motor axons with overlapping thresholds firing in different combinations. Consequently, the more stimuli that were given in a MUNE, the greater the opportunity for alternation, and the higher the estimate. It is probably because of alternation that the new computer-based MUNE techniques yield rather lower values than the original "manual" method. In an attempt to eliminate alternation we tried to obtain our sample of motor unit potentials in other ways. One was to take only one or two motor unit potentials at each of several stimulation points along the nerve, a method subsequently developed by Brown and colleagues (Kadrie et al., 1976) and termed "multiple point stimulation". The other was to collect potentials during weak voluntary contractions, but the problem here was the poor signal-to-noise ratio. In the end we came back to graded stimulation because of its speed and convenience.

First results in control subjects and later thoughts

The results in our first 20 subjects produced three interesting findings. First, there were, on average, approximately 200 motor units in the EDB muscle. Second, there was a considerable variation from subject to subject and, lastly, there did not seem to be any significant loss of motor units before the age of 60 years. So far as the between-subject variation is concerned, this has still not been examined systematically, but it is our firm impression that the results are consistent throughout the musculature. That is, a person with a large number of units in EDB will tend to have large numbers in other muscles. No doubt this will eventually be explained by the timing and duration of the genetic signals responsible for motoneuron apoptosis.

The effect of age on motor unit numbers remains an active research topic. In the Newcastle laboratories, Tomlinson and Irving (1977) counted presumptive motoneurons in the lumbosacral segments of spinal cords from several victims of sudden death and they confirmed that motoneuron populations were relatively stable up to 60 years. Beyond 60, Campbell et al. (1973) found that there was an exponential loss of motor units in EDB. We were careful to speak of "functioning" units since it was quite possible that the motoneurons were still present in the spinal cord – as happens, of course, in the dying-back neuropathies. As in younger subjects, there was considerable variation between one subject and another. Although the aging effects were so convincing in EDB, such dramatic losses were not seen in a more recent study of the same muscle in a North American population, while no reductions were seen at all in a more proximal muscle, the biceps brachii (Galea, 1996). Although other workers have used a variety of MUNE methods to demonstrate motor unit loss with age, it would not be surprising if distal muscles proved more susceptible to aging than proximal ones. Perhaps someone will have the dedication and patience to follow a cohort of subjects as they age, so as to obtain more precise information on this matter.

Other achievements of MUNE

One of the successes of MUNE, the demonstration of aging effects, has already been touched upon and will be considered more fully elsewhere in these Proceedings. Perhaps the greatest achievement of MUNE, however, has been the provision of motor unit and motoneuron numbers for a variety of limb muscles in healthy young subjects. These values, given in Table 2, are from our own and other laboratories, using a variety of methods. Bearing in mind that there are 2.5 thenar muscles supplied

TABLE 2

MUNEs IN HUMAN LIMB MUSCLES

Muscle	Incremental methods[a]	Other methods[b]
Arm		
Biceps brachii	109 ± 43 (80)[c]	
Biceps brachialis		357 ± 97 (24)
Abductor pollicis longus*	421 ± 99 (40)	
Hypothenar	411 ± 174 (41)	226 (3 studies)
Thenar (median n.)	230 ± 90 (90)	206 (8 studies)
Leg		
Vastus medialis	224 ± 112 (24)	
Tibialis anterior	256 ± 107 (22)	
Soleus*	553 ± 144 (13)	
Extensor digitorum brevis	143 ± 73 (86)	143 (5 studies)
Plantar*	381 ± 162 (26)	285 ± 187 (30)

Data from Tables 1 and 2 of McComas (1998).

[a] Values (mean ± SDs) for the incremental methods were obtained in our laboratory using the automated or manual (asterisk) variations.

[b] Values found with other methods are shown as grand means or, if only one study was involved, as the mean ± SD for that study.

[c] Numbers of muscles examined are given in parentheses.

by the median nerve, and four hypothenar muscles innervated by the ulnar nerve, then each small muscle of the hand must have rather less than 100 units, a finding in keeping with most anatomical counts in Table 1. The larger, more proximal, limb muscles have greater numbers, though the biceps brachii has a surprisingly modest population for a muscle of its size. In contrast, the soleus has a larger population than might have been anticipated, given that its only action is to plantarflex the ankle. In passing, the first recordings of human motor unit twitches, in the EDB, were an offshoot of MUNE, being made by threshold stimulation of motor axons in the deep peroneal nerve and muscle belly (Sica and McComas, 1971). These results showed there was a threefold range of contraction times for human limb muscles and, in distinction to animal studies, a lack of correlation between motor unit size, as gauged from the twitch tension, and twitch duration. Our understanding of pathophysiology is likely to be enhanced, now that Chan et al. (1998) have adopted threshold stimulation to follow the electrical and contractile properties of single motor units in the course of disease and following physiological perturbations.

In our own early experiments the ability of collateral reinnervation to compensate for partial muscle denervation was explored by comparing MUNEs with twitch tensions, and it was found that, in some instances, up to 80% of motor units could be lost before strength declined (McComas et al., 1971d). Among other implications, this remarkable result undermined the clinician's claim, still frequently heard, that the EMG is superfluous to a thorough neurological examination. The role of MUNE in motoneuron disorders will be discussed later in the symposium. It is sufficient for now to say that MUNE has enabled the rate of motoneuron loss to be determined in ALS (Dantes and McComas, 1991), while in the adult and intermediate childhood forms of SMA some motoneuron populations appear to be stable, all the losses having taken place in utero (McComas, 1987; Fehlings et al., this volume). In patients with prior poliomyelitis MUNE has revealed unexpected losses of motoneurons in limbs thought not to have been affected in the paralytic illness (McComas et al., 1997). In occasional patients with a variety of disorders, MUNE has also been instrumental in drawing attention to the existence of "silent" neuromuscular junctions (McComas et al., 1991), that is, junctions that are temporarily incapable of exciting muscle fibers. One possible explanation for this phenomenon is that the parent motoneurons have become dysfunctional and that the synaptic changes are secondary to events in the cell bodies. Since silent synapses are present in nearly all patients with severe hyperthyroidism (Fig. 2), the development of an animal model should be feasible and should lead to an understanding of the cellular mechanisms involved.

Finally, the usefulness of MUNE in the diagnostic EMG clinic is a topic that is now ready for discussion, since some clinics have now had many years of experience in applying this methodology to patients with a wide array of disorders.

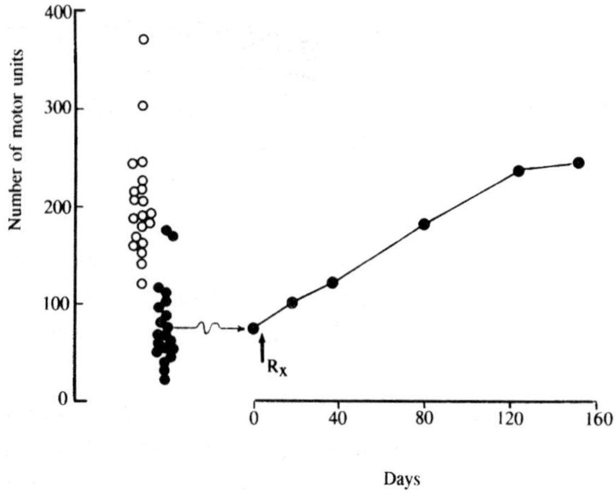

Fig. 2. *Left:* MUNE values in EDB muscles of 20 healthy control subjects (open circles) and 20 patients with severe hyperthyroidism. *Right:* Recovery of MUNE values in one patient following treatment. Data of McComas et al. (1974).

Why was MUNE neglected until recently?

The answer to this question came from a foray into the field of muscular research. One of our team, Malcolm Campbell, had a special interest in myotonic dystrophy, and it was at his suggestion that we performed MUNEs on some patients with this condition (McComas et al., 1971a). Much to our surprise, the first value was considerably reduced and the subsequent estimates on other patients were similarly diminished. We then looked at the EDB muscles of patients with Duchenne and limbgirdle dystrophies, and found losses in the majority (McComas et al., 1971e). It was natural to wonder if the dystrophic features in the muscles were secondary to some type of dysfunction in their motoneurons. Consistent with such a view were the dystrophic-like changes that could be found in denervated muscles. Also, the recent cross-innervation experiments of Buller et al. (1960) had shown that the physiological properties of the muscle fibers were under the control of the motoneuron. Finally, in both Duchenne and myotonic dystrophy, the central nervous system was clearly affected because of the mental retardation in the former and the intellectual degeneration in the latter.

We published the "sick motoneurone" hypothesis in 1971 (McComas et al., 1971c) but, while many workers in the field were interested and prepared to explore the hypothesis with their own experiments, there were others, including some of our very own colleagues, who were bitterly opposed. In their view, not only was the hypothesis wrong, but all the MUNE results which had led to it must have been erroneous. Two other groups then introduced their own modifications of the original MUNE method. Both groups used the EDB muscle for their experiments and the motor unit potentials were obtained by graded stimulation, just as in our own studies. In truth, the modification of Ballantyne and Hansen (1974) *was* an advance, since these authors used a computer to store the response templates and, by subtracting each template from the next largest, were able to extract the waveforms of the individual, putative, motor unit potentials. In addition, by measuring response areas rather than amplitudes, their results would have been less affected by temporal dispersion. The other modification was by Panayiotopoulos et al. (1974), who claimed that they could improve the sensitivity of MUNE by projecting and superimposing single traces, recorded on 35 mm film. However, inspection of their figures threw doubt on these claims since the purported small potentials were often comparable to the noise in their records. Ironically, both groups confirmed that there were losses of motor units in myotonic dystrophy

(Ballantyne and Hansen, 1975; Panayiotopoulos and Scarpalezos, 1976), but they were unable to verify our findings in the other types of dystrophy. In the end, the traditionalists won the battle of pathogenesis through the intervention of the molecular biologists, though there are still parts of the dystrophy story that are missing. All was not lost, however, for the concept of "sick" neurons in neurological disorders has become firmly accepted (Isaacson, 1993), and the identities of several trophic factors, secreted by the motoneuron and acting on the muscle fiber, are now known. Further, it was through MUNE that the first hard evidence for the existence of genetic "anticipation" in myotonic dystrophy was produced (McComas et al., 1978).

Had MUNE not been applied to muscular dystrophy, we are sure that it would have been accepted much sooner. As a tactical manoeuvre, it would have been better to have concentrated on peripheral neuropathies and disorders of the motoneurons themselves, as Ballantyne and Hansen subsequently did. However, by this time the damage had been done and their later papers did not attract the attention that they deserved. That MUNE survived at all was due, in part, to a series of methodological studies by Brown, in which several new approaches were described and the small muscles of the hand were examined. Through Brown's work, multiple point stimulation, spike-triggered averaging, and F-wave analysis were all employed as alternative methods (Kadrie et al., 1976; Brown et al., 1988; Stashuk et al., 1994). Rather later, Daube (1988, 1995) introduced his "statistical" method, based on Poisson analysis, and brought his organizational skills to the MUNE field, including the creation of special interest groups at scientific meetings. The transition to the modern era of MUNE was completed when Bromberg (1993) examined the reliability of MUNE and considered its application to the evaluation of patients with ALS. The newer methods, including one from our own laboratory (Galea et al., 1991), will be discussed later in the symposium, together with the applications of MUNE to the study of motoneuron disorders, and of ALS in particular.

Looking to the future

Now that MUNE has finally become established in the EMG laboratory as a valid test of muscle innervation, what may we expect from it in the future? As an aid to the diagnosis and assessment of the common neuromuscular disorders seen in the EMG clinic, it has enormous potential, and it is rather curious that, so far, only a few laboratories have put it to this use. If this neglect is because of the time that some of the MUNE methods require, our suggestion would be to use the original manual incremental method, since this takes only a few minutes and can be performed with the same arrangement of stimulating and recording electrodes as for motor nerve conduction velocity measurements. Further, this method requires no special computer software and can be performed on any EMG machine. For research studies, the original manual method, in experienced hands, still has a place, but any of the newer methods could be used instead. As will become obvious in the symposium, each has its advantages and limitations, and, although others may disagree, we do not feel that any one method is so superior as to be chosen over others, at least for now. One heartening aspect of MUNE is that the various methods yield very similar results, as Stein and Yang (1990) showed by testing the same subjects in different ways. The reliability of the MUNEs can obviously be enhanced by duplicate estimations and by examining more than one muscle in a patient with a generalized neuromuscular disorder.

In view of the very large numbers of muscles studied, and the variety of methods used, it is probable that many of the potential errors have been cancelled out and that the physiological MUNEs are actually more reliable than the anatomically-derived ones. Nevertheless, it would be interesting to see improved anatomical data, and possibly these could be obtained by treating sections of muscle nerve with labelled antibodies specific to motor or sensory axons. The fact that degeneration is occasionally limited to one or other type of axon in cases of Guillain-Barré syndrome indicates that this approach may be feasible.

As to research topics involving MUNE, one of the most important will undoubtedly be its use in monitoring the progress of ALS patients undergoing experimental therapies, and such studies will be reported in this symposium. Serial MUNEs would also be valuable in various types of peripheral neuropathy, not only for determining their natural time-courses, but also for evaluating the effects of treatment. An equally interesting, but very different type of problem, would be an analysis of the cellular mechanisms underlying the silent synapse phenomenon, using an animal model (see above). As peripheral neuromuscular problems are worked out, the application of MUNE to central nervous system questions should be considered. MUNE has already been employed to show the presence of transsynaptic motoneuron degeneration after upper motoneuron lesions (McComas et al., 1971f). It would be important to know if such degeneration could be prevented by experimental therapies, for example, by increasing the sensory input to motoneurons from skin and muscle. A second and more recent example of central MUNE application is the recognition of a developmental apraxia in patients with persisting obstetric brachial palsy (Brown et al., 2000). With such a powerful and yet simple methodology available, it is likely that many new applications will be found in the future.

Acknowledgements

We are indebted to Jane Butler for technical assistance and to the Natural Sciences and Engineering Research Council of Canada for financial support. Rebecca Newberry kindly prepared the illustrations.

References

Ballantyne, J.P. and Hansen, S. A new method for the estimation of the number of motor units in a muscle. 1. Control subjects and patients with myasthenia gravis. *J. Neurol. Neurosurg. Psychiatry*, 1974, 37: 907–915.

Ballantyne, J.P. and Hansen, S. Computer method for analysis of evoked motor unit potentials. 2. Duchenne, limb-girdle, facioscapulohumeral and myotonic muscular dystrophies. *J. Neurol. Neurosurg. Psychiatry*, 1975, 38: 417–428.

Boyd, I.A. and Davey, M.R. *Composition of Peripheral Nerves*. Livingstone, Edinburgh, 1968, pp. 1–57.

Bromberg, M.B. Motor unit estimation: reproducibility of the spike-triggered averaging technique in normal and ALS subjects. *Muscle Nerve*, 1993, 16: 466–471.

Brown, W.F., Strong, M.J. and Snow, R.S. Methods for estimating numbers of motor units in biceps-brachialis muscles and losses of motor units with aging. *Muscle Nerve*, 1988, 11: 423–432.

Brown, T., Cupido, C., Scarfone, H., Pape, K., Galea, V. and McComas, A. Developmental apraxia arising from neonatal brachial plexus palsy. *Neurology*, 2000, 55: 24–30.

Buller, A.J., Eccles, J.C. and Eccles, R.M. Interaction between motoneurones and muscles in respect of the characteristic speeds of their responses. *J. Physiol. (Lond.)*, 1960, 150: 417–439.

Campbell, M.J. and McComas, A.J. The effects of aging on muscle function. In: *Research in Muscular and Related Disorders*. London, Pitman. Abstract, 1970.

Campbell, M.J., McComas, A.J. and Sica, R.E.P. An electrophysiological investigation of dystrophia myotonica. *J. Physiol. (Lond.)*, 1970, 209: 28*P*.

Campbell, M.J., McComas, A.J. and Petito, F. Physiological changes in ageing muscles. *J. Neurol. Neurosurg. Psychiatry*, 1973, 36: 174–182.

Carlsöö, S. Motor units and action potentials in masticatory muscles. *Acta Morph. Neerl. Scand.*, 1958, 2: 13–19.

Carvalho, V.C. Study of motor units and arrangements of myons of human muscular plantaris. *Acta Anat.*, 1976, 96: 444–448.

Carvalho, V.C., Cintra, A.I.D. and Santo Neto, H. Motor units and functional anatomy of the human opponens digiti minimi. *Anat. Anz.*, 1988, 165: 65–68.

Chan, K.M., Stashuk, D.W. and Brown, W.F. A longitudinal study of the pathophysiological changes in single human thenar motor units in amyotrophic lateral sclerosis. *Muscle Nerve*, 1998, 21: 1714–1723.

Christensen, E. Topography of terminal motor innervation in striated muscles from stillborn infants. *Am. J. Phys. Med.*, 1959, 38: 65–78.

Dantes, M. and McComas, A. The extent and time-course of motoneuron involvement in amyotrophic lateral sclerosis. *Muscle Nerve*, 1991, 14: 416–421.

Daube, J.R. Statistical estimates of numbers of motor units in thenar and foot muscles in patients with amyotrophic lateral sclerosis or the residue of polio. *Muscle Nerve*, 1988, 11: 957-A.

Daube, J.R. Estimating the number of motor units in a muscle. *J. Clin. Neurophysiol.*, 1995, 12: 585–594.

Eccles, J.C. and Sherrington, C.S. Numbers and contraction-values of individual motor units examined in some muscles of the limb. *Proc. Roy. Soc. Lond., Ser. B*, 1930, 106: 326–357.

Feinstein, B., Lindegård, B., Nyman, E. and Wohlfart, G. Morphologic studies of motor units in normal human muscles. *Acta Anat.*, 1955, 23: 127–142.

Galea, V. Changes in motor unit estimates with aging. *J. Clin. Neurophysiol.*, 1996, 13: 253–260.

Galea, V., DeBruin, H., Cavasin, R. and McComas, A.J. The numbers and relative sizes of motor units estimated by computer. *Muscle Nerve*, 1991, 14: 1123–1130.

Gasser, H.S. and Erlanger, J. The nature of conduction of an impulse in the relative refractory period. *Am. J. Physiol.*, 1924, 73: 613–635.

Isaacson, O. On neuronal health. *TINS*, 1993, 16: 306–308.

Jennekens, F.G.I., Tomlinson, B.E. and Walton, J.N. The extensor digitorum brevis: histological and histochemical aspects. *J. Neurol. Neurosurg. Psychiatry*, 1972, 35: 124–132.

Kadrie, H.A., Yates, S.K., Milner-Brown, H.S. and Brown, W.F. Multiple point electrical stimulation of ulnar and median nerves. *J. Neurol. Neurosurg. Psychiatry*, 1976, 39: 973–985.

Lee, R.G., Ashby, P., White, D.G. and Aguayo, A.J. Analysis of motor conduction velocity in the human median nerve by computer simulation of compound muscle action potentials. *Electroencephalogr. Clin. Neurophysiol.*, 1975, 39: 225–237.

Leksell, L. The action potential and excitatory effects of the small ventral root fibres to skeletal muscle. *Acta Physiol. Scand.*, 1945, 10 (Suppl. 31): 1–84.

Liddell, E.G.T. and Sherrington, C.S. Recruitment and some other features of reflex inhibition. *Proc. Roy. Soc. Lond., Ser. B*, 1925, 97: 488–518.

McComas, A.J. Motor neurone disorders. "Clinical Electromyography" (W.F. Brown and C.F. Bolton, Eds.), 1987, pp. 431–451. Butterworths, Stoneham, MA.

McComas, A.J. Motor units: how many, how large, what kind? *J. Electromyogr. Kinesiol.*, 1998, 8: 391–402.

McComas, A.J., Campbell, M.J. and Sica, R.E.P. Electrophysiological study of dystrophia myotonica. *J. Neurol. Neurosurg. Psychiatry*, 1971a, 34: 132–139.

McComas, A.J., Fawcett, P.R.W., Campbell, M.J. and Sica, R. E.P. Electrophysiological estimation of the number of motor units within a human muscle. *J. Neurol. Neurosurg. Psychiatry*, 1971b, 34: 121–131.

McComas, A.J., Sica, R.E.P. and Campbell, M.J. "Sick" motoneurones. A unifying concept of muscle disease. *Lancet*, 1971c, 1: 321–325.

McComas, A.J., Sica, R.E.P., Campbell, M.J. and Upton, A.R. M. Functional compensation in partially denervated muscles. *J. Neurol. Neurosurg. Psychiatry*, 1971d, 34: 453–460.

McComas, A.J., Sica, R.E.P. and Currie, S. An electrophysiological study of Duchenne dystrophy. *J. Neurol. Neurosurg. Psychiatry*, 1971e, 34: 461–468.

McComas, A.J., Sica, R.E.P., Upton, A.R.M., Aguilera, N. and Currie, S. Motoneurone dysfunction in patients with hemiplegic atrophy. *Nature New Biol.*, 1971f, 233: 21–23.

McComas, A.J., Sica, R.E.P., McNabb, A.R., Goldberg, W.M. and Upton, A.R.M. Evidence for reversible motoneurone dysfunction in thyrotoxicosis. *J. Neurol. Neurol. Psychiatry*, 1974, 37: 548–558.

McComas, A.J., Sica, R.E.P. and Toyonaga, K. Incidence, severity and time-course of motoneurone dysfunction in myotonic dystrophy. Their significance for an understanding of anticipation. *J. Neurol. Neurosurg. Psychiatry*, 1978, 41: 882–893.

McComas, A.J., DeBruin, H. and Quartly, C. Non-transmitting synapses in human neuromuscular disorders? "Plasticity of Motoneuronal Connections" (A. Wernig, Ed.), 1991, pp. 223–229. Elsevier, Amsterdam.

McComas, A.J., Quartly, C. and Griggs, R.C. Early and late losses of motor units after poliomyelitis. *Brain*, 1997, 120: 1415–1421.

McPhedran, A.M., Wuerker, R.B. and Henneman, E. Properties of motor units in heterogeneous pale muscle (m. gastrocnemius) of the cat. *J. Neurophysiol.*, 1965, 27: 85–99.

Panayiotopoulos, C.P. and Scarpalezos, S. Dystrophia myotonia. Peripheral nerve involvement and pathogenetic implications. *J. Neurol. Sci.*, 1976, 27: 1–16.

Panayiotopoulos, C.P., Scarpalezos, S. and Papapetropoulos, Th. Electrophysiological estimation of motor units in Duchenne muscular dystrophy. *J. Neurol. Sci.*, 1974, 23: 89–98.

Santo Neto, H., Carvalho, V.C. and Penteado, C.V. Motor units of the human abductor digiti minimi. *Arch. Ital. Anat. Embriol.*, 1985, XC: 47–51.

Santo Neto, H., Carvalho, V.C. and Marques, M.J. Estimation of the number and size of human flexor digiti minimi muscle motor units using histological methods. *Muscle Nerve*, 1998, 21: 112–114.

Sherrington, C.S. Some functional problems attaching to convergence. *Proc. Roy. Soc. Lond., Ser. B*, 1929, 105: 332–362.

Sica, R.E.P. and McComas, A.J. Fast and slow muscle units in a human muscle. *J. Neurol. Neurosurg. Psychiatry*, 1971, 34: 113–120.

Stashuk, D.W., Doherty, T.J., Kassam, A. and Brown, W.F. Motor unit number estimates based on the automated analysis of F-responses. *Muscle Nerve*, 1994, 17: 881–890.

Stein, R.B. and Yang, J.F. Methods for estimating the number of motor units in human muscles. *Ann. Neurol.*, 1990, 28: 487–495.

Tomlinson, B.E. and Irving, D. The numbers of limb motor neurons in the human lumbosacral cord throughout life. *J. Neurol. Sci.*, 1977, 34: 213–219.

Wuerker, R.B., McPhedran, A.M. and Henneman, E. Properties of motor units in a heterogeneous pale muscle (m. gastrocnemius) of the cat. *J. Neurophysiol.*, 1965, 28: 85–99.

Discussion after Section I

Mark Bromberg, Salt Lake City

Thank you very much Alan for an interesting and informative presentation on the history of MUNE. It is valuable to understand how a technique evolved from the first idea, and how it progressed to a well worked out methodology. It is clear that most of the issues we will be discussing during this Symposium were the same that you considered during the early development. This is a reflection on your basic physiology background and thoroughness.

We are now going to proceed to the section on MUNE physiology that will focus on issues that have shaped the field of MUNE since your first description in 1971.

Section II

MUNE Physiology

Motor Unit Number Estimation (Supplements to Clinical Neurophysiology Vol. 55)
Editor: M.B. Bromberg

Chapter 2

Axon excitability in motor unit number estimation

Timothy J. Doherty[a,*], Daniel W. Stashuk[b] and William F. Brown[c]

[a]*Department of Physical Medicine and Rehabilitation, University of Western Ontario, London, ON N6A 1Y6, Canada*
[b]*Department of Systems Design Engineering, University of Waterloo, Waterloo, ON N2L 3G1, Canada*
[c]*Department of Neurology, Tuft's University, Boston, MA, USA*

Introduction

A number of electrophysiological techniques have been developed to estimate the numbers of motor units (MUs) in human muscles (McComas, 1991; Doherty et al., 1995; Shefner, 2001). The original incremental stimulation (IS) technique (McComas et al., 1971), and the majority of subsequently developed techniques, use submaximal electrical stimulation of the peripheral nerve to obtain the sample of MU responses from which to calculate the average surface-detected MU action potential (S-MUP) size. The MU number estimate (MUNE) is then calculated by dividing the amplitude or area of the maximum compound muscle action potential (CMAP) by the corresponding average S-MUP value.

A number of underlying assumptions govern the response of the motor axon to percutaneous stimulation. The extent to which they impact the performance and validity of MUNE techniques, and in particular the IS and multiple point stimulation (MPS) techniques, will be reviewed (Doherty and Brown, 1993).

Fundamental assumptions

The validity of the IS technique, including subsequent modifications, and the MPS technique in particular, are dependent on the following assumptions:

1. All-or-nothing responses representing S-MUPs can be obtained and detected with graded percutaneous threshold stimulation of the peripheral nerve to a given muscle or muscle group.
2. Stimulation thresholds of at least the lowest threshold motor nerve fibers are sufficiently separate so that finely graded increases in stimulus intensity excites either single nerve fibers (MPS technique) or a succession of higher threshold motor nerve fibers (IS technique). This results in successive quantal additions to the size of the CMAP through the addition of associated S-MUPs.
3. The MUs activated by stimulating the first few motor nerve fibers (1–10) produce S-MUPs that

**Correspondence to*: Dr. T.J. Doherty, Department of Physical Medicine and Rehabilitation, The University of Western Ontario, St Joseph's Health Care, 21 Grosvenor St., London, ON N6A 1Y6, Canada.
Tel.: (519) 646-6100x65975, Fax: (519) 646-6174.
e-mail: tim.doherty@sjhc.london.on.ca

doi: 10.1016/S1567-424X(03)00002-3

are representative of the different sizes of S-MUPs that sum to form the maximum CMAP for the muscle or muscle group being studied.

Assumption 1: Threshold percutaneous stimuli activate single motor axons

The IS and MPS techniques are dependent on the ability of percutaneous stimulation to excite motor axons, either singly (MPS), or successively in response to progressively higher stimulus intensities (IS). The evidence that a single motor nerve fiber can be activated and its S-MUP detected, in response to graded electrical stimulation, is well established and based on the following observations:

a) Small increments and decrements in the stimulus intensity delivered to a motor nerve are matched by the appearance and disappearance of an "all-or-nothing" potential corresponding to the surface (or intramuscularly) detected MUAP generated by that specific motor nerve fiber (Bergmans, 1970; McComas et al., 1971; Kadrie et al., 1976; Doherty and Brown, 2002). In the few studies where twitch force has been recorded simultaneously from the same muscle, force recordings respond in the same all-or-nothing fashion with graded threshold stimuli (Fig. 1) (Stein and Yang, 1990; Doherty and Brown, 1997).
b) Putative S-MUPs exhibit no fractionation or other change in shape or size (except under pathological conditions), such as might indicate the presence of two or more motor nerve fibers with similar thresholds (Doherty and Brown, 1993, 1994) (Fig. 2).
c) In instances where an F-response occurs (well under 10% of stimuli in healthy motor nerve fibers) the shape and size of the F-response are identical to the direct S-MUP (Doherty and Brown, 1993, 1994).

Based on the above evidence, it is well established that at least the lowest threshold single motor axons can be activated in isolation and that the evoked potentials represent the responses from single MUs.

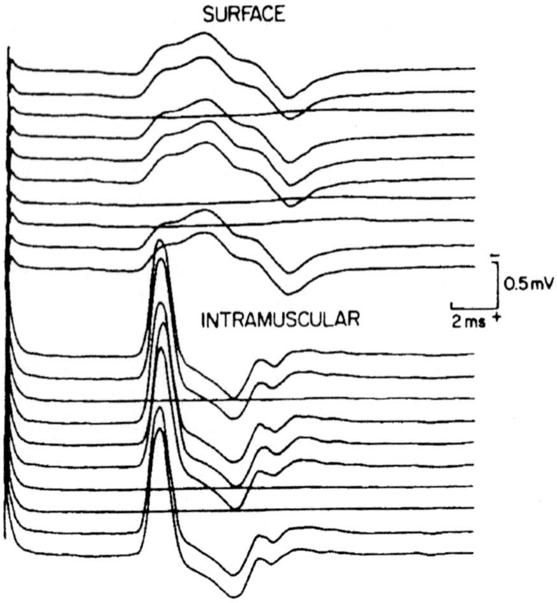

Fig. 1. All-or-none surface and intramuscular detected thenar motor unit action potentials in response to graded threshold stimulation of median nerve at wrist. *Note:* in each case an identical all-or-nothing response is present in the surface and intramuscular recording with no fractionation upon repeated stimulation.

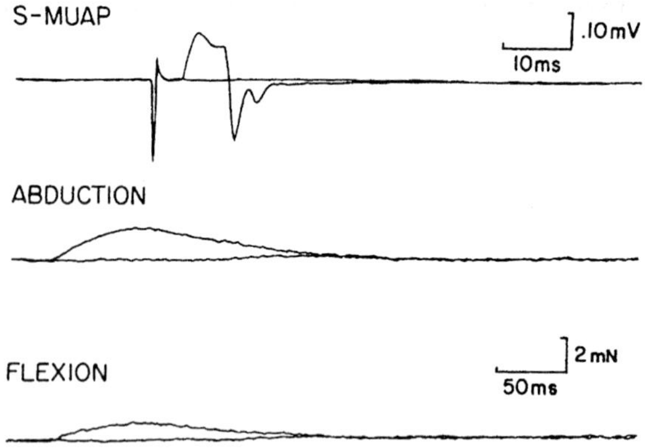

Fig. 2. All-or-none surface-detected thenar motor unit action potential and associated twitch force records from abduction and flexion vector.

Assumption 2: Stimulation thresholds of motor axons remain separate with graded stimuli

The IS technique involves the application of successive, manually adjusted, graded electrical stimuli to the motor nerve. It is assumed that each resulting step increment or fluctuation in the compound potential (usually 10 or more steps), in response to progressively higher intensity stimuli, corresponds to the activation of an additional motor axon and its S-MUP (McComas et al., 1971). This being the case, the average MU size can be determined by simple division of the CMAP amplitude or area by the number of steps. For this assumption to be considered valid, the separation in stimulus thresholds must be such that graded stimuli excite axons one-by-one with successively higher threshold motor nerve fibers in an orderly and reproducible manner.

It turns out however, that motor nerve fiber thresholds frequently overlap with one another, even at the lowest motor threshold. Such an overlap of thresholds is not surprising given the numbers of motor nerve fibers innervating a muscle (for example, as many as 100 per healthy intrinsic hand muscle). Further, thresholds are not finite values, but represent ranges of stimulus intensities over which the probability of an "all" response of an S-MUP increases from 0 to 100% as the stimulus intensity is increased (Brown and Milner-Brown, 1976; Milner-Brown and Brown, 1976) (Fig. 3). When thresholds of two or more motor nerve fibers overlap at a specific stimulus intensity, trains of stimuli, if carried out long enough, will evoke $2^n - 1$ incremental steps in the response, where n is the number of motor nerve fibers whose thresholds overlap at that stimulus intensity (Fig. 4). These steps, or *alternations*, represent various combinations of S-MUPs, which in turn represent stimulus-to-stimulus variations in the number of MUs that fire in response to a given stimulus. The number of alternations may greatly exceed the actual number of motor nerve fibers responsible for the increments; for example, seven combinations can result from only three motor nerve fibers with overlapping thresholds (Brown and Milner-Brown, 1976; Milner-Brown and Brown, 1976). This in turn can lead to substantial underestimation of the mean S-MUAP size, and overestimation of the MUNE value. McComas and colleagues discussed this potential source of error in the original MUNE description, and suggested that its presence could be recognized on occasion, but with greater difficulty as the stimulus intensity was increased beyond the first two or three steps. The problem

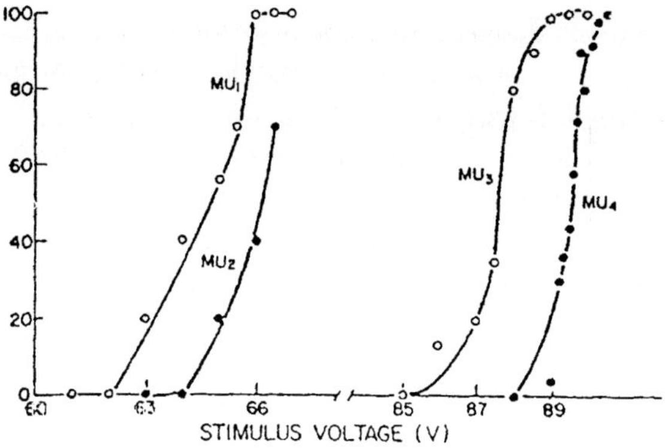

Fig. 3. Excitability curves of three motor units (MUs) form two normal subjects and one MU from a patient with diabetic neuropathy. Fifty stimuli were applied to the median (MU1, MU2), ulnar (MU3) and peroneal nerves at fixed voltages. The voltage was increased in 0.2–0.5 V steps until the firing probability was 100%. MU2 was not completed because of change in the subjects position (see text).

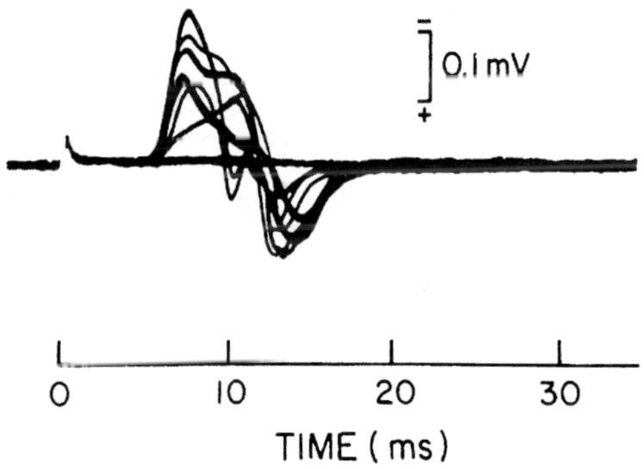

Fig. 4. Fluctuations or alternations in the amplitude of the thenar compound muscle action potential in response to 100 constant intensity stimuli delivered to the median nerve at the wrist. The observation of seven steps in response to the 100 stimuli made it highly probable that three motor axons with overlapping thresholds were responsible for all of the fluctuations (see text).

of alternation led to modifications to the IS technique (Ballantyne and Hansen, 1974; Panayiotopoulos et al., 1974; Galea et al., 1991) and the development of other techniques designed to avoid alternation entirely. These include the MPS (Doherty and Brown, 1993), F-response (Stashuk et al., 1994), and spike-triggered averaging (STA) techniques (Brown et al., 1988). In contrast, the statistical technique relies on alternation (Daube, 1988, 1995). In general, MUNE values from the methods designed to account for or avoid alternation are somewhat lower than those based on the original IS techniques (McComas, 1998).

The presence of alternation by no means invalidates the IS technique. It is important to appreciate that alternation can occur whenever motor threshold values overlap, and therefore comes into play with the MPS technique and its modifications. One must however be aware of its presence with the IS technique in particular, and recognize that even in experienced hands it is likely impossible to completely avoid.

Assumption 3: There is no systematic relationship between stimulus intensity and S-MUP size or latency

In order for any MUNE technique to be considered valid, the sample of S-MUPs used to calculate the mean S-MUP size should accurately represent the relative numbers of S-MUPs of different sizes that sum to form the maximum CMAP. With regard to electrical stimulation of peripheral nerves, classical studies of the relative excitabilities of nerve fibers suggested that the largest fibers with the most rapid conduction velocities had the lowest thresholds for electrical stimulation (Erlanger and Gasser, 1937). These differences, however, were most true between major classes of nerve fibers and less so within a class, such as within the class of alpha motor axons. Furthermore, these studies were carried out using direct stimulation of amphibian peripheral nerve, and whether these same conclusions are valid for percutaneous stimulation of a human mixed nerve is questionable.

Clinical data from our studies that of others suggest that percutaneous electrical stimulation provides an unbiased sample from which to determine mean S-MUP size and a MUNE:

a) A wide range of S-MUP sizes and relative latencies are present in the population of responses obtained by MPS and IS techniques (McComas et al., 1971; Doherty and Brown, 1993). These distributions are similar to those obtained using voluntary contraction and the F-response technique (Fig. 5) (Doherty and Brown, 1993; Doherty et al., 1994). In support is the finding that the distribution of thenar MU twitch tensions is similar when obtained by MPS and intraneural stimulation of the median nerve (Thomas et al., 1990; Doherty and Brown, 1997).

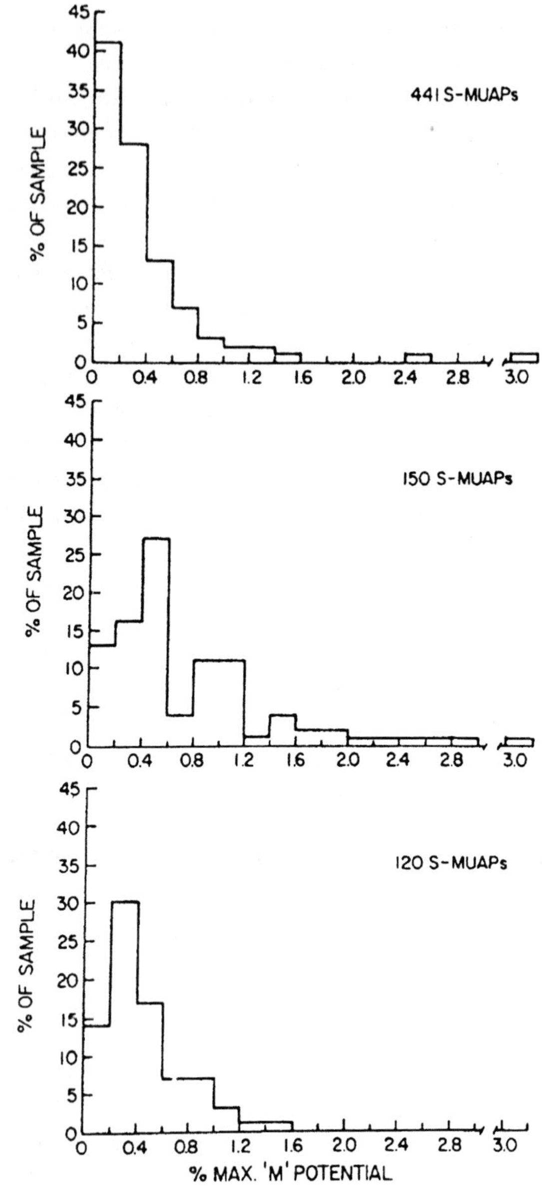

Fig. 5. Distribution of median innervate thenar S-MUP sizes as collected by multiple point stimulation (top panel), the F-response (middle panel) and spike-triggered averaging (bottom panel). *Note:* regardless of the method of collection, relatively greater numbers of small S-MUPs are present.

b) With both the IS technique and the automated IS technique, the mean size of the lowest and highest threshold responses did not differ (McComas et al., 1971; Galea et al., 1991).
c) Collision studies revealed that the probability of stimulating the same population of motor fibers at two separate sites of stimulation, as one would expect if a direct relationship existed between stimulus intensity and axon size, was little better than by chance (McComas et al., 1971; Doherty and Brown, 1993).

Summary

Percutaneous electrical stimulation is capable of exciting single motor axons and obtaining an unbiased sample of S-MUPs from which to derive a MUNE. Alternation, recognized at the outset by McComas and colleagues, has been problematic for the IS technique. This has prompted the development of other techniques including an automated IS method that tests statistically for alternation, the MPS technique and its modifications, the STA technique, and a statistical technique. Further investigation is required regarding the extent to which the above arguments hold true in pathologic disorders affecting the MU, especially ALS.

References

Ballantyne, J.P. and Hansen, S. A new method for the estimation of the number of motor units in a muscle. I. Control subjects and patients with myasthenia gravis. *J. Neurol. Neurosurg. Psychiatry*., 1974, 37: 907–915.

Bergmans, J. *The physiology of single human nerve fibres*. Vander, Catholic University of Louvain, Belgium, 1970.

Brown, W.F. and Milner-Brown, H.S. Some electrical properties of motor units and their effects on the methods of estimating motor unit numbers. *J. Neurol. Neurosurg. Psychiatry*, 1976, 39: 249–257.

Brown, W.F., Strong, M.J. and Snow, R. Methods for estimating numbers of motor units in biceps-brachialis muscles and losses of motor units with aging. *Muscle Nerve*, 1988, 11: 423–432.

Daube, J.R. Statistical estimates of number of motor units in thenar and foot muscles in patients with amyotrophic lateral sclerosis or the residue of poliomyelitis. *Muscle Nerve*, 1988, 11: 957.

Daube, J.R. Estimating the number of motor units in a muscle. *J. Clin. Neurophysiol*., 1995, 12: 585–594.

Doherty, T.J. and Brown, W.F. The estimated numbers and relative sizes of thenar motor units as selected by multiple point stimulation in young and older adults. *Muscle Nerve*, 1993, 16: 355–366.

Doherty, T.J. and Brown, W.F. A method for the longitudinal study of human thenar motor units. *Muscle Nerve*, 1994, 17: 1029–1036.

Doherty, T.J. and Brown, W.F. Age-related changes in the twitch contractile properties of human thenar motor units. *J. Appl. Physiol*., 1997, 82: 93–101.

Doherty, T.J. and Brown, W.F. Motor Unit Number Estimation. In: Brown, W.F., Bolton, C.F., Aminoff, M.J. (Eds), *Clinical Neurophysiology and Neuromuscular Disease*. Philadelphia, W.B. Saunders, 2002, 274–290.

Doherty, T.J., Komori, T., Stashuk, D.W., Kassam, A. and Brown, W.F. Physiological properties of single thenar motor units in the F-response of younger and older adults. *Muscle Nerve*, 1994, 17: 860–872.

Doherty, T., Simmons, Z., O'Connell, B., Felice, K.J., Conwit, R., Chan, K.M., Komori, T., Brown, T., Stashuk, D.W. and Brown, W.F. Methods for estimating the numbers of motor units in human muscles. *J. Clin. Neurophysiol*., 1995, 12: 565–584.

Erlanger, J. and Gasser, H.S. *Electrical signs of nervous activity* University of Pennsylvania Press, Philadelphia, 1937.

Galea, V., de Bruin, H., Cavasin, R. and McComas, A.J. The numbers and relative sizes of motor units estimated by computer. *Muscle Nerve*, 1991, 14: 1123–1130.

Kadrie, H.A., Yates, S.K., Milner Brown, H.S. and Brown, W.F. Multiple point electrical stimulation of ulnar and median nerves. *J. Neurol. Neurosurg. Psychiatry*., 1976, 39: 973–985.

McComas, A.J. Motor unit estimation: methods, results, and present status. *Muscle Nerve*, 1991, 14: 585–597.

McComas, A.J. Motor units: how many, how large, what kind? International Society of Electrophysiology and Kinesiology. *J. Electromyogr. Kinesiol*., 1998, 8: 391–402.

McComas, A.J., Fawcett, P.R., Campbell, M.J. and Sica, R.E. Electrophysiological estimation of the number of motor units within a human muscle. *J. Neurol. Neurosurg. Psychiatry*., 1971, 34: 121–131.

Milner-Brown, H.S. and Brown, W.F. New methods of estimating the number of motor units in a muscle. *J. Neurol. Neurosurg. Psychiatry*., 1976, 39: 258–265.

Panayiotopoulos, C.P., Scarpalezos, S. and Papapetropoulos, T. Electrophysiological estimation of motor units in Duchenne muscular dystrophy. *J. Neurol. Sci*., 1974, 23: 89–98.

Shefner, J.M. Motor unit number estimation in human neurological diseases and animal models. *Clin. Neurophysiol*., 2001, 112: 955–964.

Stashuk, D.W., Doherty, T.J., Kassam, A. and Brown, W.F. Motor unit number estimates based on the automated analysis of F-responses. *Muscle Nerve*, 1994, 17: 881–890.

Stein, R.B. and Yang, J.F. Methods for estimating the number of motor units in human muscles. *Ann. Neurol*., 1990, 28: 487–495.

Thomas, C.K., Johansson, R.S., Westling, G. and Bigland-Ritchie, B. Twitch properties of human thenar motor units measured in response to intraneural motor-axon stimulation. *J. Neurophysiol*., 1990, 64: 1339–1346.

Motor Unit Number Estimation (Supplements to Clinical Neurophysiology Vol. 55)
Editor: M.B. Bromberg

Chapter 3

Issues in motor unit number estimation

Michael P. Slawnych*

Faculty of Medicine, Health Sciences Centre, University of Calgary, 3330 Hospital Drive N.W., Calgary, AB T2N 4N1, Canada

Introduction

"*By a small sample we may judge of the whole piece*" Cervantes

Since first being introduced by McComas and Fawcett (1971), much attention has been directed towards developing techniques aimed at estimating the number of motor units (MUs) in nerve/muscle systems. To date, all of the existing techniques are based on a sampling procedure in which two pieces of information are required:

1. the summated response of all of the MUs, and
2. the mean MU response, which is usually calculated by examining a relatively small number of MUs.

These responses are generally measured in terms of the amplitudes or areas of their associated potential waveforms, although tension measurements have also been used (Stein and Yang, 1990; Arasaki et al., 1997). Given the summated and mean responses, the MU number estimate (MUNE), designated as N, is simply calculated as follows:

$$N = \frac{M}{m}, \tag{1}$$

where M is the amplitude (or corresponding area or tension) of the summated response and m is mean motor unit action potential (MUAP) amplitude (or corresponding area or tension). The summated response is easily obtained by electrically stimulating the nerve at supra-maximal levels. This results in the near-synchronous activation of the entire MU pool, with the associated electrical response being termed the maximal compound muscle action potential (CMAP). The acquisition of the representative MU sample, on the other hand, is not as straightforward, and has been approached in a number of different ways. The aim of this paper it to address some of the main issues associated with current MUNE techniques.

Sampling errors

As stated above, all of the existing estimation techniques are based on a sampling procedure. Hence, the MUNEs are associated with an inherent sampling error. We developed a computer model to examine this sampling error (Slawnych et al., 1997)

**Correspondence to*: Michael P. Slawnych, PhD, Health Sciences Centre, University of Calgary, 3330 Hospital Drive N.W., Calgary, AB T2N 4N1, Canada. Tel.: 403-220-2219, Fax: 403-210-8140.
e-mail: msplawny@ucalgary.ca

doi: 10.1016/S1567-424X(03)00003-5

in which the following parameters could be varied: the number of motor units in the muscle (termed the population size), the number of motor units in the representative sample (termed the sample size), the type of motor unit amplitude distribution used to represent the MU population, and the number of observations (i.e. the number of times in which the estimate is calculated, with a new random sample being selected each time).

Figure 1 shows two specific amplitude distributions, one representing a normal muscle and one representing a neurogenic muscle. Specifically, under normal conditions, the majority of the motor unit potentials have small amplitudes, although there are some potentials with larger amplitudes (Brown, 1984). Conversely, in a muscle undergoing a neurogenic disease process, the amplitudes of the motor unit potentials shift to higher values, reflecting the reinnervation process that usually takes place. These distributions were used to obtain the data shown in Fig. 2. It is not surprising to see that the estimation error decreases with increased sample size and increases with increased population size. However, it is interesting to observe that in general the estimates are larger than the actual number of MUs, and that this over-estimation error decreases as a function of sample size. It is also interesting to observe that the distribution modeling a normal muscle yields much higher estimation errors than those associated with the

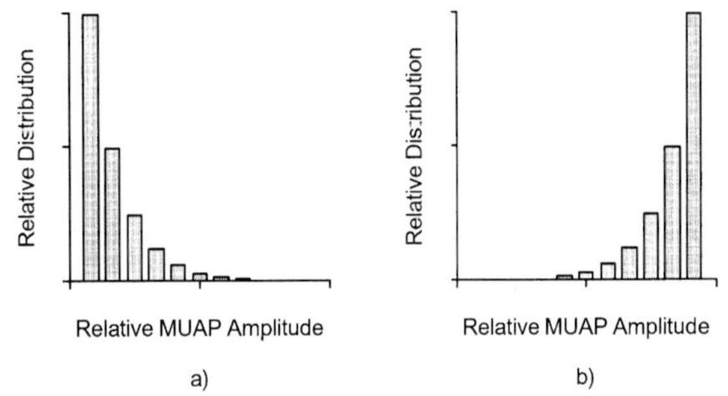

Fig. 1. Amplitude distributions used to represent: (a) normal; and (b) neurogenic muscles.

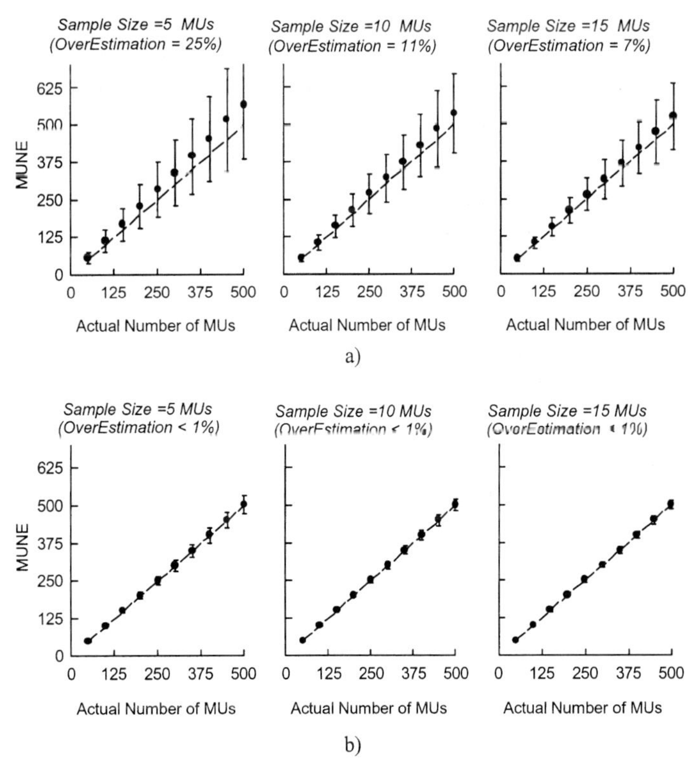

Fig. 2. Estimation error (expressed in terms of a standard deviation) as a function of population and sample size. (a) Data obtained using the distribution representing normal muscle. (b) Data obtained using the distribution representing neurogenic muscle.

distribution modeling a neurogenic muscle. In addition, neurogenic disease processes are associated with motor unit loss, hence reducing the population size, which in turn should act to further reduce the estimation error. It is important to note that the error values shown in Fig. 2 are only estimates of the actual errors since the distribution functions for the MU amplitudes are not explicitly known.

Temporal registration

Up to this point, the representation issue has only been considered in the context of how well the amplitude or area of the MU sample is representative of the entire MU population. However, there is a second component to the representation issue, namely temporal registration. Generally speaking, individual MUAPs tend to be biphasic or triphasic in nature. Therefore, in calculating the mean MU amplitude or area, it is important to maintain the proper temporal relationships of individual MUAPs with respect to each other. That is, phase cancellation will play a role in determining the mean MU amplitude or area.

Not all of the estimation techniques take temporal dispersion into account. In particular, with the increment counting technique and its derivatives, the temporal alignment of the individual MUAPs with respect to the M-wave potential is preserved, and is taken into account when calculating the average MUAP amplitude. However, techniques such as multiple point stimulation and those that use voluntary muscle activation to obtain the MU sample do not provide any temporal information in terms of how individual MUAPs should be aligned with respect to the M-wave potential. Therefore, in order to arrive at a MUNE value, it is assumed that the individual MUAPs summate in an algebraic manner. However, when the peaks of the MUAPs do not coincide with one another, the amplitude of the M-wave potential will be lower than the sum of the amplitudes of its constituent MUs. This results in an under-estimation of the MUNE value in the muscle.

Interestingly, Loof evaluated a similar problem that involved the temporal alignment of individual muscle fiber action potentials to their associated MUAP (Loof, 1986). Each muscle fiber action potential was aligned to the MUAP on the basis of the maximum correlation value between these two signals. While this approach could readily be extended to our problem of aligning MUAPs to the M-wave, there is no guarantee that the delay that yields the maximum correlation corresponds with the actual delay of the MUAP with respect to the M-wave. Specifically, let us assume that we are examining a muscle in which the shape of each MUAP is identical, but the latencies are not (i.e. each MU is associated with a different conduction velocity). Using Loof's correlation approach, the alignment of each MUAP with respect to the M-wave potential would be identical. This is clearly incorrect. While this example oversimplifies the actual conditions, it nonetheless illustrates the shortcomings of this approach. It should also be noted that Fang and colleagues have developed a neural network based approach to obtain temporal registration (Fang et al., 1996).

Linearity

In calculating the MU estimate using Eq. (1), it is assumed that the individual MUAPs summate in a linear fashion to yield the maximal evoked response. This translates to the following:

$$M(t) = \sum_{j=1}^{N} a_j(t), \qquad (2)$$

where $M(t)$ is the maximal CMAP response, $a_j(t)$ is the jth MUAP and N is the number of MUs. However, the contribution of a particular MU to the compound muscle potential depends on a number of factors, including muscle conductivity. Hence, Eq. (2) should be re-written as follows:

$$M(t) = \sum_{j=1}^{N} w_j \cdot a_j(t), \qquad (3)$$

where w_j is a weighting factor.

Parry et al. (1977) evaluated the influence of muscle conductivity on the MU estimates using both modeling and experimental studies. In particular, they modeled the muscle system in terms of a number of parallel MUs. Each MU was represented as a series combination of a voltage source and a source conductance, and was switched into the circuit only when it was active (Fig. 3a). Using this model, they predicted that the contribution of any given MU to the recorded surface potential decreased as a function of the number of active MUs (Fig. 3b). That is, the individual MUAPs did not summate in a linear fashion to yield the M-wave potential. The model explained this non-linearity in terms of a progressive increase in muscle conductivity as increased numbers of MUs are activated. They also demonstrated this non-linearity experimentally by recording the contribution of a number of MUs at both low stimulation levels (at which only a few MUs are active) and at supra-maximal stimulation levels (at which the entire MU population is active). On average, Parry and colleagues found that the MUAP amplitudes decreased by 20%, thus effectively leading to the underestimation the number of MUs in the muscle. However, it should be noted that there is some variability associated with the amplitude of the M-wave, and hence it is difficult to quantify the exact contribution of any given MU to the M-wave response. Secondly, the model employed by Parry and colleagues grossly over-simplifies the actual muscle system. In particular, they treat each MU as a lumped element consisting of purely resistive impedances, and assume that all of the MUs are in parallel with one another. Using computer models, Gielen et al. (1986) and Roth (1988) have shown that detailed anatomical parameters play an important role in the evolution of the recorded muscle potential and hence must be taken into account by any model of the muscle system. Interestingly, Roth and colleagues found that changes in the impedance of the muscle fiber membrane (and hence the conductivity of the MU) do not significantly influence the recorded potential. Therefore, at the present time, the role that muscle conductivity plays on the validity of the MU estimate remains uncertain.

Discussion

The purpose of this paper was to examine some of the current issues in motor unit number estimation. Of these, the sampling issue has received the

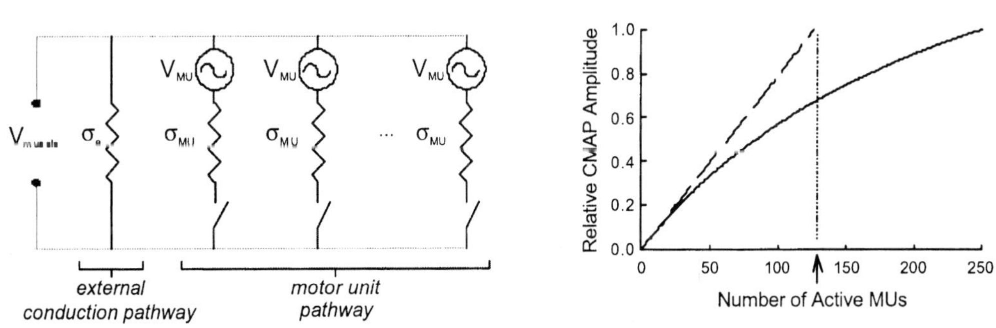

Fig. 3. (a) The model used by Parry and colleagues to represent the muscle system. Each MU represented is represented as a series arrangement of a voltage generator and a source conductance, and is switched into the circuit as it is activated. The muscle also has its own intrinsic conductance, which is represented by σ_{MU}. (b) The contribution of MU_1 (that is, the first MU to be activated) to the overall muscle potential as a function of the number of active MUs. This effectively results in the underestimation of the MUNE (e.g. 130 instead of the desired value of 250 for this particular example).

most attention. One obvious way of eliminating the sampling error would be to extend the sampling procedure to include all of the constituent MUs. However, this is not a viable approach since it becomes progressively more difficult to detect the activation of successive MUs. Sampling error would also not be a concern if all of the MUAPs were identical to one another. Unfortunately, there are several reasons why this is not the case. Firstly, there may be a large variation in the number of muscle fibers comprising each MU. Secondly, the fibers from each MU occupy a unique sub-space of the muscle. Hence, more superficial MUs make a larger contribution to surface recorded potentials than more distant MUs. In an effort to eliminate this inequality, some investigators have proposed that the recording location be removed from a site directly overlying the muscle and placed more remotely (Wee and Ashley, 1990). While volume conducted activity from other muscles may corrupt the activity originating from the muscle of interest, this idea warrants further attention, particularly if the ultimate goal of MU number estimation is to facilitate the early detection of muscle denervation that is manifested by a decreased number of motor units.

References

Arasaki, K., Tamaki, M., Hosoya, Y. and Kudo, N. Validity of electromyograms and tension as a means of motor unit number estimation. *Muscle Nerve*, 1997, 20: 552–560.

Brown, W.F. *The Physiological and Technical Basis of Electromyography*. Boston, Butterworths, 1984.

Fang, J., Shahani, B.T. et al. Motor unit estimate by spatial-temporal summation of single motor unit potentials (Abstract). *Muscle Nerve*, 1996, 19: 1203.

Gielen, F., Cruts, H. et al. Model of electrical conductivity of skeletal muscle based on tissue structure. *Med. Biol. Eng. Comput.*, 1986, 24(1): 34–40.

Loof, Y. Model for decomposition of the motor unit potential. I: the algorithm. *Med. Biol. Eng. Comput.*, 1986, 24: 506–512.

McComas, A.J., Fawcett, P.R.W. et al. Electrophysiological estimation of the number of motor units within a human muscle. *J. Neurol. Neurosurg. Psychiatry.*, 1971, 34: 121–131.

Parry, D.J., Mainwood, G.W. et al. The relationship between surface potentials and the number of active motor units. *J. Neurol. Sci.*, 1977, 33: 283–296.

Roth, B.J. The electrical potential produced by a strand of cardiac muscle: a bidomain analysis. *Ann. Biomed. Eng.*, 1988, 16(6): 609–637.

Slawnych, M., Laszlo, C. et al. Motor unit number estimation – sample size considerations. *Muscle Nerve*, 1997, 20(1): 22–28.

Stein, R.B. and Yang, J.F. Methods for estimating the number of motor units in human muscles. *Ann. Neurol.*, 1990, 28(4): 487–495.

Wee, A.S. and Ashley, R.A. Volume-Conducted or 'far-field' compound action potentials originating from the intrinsic-hand muscles. *Electromyogr. Clin. Neurophysiol.*, 1990, 30(6): 325–333.

Discussion after Section II

Clifton Gooch, New York, NY

It seems reasonable to assume that the effect of phase cancellation results in an underestimate of the total motor unit numbers, and the effect applies to many of the MUNE techniques. My first question is, can the magnitude of this effect be estimated by comparing motor unit numbers derived electrically by waveform analysis to numbers derived by twitch tension analysis?

Timothy Doherty, London, Ontario

Let me tell you what I know about such comparisons. Stein and Yang (*Annals of Neurology*, 1990, 28: 487–495) compared MUNE values based on force measures and surface-detected motor unit potentials in thenar muscles. Single units were elicited by intramuscular motor nerve stimulation, percutaneous stimulation, and voluntary activation. Their data showed that if you use area measures and compared MUNE values derived from surface-detected motor unit action potentials to force measures, the degree of phase cancellation is not as much of an issue (about 10% difference) compared to using peak measures. Our experience with the multiple point stimulation technique with thenar muscles is similar, and I will show the data in the next presentation.

Mike addressed some of the issues. If we use area values and perform a simple summation and mathematical average, we get a value that is only about 4–5% different than taking data point by data point and averaging waveforms. However, if we use peak-to-peak values and take a simple arithmetic average, and compare it to the maximum CMAP potential, the differences based on phase cancellation are as high as 15–20%.

Clifton Gooch, New York, NY

I think your points about no phase cancellation with the monophasic force responses are well taken. That being said, I think there is evidence that incremental force responses, or force responses due to single motor units, do not necessarily summate in a linear fashion. Nonlinearity in force measures is something that will have to considered, and may in the end negate any gains in terms of no phase cancellation.

Jasper Daube, Rochester, Minnesota

When you discussed this issue Mike, you really put together three different considerations. One consideration is the error that occurs in a waveform when you have a positive component that is being added to a negative waveform. You are canceling part of one (positive) by the other (negative). A second consideration is latency differences that represent a different kind of change than adding positive components. A third consideration is whether you are measuring waveform amplitude or area. If you are measuring area, many of the issues you described are no longer issues; latency differences do not have an effect, nor does phase cancellation. I do not have an answer when waveforms contain positive components, and I am wondering whether Mike has a thought about ways of dealing with the positive component?

Michael Slawnych, Calgary, Alberta

I do not know if I can add anything, other that to clarify what you said. You mentioned linearity, but I believe you are not referring to a linearity issue but to a phase cancellation issue. I am viewing it in a different context. By linearity, I am referring to the fact that each motor unit makes the same contribution to the compound muscle response, irrespective of how many motor units are active. By phase cancellation, I am referring to adding multiphasic potentials displaced in time due latency differences from temporal dispersion of the constituent motor unit action potentials.

My initial thoughts are that there will be some level of phase cancellation because even with a predominately negative waveform, because there may be positive components, and there will be some degree of temporal dispersion.

Timothy Doherty, London, Ontario

I would like to add that with the original incremental stimulation technique, these issues are dealt with in a physiologically appropriate manner. Stimulation at the same site on the nerve means that individual waveforms are contributing to the maximum CMAP as they originally would with regard to phase cancellation – positive, negative, peak alignment, and so on. These only become issues in techniques that lose the original temporal relationship, such as the multiple point stimulation or spike triggered averaging techniques. With these other techniques, reasonable modifications can be made to alignment individual waveforms as close as possible to the way they would have originally contributed to the CMAP wave, based on their temporal dispersion. Although the issue does exist, I do not know if phase cancellation is as much of an issue because it happens within the maximum CMAP. So, it may not necessarily be something we have to eliminate, but we need to make sure that it is not a bias that occurs in disease states that systematically pushes our MUNE one way or another.

Daniel Stashuk, Waterloo, Ontario

I would like to comment in regard to phase cancellation. Tim mentioned that techniques like multiple point stimulation and spike triggered averaging suffer from not having the proper alignment of individual units that they would have as they contribute to the CMAP. Michael showed sophisticated models to accomplish or compensate for lack of knowing the exact temporal relationships. The multiple point stimulation software Tim referred to does try to overcome this by aligning individual waveforms to the onset of the negative peak. If the electrodes are positioned over the motor point and you use onset alignment, latency differences between the different motor units are compensated for quite well. So, simple alignment and averaging of each individual SMUP goes a long way to having the mean SMUP contain the same amount of phase cancellation, or maybe a representative amount of phase cancellation, as would occur in the CMAP.

Clifton Gooch, New York, NY

My other question is whether anyone has done a histological cross-sectional analysis of the fibers in peripheral nerves that we typically test, and compare the results to motor units that are obtained by multiple point or incremental stimulation or other techniques to determine whether there is basis?

Alan McComas, Hamilton, Ontario

I cannot give a complete answer. In our 1971 paper, we looked at two specimens of deep peroneal nerve and counted the number of fibers and measured their diameters. The problem was that some nerve fibers pass through the extensor digitorum muscle and on to the interosseous muscles, leading to an anatomical overestimate. Another problem is that sometimes there is not a clear separation of large from smaller diameter fibers, leading to a unimodal distribution. Having said all that, it does need to be done again.

I would like to make two comments. First, I agree with everything Tim said about possible bias between stimulus intensity and motor unit size. I would mention that in certain muscles with a long length of peripheral nerve to work with, one can apply collision techniques to look at this issue. If it is the biophysical properties of the axon that is determining its excitability, then regardless of where you stimulate along the nerve, you should always preferentially excite that axon and its neighbors. In fact, that does not work out.

Second, my comment for Michael is that in your modeling of the neuropathic motor unit population, it appears as if, in addition to the large units which we are all familiar with, there is a population of normal-sized units, or even units smaller than normal because they are decompensating and presumably about to disappear.

Daniel Stashuk, Waterloo, Ontario

I have a question for Michael with regard to linearity. As the number of activated motor units increases, the contribution of individual motor units seem to decrease. Could that be because there is a greater chance of phase cancellation as more motor units are active, or is it really a nonlinear change in tissue characteristics?

Michael Slawnych, Calgary, Alberta

I think if you look at the technique that Parry and colleagues used (*J. Neurol. Sci.*, 1977; 33: 283–296) phase cancellation is not really an issue. They were able to isolate a single motor unit and measure its contribution when practically no motor units are active and when almost all motor units are active. Phase cancellation did not really play a role in the way that their experiment was set up. Does that answer your question?

Jasper Daube, Rochester, Minnesota

I did not understand the term "linearity" a little while ago, and I now know what you are referring to. My problem is that what you said makes no sense. What I like about what Alan described is simple and direct. When you say you add something in and it does not contribute, it makes no sense, so I wonder whether that paper was any good?

Section III

Stimulation MUNE Techniques

Motor Unit Number Estimation (Supplements to Clinical Neurophysiology Vol. 55)
Editor: M.B. Bromberg

Chapter 4

Multiple point stimulation and F-response MUNE techniques

Timothy J. Doherty[a,*], Daniel W. Stashuk[b] and William F. Brown[c]

[a]Department of Physical Medicine and Rehabilitation, The University of Western Ontario, St. Joseph's Health Care, 21 Grosvenor St., London, ON N6A 1Y6, Canada
[b]Department of Systems Design Engineering, The University of Waterloo, Waterloo, ON N2L 3G1, Canada
[c]Department of Neurology, Tuft's University, Boston, MA, USA

Introduction

Amyotrophic lateral sclerosis (ALS) and many inherited and acquired peripheral neuropathies result in progressive losses of motor axons and motor units (MUs). It is desirable to have reliable and sensitive techniques for estimating the numbers of MUs in a muscle group to provide a direct means to assess the severity, course, and responsive to treatment for these disorders. Several techniques now exist for estimating the number of MUs in a muscle or muscle group (Shefner, 2001; Doherty and Brown, 2002). They are referred to as motor unit number estimation (MUNE) techniques, and all rely on the same basic premise: the number of MUs in a muscle can be determined by dividing the size of the maximum compound muscle action potential (CMAP) by the average size of a representative sample of surface-detected MU action potentials (S-MUPs).

McComas et al. (1971) described the first electrophysiologic MUNE technique. As initially described for the extensor digitorum (EDB) muscle, successive, manually adjusted electrical stimuli were applied to the deep peroneal nerve at a single site close to the ankle through a bipolar surface electrode. With progressive increases in the stimulus intensity beyond motor threshold, incremental increases in the CMAP were detected. Each successive increment in the CMAP, as the stimulus intensity was increased, was considered to represent the addition of another single S-MUP as the activation threshold of its corresponding motor axon was reached. The stimulus was increased until there were 8–10 steps in the CMAP. The average S-MUP size was derived by dividing the negative peak or peak-to-peak amplitude of the CMAP by the number of component quantal steps. The estimate of the number of MUs in the EDB muscle (MUNE) was obtained by dividing the size of the maximum CMAP, evoked by supramaximal stimulation of the nerve at the same site, by the average S-MUP size. The technique was later applied to the intrinsic hand muscles (Brown, 1972; Sica et al., 1974).

It is well established that excitation of single motor axons and detection of their S-MUPs

*Correspondence to: Dr. T.J. Doherty, Department of Physical Medicine and Rehabilitation, The University of Western Ontario, St. Joseph's Health Care, 21 Grosvenor St., London, ON N6A 1Y6, Canada.
Tel.: (519) 646-6100x65975, Fax: (519) 646-6174.
e-mail: tim.doherty@sjhc.london.on.ca

doi: 10.1016/S1567-424X(03)00004-7

in response to graded percutaneous stimulation is entirely possible (Bergmans, 1973; Kadrie et al., 1976; Doherty and Brown, 1993). However, the phenomenon of alternation, or overlapping motor axon stimulation thresholds at a given stimulus intensity, has remained problematic for the original manual incremental stimulation (IS) technique (cf. Doherty et al., 2002, this volume). Therefore, multiple point stimulation (MPS) and the F-response techniques, among others, were established as a means of collecting a sample of S-MUPs, free of alternation, from which a MUNE could be derived. This paper will discuss the theoretical basis of the MPS and F-response techniques, their application to MUNE, pros and cons of each, and directions for future research.

Multiple point stimulation technique

In the original description of MPS (Doherty and Brown, 2002), the motor nerve was stimulated at several sites along its course, and at each site accepting as a single S-MUP only the "all" response of the first motor nerve fiber excited at that site (Fig. 1). Ten or more S-MUPs were collected from as many stimulus sites to provide a sample from which to derive the average S-MUP. Because MPS requires access to at least 50–100 mm of the motor nerve proximal to the muscle, the method is best applied to distal muscles including:

1. The median innervated thenar group.
2. The ulnar innervated hypothenar group.
3. The first dorsal interosseous/adductor pollicis muscle group.
4. The extensor digitorum brevis muscle.
5. In some instances more proximal muscles such as the anterolateral compartment muscles of the lower leg can be assessed. However, in most cases it is difficult to collect an adequate number of S-MUPs from the short segment of available nerve.

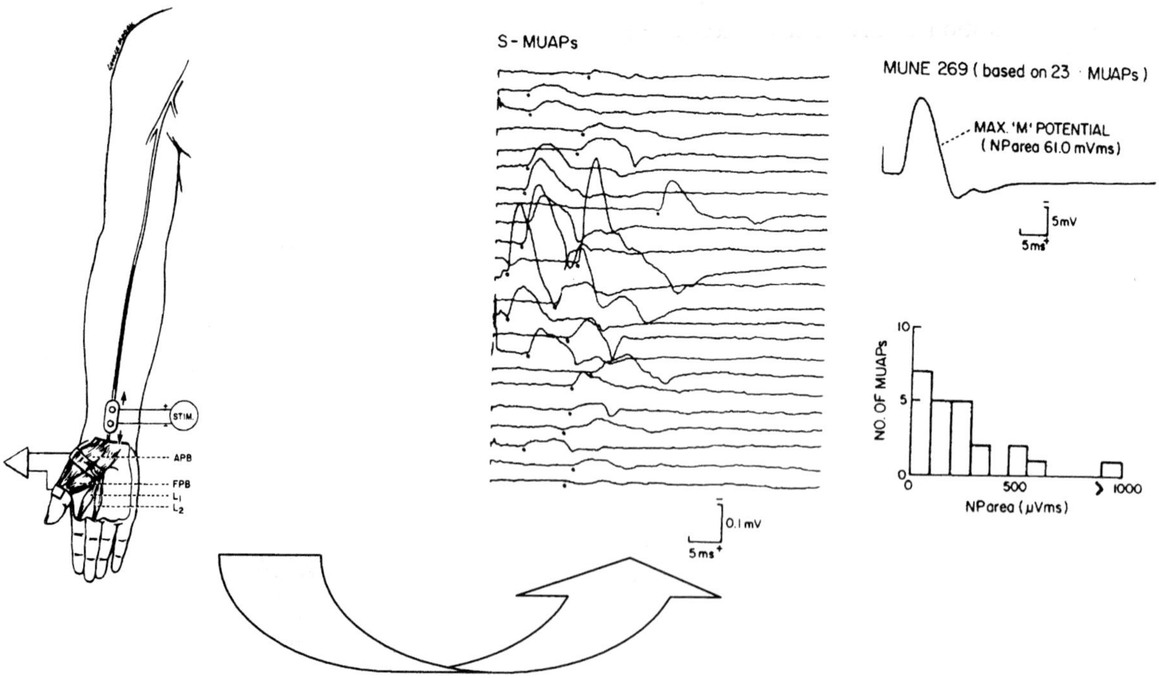

Fig. 1. Multiple point stimulation MUNE technique. *Left panel:* Recording and stimulating electrode arrangement for median nerve-thenar muscle group. *Middle panel:* Sample of 23 single motor unit potentials (S-MUPs). *Note:* Initial negative onset for most S-MUPs, and variation in onset latencies reflecting different sites of stimulation along median nerve. *Right panel:* Maximum M-potential in healthy control subject with MUNE value of 269. Histogram shows range of S-MUP sizes.

Methods: MPS applied to thenar muscles

Recording and ground electrodes

We have used self-adhering, commercially available electrodes, cut in strips approximately 1 × 3 cm, for detecting surface EMG signals. The active electrode is positioned transversely, in close proximity to the innervation zone of as many of the median innervated thenar MUs as possible. The reference electrode is located over the metacarpal phalangeal joint of the thumb. A ground electrode is placed over the back of the hand. The thumb is immobilized by tape to the side of the hand to minimize movement artifact. Surface signals are acquired with a band-width of 0.5–2 Hz to 5 kHz. With this position arrangement, S-MUPs voluntarily or electrically evoked are usually simple, bi-phasic, negative–positive potentials and the maximum M-potential has a corresponding initial negative deflection (Fig. 1).

At the outset of the study, single, supramaximal stimuli are delivered to the median nerve at the wrist and the position of the "active" electrode is adjusted in such a manner so as to maximize the negative peak amplitude and minimize the rise time of the maximum M-potential.

Finding suitable S-MUPs

In normal subjects, stimulation is carried out at 1 Hz with 50–100 μs pulses, using a commercially available hand-held stimulator with the cathode distal (Dantec Corp., model 13L26 or equivalent is suitable). Beginning with a stimulus site just proximal to the thenar motor point, the stimulus intensity is increased to the level at which the first single, reproducible, all-or-nothing S-MUP free of any indication of alternation, is found. Should it prove impossible to identify a suitable S-MUP, free of any indication of alternation at this site, the stimulating electrode is slightly moved to a new site. With practice, only a slight change in the pressure applied to the stimulator, or slightly rolling the stimulator over the nerve, will result in the ability to collect a suitable S-MUP, free of alternation. This process is repeated until 10 or more responses meeting the criteria for single S-MUPs are collected from various sites, stored and viewed on a rastered display.

Template subtraction

Special software has been developed that allows for template subtraction such that the "null" response may be stored and subtracted from the "all" response. This allows for subtraction of any stimulus or other artifact within the "null" response from the "all" response, and allows a better and more accurate indication of the onset and negative peak area of the corresponding S-MUP. Template subtraction, for the foregoing reasons, also makes it possible to stimulate the median nerve very close to the motor point (within 10–20 mm of the "active" electrode). Additionally, template subtraction allows the experienced operator to obtain S-MUPs corresponding to the second and sometimes even third or fourth successively higher threshold motor nerve fibers at a single site of stimulation. This latter approach greatly speeds up the acquisition and increases the number of S-MUPs in the sample.

In healthy controls, it is usually possible to collect 15 or more separate and distinct S-MUPs from the median nerve with stimulus sites between the distal forearm and motor point and again between the axilla and elbow. In the latter sites, it is important to avoid stimulating the ulnar nerve as it supplies part of the flexor pollicis brevis as well as several other nearby muscles whose S-MUPs might well be picked up by the recording electrodes. Stimulation of the median nerve in the proximal two-thirds of the forearm is generally unsatisfactory as the nerve lies too deep to stimulate comfortably or without producing so much movement and volume conducted EMG activity from the forearm muscles as to make the acquisition of single median innervated thenar S-MUPs impossible. An experienced operator can collect the sample of 15–20 S-MUPs in about 20 min.

Calculation of the MUNE

For each S-MUP, the onset and peak amplitudes are automatically selected, and the latency, negative peak, positive peak, negative peak duration, and negative peak area are determined.

One problem posed by the MPS, F-response and spike-triggered averaging techniques is that the relative latencies to the onsets and peaks for the various S-MUPs, as originally occurred when the maximum M-potential was obtained, are unknown. Such differences are naturally incorporated within the sum of the S-MUPs when the sample is collected at a single site of stimulation as is the case with both the original manual IS method and the subsequently developed statistical method (McComas et al., 1971; Daube, 1988). Our solution to this problem was to develop software that temporally aligns the onsets of all of the S-MUPs to the same latency value before they are averaged data point by data point. This produces a mean S-MUP template that best represents the effects of various phase cancellation and summation that occurred in the maximum M-potential. We feel, this method represents a reasonable approximation of how S-MUPs naturally sum in the CMAP especially when the maximum CMAP is collected as close to the motor point as possible (Doherty et al., 1993; Doherty and Brown, 2002). Mean values for younger and older subjects from our laboratory are shown in Table 1.

Assumptions underlying MPS

The MPS technique is based on a number of assumptions:

1. Threshold nerve stimulation is capable of reliably exciting a single motor nerve fiber.
2. A sufficiently large sample of S-MUPs can be selected by MPS to provide a meaningful and reliable measure of the mean S-MUP size from which to derive a MUNE.
3. The sample of S-MUPs collected by threshold stimulation is representative of the relative numbers of S-MUPs of different sizes for the population of S-MUPs that contributed to the maximum M-potential.

As with the manual IS technique, the evidence for the unitary nature of the S-MUPs in response to threshold stimulation is provided by their clear all-or-nothing characteristic in both surface and intramuscular signals. Additionally, with repeated stimuli there is no fractionation of the potentials as would suggest a compound potential corresponding to the stimulation of two or more motor axons simultaneously (Bergmans, 1973; Feasby and Brown, 1974; Doherty and Brown, 1993, 1994). The occasional presence of F-responses identical in size and shape to the direct response also provides evidence that a single motor axon has been stimulated. The low probability of obtaining an F-response, however, prevents its use as an absolute criterion that a single motor axon has been stimulated.

With regard to sample size, our studies in control subjects suggest that the mean S-MUP size can be calculated from a sample of 10 S-MUPs (Doherty and Brown, 1993). This is easily obtained for distal muscles with 50–100 mm of accessible nerve (thenar, hypothenar, EDB muscles). Obviously, for this or any other MUNE method, increasing

TABLE 1

MEAN VALUES ± SD FOR THENAR MUNE VALUES FROM THE MPS AND F-RESPONSE TECHNIQUES

MUNE technique	MUNE (value ± SD)	
	Young age	Older age (>65 years)
Multiple point stimulation		
Peak–peak amplitude	206 ± 58	104 ± 45
Negative peak area	288 ± 95	139 ± 68
F-response		
Negative peak area	245 ± 105	

the sample size may result in a sample that better represents the population of S-MUPs that contributed to the maximum M-potential and, in so doing, potentially increase the reliability and validity of the MUNE.

The degree to which MPS provides an unbiased sample of S-MUPs, representative of the relative numbers of S-MUPs of different sizes within the maximum M-potential, is perhaps more contentious. Classical studies based on direct stimulation of bared amphibian nerve trunks suggested that the larger, faster conducting fibers possessed lower thresholds for stimulation than the smaller, more slowly conducting fibers (Erlanger and Gasser, 1937). This was most true, however, when comparing different classes of nerve fibers and less so for a given class, such as in this case the alpha motor neurons. Kadrie et al. (1976) reported a rank ordering of median-innervated thenar S-MUPs with graded, low threshold percutaneous stimulation at a single site, such that the amplitudes of the lower threshold S-MUPs were less than those of subsequently evoked S-MUPs. These results were not supported in the original description of the manual incremental technique (McComas et al., 1971), nor in a more recent study in which the areas of the first and last of 20 step increases in the CMAP evoked by computer based IS were similar for both the thenar and EDB muscles (Galea et al., 1991).

Our own experience with threshold stimulation suggests that MPS provides an unbiased sample from which to derive a MUNE. This conclusion is based on several observations:

1. There is a wide range of S-MUP sizes and relative latencies in the sample collected from individual trials and across subjects (Doherty and Brown, 1993).
2. The size distribution of S-MUPs for individual trials mirrors the distribution for pooled subjects (Doherty and Brown, 1993).
3. Thenar MU twitch tensions are similar when samples are obtained with MPS (Doherty and Brown, 1997) are compared with samples obtained using intraneural microstimulation, intramuscular stimulation and spike-triggered averaging (Stein and Yang, 1990; Thomas et al., 1990).
4. Similar mean S-MUP sizes and MUNEs are obtained when MPS is directly compared with other methods for obtaining a sample of S-MUPs (spike-triggered averaging, F-response) (Doherty and Brown, 1993).
5. Collision experiments reveal that the likelihood of exciting the same motor axon at two separate sites along the nerve is only slightly greater than chance alone (Doherty and Brown, 1993).

Although MPS does not appear to provide a *biased* sample of MUs with regard to S-MUP size, MU force or relative latency, the selection of motor axons with low threshold stimulation does not occur entirely randomly. Recent observations suggest that for many sites of stimulation, one, or in some cases, several motor axons exhibit habitually lower thresholds than other motor axons (Doherty and Brown, 1994; Chan et al., 1998a, 1999). That is, for a given median nerve in a healthy control, the probability of stimulating any given motor axon is not 1 in 300, but considerably less for those axons located close to the stimulating electrode. As result, many of the same motor axons (MUs) may be found and excited time and time again in serial studies by threshold stimulation delivered at precisely the same site along the nerve.

The evidence that S-MUPs found in serial studies are generated by the same motor axon is based on their identical size, shape, latency, and in some cases twitch and tetanic tension in serial studies. The range of S-MUP sizes, MU twitch tensions, and latencies of this subset of motor axons does not appreciably differ however from that of the whole population. Thus, while this represents a subset of the whole population, it is an unbiased subset that remains representative of the whole population. This phenomenon has been exploited to follow individual MUs serially in patients with ALS (Chan et al., 1998b) and has provided a method to longitudinally follow physiologic responses to training in single MUs (Chan et al., 1999).

Advantages and disadvantages of MUPs

Advantages

Advantages of MPS as compared with other methods of deriving MUNEs include:

1. The average S-MUP size is based on the surface potentials generated by "true" single MUs and not a statistical estimate of S-MUP size or an estimate derived by algorithms designed to correct for alternation.
2. There is no alternation.
3. Near-motor-threshold stimuli are well tolerated.
4. The operator can readily identify other pathological properties of motor nerve fibers such as repetitive firing or decrements in the size of S-MUPs in response to repetitive stimulation. The latter are common in ALS and other rapidly developing axonal neuropathies where failures in neuromuscular transmission are common. It is important to realize that the latter may pass unrecognized and may represent an important potential source of error in both the manual IS and statistical methods for estimating motor unit numbers.

Disadvantages

The most important disadvantage of MPS is that it is not a hands-off technique. MPS requires skill on the part of the operator if a sufficient number of suitable motor nerve fibers with thresholds with clearly distinct thresholds are to be found within a reasonable time period (generally within 20 min). These skills include:

1. Learning to recognize the "all-or-nothing" change in the surface EMG signal associated with near threshold stimulation of a single motor nerve fiber while at the same time recognizing "alternation" and other errors which might lead to mistakes in properly identifying stimulation of single MUs.
2. Electromyographers must acquire, through experience and hands-on teaching, the requisite sensitivity and manual skill to satisfactorily carry out MPS. They must learn for example, to closely coordinate the position and pressure of the stimulating electrode with the changes observed in the surface EMG signal in response to fine changes in the stimulus intensity. The skills required are very similar to those required for carrying out stimulated single-fiber EMG.
3. Learning the "art" of searching along the course of the motor nerve for suitable low threshold, motor nerve fibers. This often involves making small adjustments in the position of the stimulating electrode by moving the electrode distally and proximally along the course of the nerve or even laterally while making fine changes in the pressure applied to the electrode, coupled with slight changes in the stimulus intensity. Once a suitable candidate single motor axon/S-MUP has been found, the operator must learn to hold the stimulating electrode steadily enough to acquire the requisite S-MUP.

MPS is much easier once electromyographers learn how to acquire successively higher threshold S-MUPs at single sites of stimulation and in some situations even learning how to acquire satisfactory S-MUPs in the face of "alternation".

The challenge of finding suitable single motor nerve fibers is greatest in young and healthy motor nerves, probably because there are many more motor nerve fibers (about 100 per intrinsic hand muscle). As well, the task is made more difficult as the thresholds of these motor nerve fibers often overlap even close to motor threshold. However, the task of finding suitable motor nerve fibers for stimulation is much easier in older subjects and patients with various motor neuropathies and motor neuronopathies because there are fewer motor nerve fibers, and more importantly, their thresholds are often more widely separated from one another. Indeed, in some patients the number of surviving motor nerve fibers is so low and the differences between their thresholds so great as to make it possible to "count" all the motor nerve fibers present by simply increasing the stimulus intensity of successive stimuli and activating successively higher threshold motor nerve fibers.

F-response technique

A second method of deriving a MUNE, free of alternation, is to draw on the pool of single S-MUPs in the population of F-responses elicited by a train of stimuli delivered to the motor nerve (Doherty et al., 1994; Stashuk et al., 1994). From such a pool of single S-MUPs in the F-response, an average S-MUP size may be calculated and divided into the maximum CMAP. For this method to be acceptable, however, it must be shown that the sample of S-MUPs so collected are indeed representative of the relative numbers of S-MUPs of different sizes and conduction velocities in the muscles group. Furthermore, the method should be well tolerated and conveniently carried out.

Methods: F-response technique applied to thenar muscles

Recording and ground electrodes

The F-response method, as with the manual IS method and MPS, is best applied to distal muscles. For the median innervated thenar muscles, the electrode arrangement and amplifier band-pass is the same as that described earlier for MPS. We have described both "manual" and "automated" methods of deriving a MUNE with the F-response (Doherty et al., 1994, 1995; Stashuk et al., 1994).

Manual and automated F-response detection

To collect a sufficient number of F-responses that meet the criteria for S-MUPs, at least 200–300 successive stimuli must be applied to the motor nerve distally (e.g. the wrist for the median innervated thenar muscles). In control subjects, the stimulus frequency is 2 Hz and is of sufficient intensity to evoke a direct thenar M-potential 10–30% of the maximum CMAP. Usually, such a train of stimuli is sufficient to obtain a population of F-responses containing at least 10 separate and distinct S-MUPs from which the mean S-MUP size may be calculated. At times, however, depending on the firing probability for F-responses in a given subject, a single site of stimulation proves insufficient to obtain enough S-MUPs to derive a MUNE. In these cases, a second or perhaps even a third site of stimulation must be chosen, at which additional trains of stimuli must be delivered to obtain the requisite number of S-MUPs from which to derive a MUNE. This strategy may also be used to obtain two or more independent MUNEs from which an average MUNE can be calculated as put forward by Galea et al. (1991).

We have developed computer-based algorithms to extract putative S-MUPs from the F-response (Stashuk et al., 1994). The first step in the process is to interpolate the baseline of each F-response in the train, using information contained in the positivitythat immediately precedes and follows each F-response. The interpolated baseline of each response is in turn subtracted from the corresponding F-response to obtain a response as free as possible of any baseline displacement. This initial processing makes it subsequently easier, either with simple visual comparison for the "manual" method or with computer algorithms for the automated method, to compare and sort out from all the F-responses those that represent single MUs.

Using the "manual", visual comparison method, each putative S-MUP extracted from the F-response is compared with all other responses and those that are identical in size, shape and latency are grouped. In our studies, F-responses identical in size, shape and latency that occurred on two or more occasions were considered to represent single MUs. Those that occur in isolation are considered to represent either compound F-responses (two or more MUs in combination), or F-responses generated by MUs with very low firing probability (i.e. fired once, or less than 0.67% in response to train of 300 stimuli). With the automated method, putative S-MUPs are compared with all of the extracted F-responses and template-matching algorithms are used to cluster identical S-MUPs into groups based on size, shape and latency criteria. A representative S-MUP from each group of identical responses, the members of which are considered to represent S-MUPs produced by the same MU, is then chosen. The sample of representative S-MUPs (10 or more) is then averaged on a data-point by data-point basis (as described for MPS) to derive a mean S-MUP size. This is then divided into the maximum CMAP to calculate the MUNE. Additionally, with the inclusion of the distance from the site of stimulation to the cervical cord, in the case of the thenar or hypothenar muscles, it is possible to calculate axonal conduction velocities from the F latency values (Doherty et al., 1994).

Assumptions underlying F-response technique

The appropriateness of drawing upon a sample of S-MUPs extracted from the F-response as a method of deriving a MUNE is based on the following assumptions:

1. It is possible manually, or with an automated program, to extract a sample of S-MUPs from the F-response that represents the activity of single MUs.
2. Such a sample is representative of the relative numbers of S-MUPs of different sizes and latencies for the whole population of S-MUPs in the muscle group in both health and disease.
3. The preceding are independent of the stimulus intensity at which the F-responses are collected.

With the above described methods, in order for an F-response to be considered as representing a single MU, it must occur with identical size, shape and latency on two or more occasions (Feasby and Brown, 1974; Doherty et al., 1994). This assumption is based on our own and other's observations that in healthy controls the chance of an F-response occurring in any one MU rarely exceeds 10% and is usually on the order of 1 in 50 to 1 in 100 (mean $1.6 \pm 1.5\%$ SD in our studies on the median innervated thenar muscles in controls). Provided the chance of an F-response occurring in any single MU is truly independent of the chance of an F-response in any other MU, the chance of seeing any particular combination of two or more MUs in the F-response should equal the product of the chances of an F-response in each of the individual MUs.

For example, in the case of two MUs, each with a 1 in 10 chance of an F-response, the combination might be expected to occur once in 100 stimuli, or 2–3 times in 200–300 stimuli (the typical number of stimuli used in our method). However, as pointed out for controls, the probability of an F-response occurring in any one MU seldom approaches 10%, most with occurrence rates of 1–3 in 100. Therefore, provided that the chances that F-responses in different MUs are truly independent, the likelihood of a compound F-response being accepted as representing a single MU is exceedingly low (1–2 times per 1000 trials).

In some pathologic conditions, however, such as ALS or occasionally in the recovering stages of the Guillain–Barré syndrome, the chance of an F-reponse occurring in any one MU is much higher (possibly greater than 50%). In such cases, taking the above into account, the combination of two or more MUs masquerading as a single MU might be expected to be quite high. Obviously, if such combinations were accepted as representing S-MUPs (single MUs), the average S-MUP size would be distorted and the MUNE erroneous. This potential source of error needs to be considered in applying this method in such circumstances. However, under most conditions it is very reasonable to consider that a sample of S-MUPs extracted as described from the F-response represent the activity of single MUs.

In our experience, S-MUPs drawn from the F-response, meeting the criteria for single MUs, vary widely in size and their size distributions are similar to those collected from the same subjects with MPS or spike-triggered averaging methods (Doherty et al., 1993, 1994, 1995; Fig. 2). Additionally, the latencies for single S-MUPs in the F-response vary widely in control subjects and their calculated conduction velocities are similar to the ranges of conduction velocities published based on other methods (Ingram et al., 1987; Dengler et al., 1988; Dengler et al., 1992). In our studies, both the size and latency of S-MUPs were independent of the stimulus intensity between 10 and 30% of the maximum M-potential. Thus, at

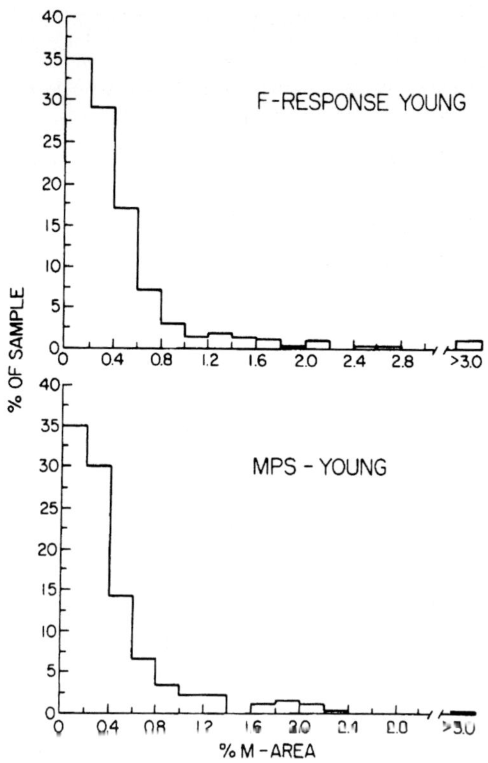

Fig. 2. The distribution of the size (negative peak area) of single motor unit potentials collected by the MPS and F-response techniques. *Note:* Similar distributions, including relatively large number of small potentials, from both techniques.

TABLE 2

ADVANTAGES AND DISADVANTAGES OF THE MPS AND F-RESPONSE METHODS

Multiple point stimulation technique

Advantages
1) Applicable to any EMG system in basic form
2) Non-invasive
3) Threshold stimuli well tolerated
4) Ability to recognize pathologic features of S-MUAP (e.g. decrement, repetitive firing)
5) Minimal patient cooperation required

Disadvantages
1) Requires considerable operator skill and experience
2) Not applicable to proximal muscles
3) S-MUAPs not collected at a single site of stimulation

F-response technique

Advantages
1) Non-invasive
2) Requires little operator skill
3) Provides additional information about axonal conduction velocity
4) Minimal patient cooperation required

Disadvantages
1) Requires special software
2) May be time consuming
3) Patients may not tolerate multiple stimuli
4) Not applicable to proximal muscles

least for controls, there appears to be no bias in the sample of S-MUPs drawn from the F-response. As noted above, however, in some pathologic conditions a subset of MUs may have a much higher probability of firing an F-response, thus, leading to a potentially biased sample of S-MUPs. This has not been systematically investigated to date in specific disorders.

Advantages and disadvantages of F-response technique

The advantages and disadvantages of the F-response technique are outlined in Table 2. The major advantages of the F-response technique are that it is a "hands-off" technique and that it provides information related to latency and conduction velocity. The disadvantages include the need for specialized software and that in some cases very few F-responses meeting the criteria for S-MUPs are obtained.

Summary

Both MPS and the F-response techniques provide what appears to be a representative sample of S-MUPs from which to derive a MUNE. While MPS in its basic form can be carried out on any EMG system, specialized software that allows for template subtraction and the calculation of an average S-MUP waveform are important additions and improve efficiency and validity, respectively. Future work is required to determine the reliability and precision of MPS in specific clinical conditions – both of which are important in order for MPS or any other MUNE method to be accepted as useful clinical outcomes.

References

Bergmans, J. Physiologic observation of single human nerve fibres. "*Electromyography and Clinical Neurophysiology*" (J.E. Desmedt, Ed.), 1973, pp. 89–127. Karger, Basel.

Brown, W.F. A method for estimating the number of motor units in thenar muscles and the changes in motor unit count with ageing. *J. Neurol. Neurosurg. Psychiatry*, 1972, 35: 845–852.

Chan, K.M., Doherty, T.J., Andres, L.P., Porter, M.M., Brown, T. and Brown, W.F. Longitudinal study of the contractile and electrical properties of single human thenar motor units. *Muscle Nerve*, 1998a, 21: 839–849.

Chan, K.M., Stashuk, D.W. and Brown, W.F. A longitudinal study of the pathophysiological changes in single human thenar motor units in amyotrophic lateral sclerosis. *Muscle Nerve*, 1998b, 21: 1714–1723.

Chan, K.M., Andres, L.P., Polykovskaya, Y. and Brown, W.F. The effects of training through high-frequency electrical stimulation on the physiological properties of single human thenar motor units. *Muscle Nerve*, 1999, 22: 186–195.

Daube, J.R. Statistical estimates of number of motor units in thenor and foot muscles in patients with amyotrophic lateral sclerosis or the residue of poliomyelitis, *Muscle Nerve*, 1988, 11: 957.

Dengler, R., Stein, R.B. and Thomas, C.K. Axonal conduction velocity and force of single human motor units. *Muscle Nerve*, 1988, 11: 136–145.

Dengler, R., Kossev, A., Wohlfahrt, K., Schubert, M., Elek, J. and Wolf, W. F waves and motor unit size. *Muscle Nerve*, 1992, 15: 1138–1142.

Doherty, T., Simmons, Z., O'Connell, B., Felice, K.J., Conwit, R., Chan, K.M., Komori, T., Brown, T., Stashuk, D.W. and Brown, W.F. Methods for estimating the numbers of motor units in human muscles. *J. Clin. Neurophysiol.*, 1995, 12: 565–584.

Doherty, T.J. and Brown, W.F. The estimated numbers and relative sizes of thenar motor units as selected by multiple point stimulation in young and older adults. *Muscle Nerve*, 1993, 16: 355–366.

Doherty, T.J. and Brown, W.F. A method for the longitudinal study of human thenar motor units. *Muscle Nerve*, 1994, 17: 1029–1036.

Doherty, T.J. and Brown, W.F. Age-related changes in the twitch contractile properties of human thenar motor units. *J. Appl. Physiol*, 1997, 82: 93–101.

Doherty, T.J. and Brown, W.F. Motor Unit Number Estimation: Methods and Applications. In Brown, W.F., Bolton, C. F. and Aminoff, M.J. (Eds) *Clinical Neurophysiology and Neuromuscular Disease*. Philadelphia, W.B. Saunders, 2002, 274–290.

Doherty, T.J., Stashuk, D.W. and Brown, W.F. Determinants of mean motor unit size: impact on estimates of motor unit number. *Muscle Nerve*, 1993, 16: 1326–1331.

Doherty, T.J., Komori, T., Stashuk, D.W., Kassam, A. and Brown, W.F. Physiological properties of single thenar motor units in the F-response of younger and older adults. *Muscle Nerve*, 1994, 17: 860–872.

Erlanger, J. and Gasser, H.S. *Electrical signs of nervous activity*. Philadelphia, University of Pennsylvania Press, 1937.

Feasby, T.E. and Brown, W.F. Variation of motor unit size in the human extensor digitorum brevis and thenar muscles. *J. Neurol. Neurosurg. Psychiatry*, 1974, 37: 916–926.

Galea, V., de Bruin, H., Cavasin, R. and McComas, A.J. The numbers and relative sizes of motor units estimated by computer. *Muscle Nerve*, 1991, 14: 1123–1130.

Ingram, D.A., Davis, G.R. and Swash, M. Motor nerve conduction velocity distributions in man: results of a new computer-based collision technique. *Electroencephalogr. Clin. Neurophysiol.*, 1987, 66: 235–243.

Kadrie, H.A., Yates, S.K., Milner-Brown, H.S. and Brown, W.F. Multiple point electrical stimulation of ulnar and median nerves. *J. Neurol. Neurosurg. Psychiatry*, 1976, 39: 973–985.

McComas, A.J., Fawcett, P.R., Campbell, M.J. and Sica, R.E. Electrophysiological estimation of the number of motor units within a human muscle. *J. Neurol. Neurosurg. Psychiatry*, 1971, 34: 121–131.

Shefner, J.M. Motor unit number estimation in human neurological diseases and animal models. *Clin. Neurophysiol*, 2001, 112: 955–964.

Sica, R.E. P., McComas, A.J. and Upton, A.R.M. Motor unit estimation in small muscles of the hand. *J. Neurol. Neurosurg. Psychiatry*, 1974, 37, 55–67.

Stashuk, D.W., Doherty, T.J., Kassam, A. and Brown, W.F. Motor unit number estimates based on the automated analysis of F-responses. *Muscle Nerve*, 1994, 17: 881–890.

Stein, R.B. and Yang, J.F. Methods for estimating the number of motor units in human muscles. *Ann. Neurol.*, 1990, 28: 487–495.

Thomas, C.K., Johansson, R.S., Westling, G. and Bigland-Ritchie, B. Twitch properties of human thenar motor units measured in response to intraneural motor-axon stimulation. *J. Neurophysiol.*, 1990, 64: 1339–1346.

Motor Unit Number Estimation (Supplements to Clinical Neurophysiology Vol. 55)
Editor: M.B. Bromberg

Chapter 5

Adapted multiple point stimulation MUNE technique

F.C. Wang[a,]*, O. Bouquiaux[a], V. De Pasqua[a],
A. Maertens de Noordhout[b] and P.J. Delwaide[b]

[a]*University Department of Physical Medicine and Rehabilitation, B-4000 Liège, Belgium*
[b]*University Department of Neurology, B-4000 Liège, Belgium*

Introduction

Before developing our adapted multiple point stimulation (AMPS) technique, we tried the incremental stimulation technique initially proposed by McComas et al. (1971) and the multiple point stimulation (MPS) technique (Doherty and Brown, 1993). However, in our practice, neither was completely satisfactory. The original McComas technique was faced with the phenomenon of alternation, while with the MPS technique it was sometimes not possible to evoke 10 distinct motor unit potentials at 10 different stimulation points along the accessible course of the nerve, particularly in patients with severe axonal loss. These difficulties prompted us to seek an alternative technique, which would be non-invasive, fast and easily applicable in most clinical situations.

Methods

The principle of AMPS was initially reported by Kadrie et al. (1976). Electrode placement, recording and stimulation settings have been presented in detail (Wang and Delwaide, 1995). In this method, incremental stimulation is applied at distinct points along the median nerve between the wrist and the elbow to collect the sample of 10 motor units needed to estimate the mean motor unit size. Incremental stimulation (50 μs stimulation duration, weak intensity gradually increased by increments of 0.1–0.5 mA) is used to allow sequential activation of individual motor axons. At each stimulation point, two or three surface motor unit potentials (SMUP) are successively evoked, and the resultant compound motor response is selected only if SMUPs are free of alternation. By dividing the maximum M-potential size by the average SMUP size, a motor unit number estimate (MUNE) is obtained.

Each SMUP is randomly incorporated in the estimation. However, to avoid alternation and ensure that any increment of the motor response corresponds to the activation of one single motor unit, specific criteria have to be met. SMUP have to be evoked with distinct thresholds, in an all-or-nothing fashion, with no fractionation of the compound motor responses to successive identical stimuli, and in an orderly and reproducible manner. Predominantly positive SMUP are eliminated as they are supposed to be elicited from distant muscles.

*Correspondence to: Dr. F.C. Wang, Department of Physical Medicine and Rehabilitation, CHU Sart Tilman, B35, B-4000 Liège, Belgium.
Tel.: 32-4-366-76-44, Fax: 32-4-366-72-30.
e-mail: fc.wang@chu.ulg.ac.be

doi: 10.1016/S1567-424X(03)00005-9

Except for the first SMUP evoked at each selected stimulation point, the precise morphology of successive SMUP is not visualized, due to the summation of an additional one or two units. It is theoretically possible that the same SMUP could be recorded twice, from two different stimulation points, because their morphology might not be recognizable. To ensure that selected SMUP are different, the morphology of individual SMUP is reconstructed by subtracting from each compound motor response the preceding one obtained from the same stimulus site with a lower intensity. This reconstruction takes place automatically when point-by-point differences are measured between successive digitized traces (Wang and Delwaide, 1995).

Validity of the AMPS technique

Reproducibility

In 10 normal subjects, thenar MUNE as well as average SMUP size estimates were evaluated twice with the AMPS method by the same examiner on two successive days. Coefficients of variation between results from both trials were 10.4% for MUNE values and 9.5% for average SMUP size (Wang and Delwaide, 1995).

Comparison with other MUNE techniques

In 54 control subjects, the AMPS and F-response techniques (Stashuk et al., 1994) were compared. Results obtained with both techniques were very similar, with correlation coefficients of 0.83 ($P < 0.001$) for MUNE and 0.62 ($P < 0.001$) for average SMUP sizes (Wang and Delwaide, 1995).

Thenar MUNE values obtained with AMPS in control subjects (Wang and Delwaide, 1995) were close to those reported with other MUNE techniques (Brown, 1972; Sica et al., 1974; Lee et al., 1975; Milner-Brown and Brown, 1976; Daube, 1988; Galea et al., 1991; Doherty and Brown, 1993; Stashuk et al., 1994).

AMPS advantages and disadvantages

Advantages

The AMPS technique is easily applied in clinical practice. It does not require specific recording systems or software and can be completed in about 15 min. It was possible to obtain a MUNE in all 70 volunteers studied without technical failures. The AMPS technique is non-invasive and painless as only surface electrodes and low stimulation intensities are used.

Disadvantages

AMPS is not a hands-off technique, and the skill of the practitioner has to be taken into account. A subjective bias in recognition of new SMUP is possible. This technique is limited to superficial muscles with a long accessible segment of nerve (thenar and hypothenar muscles, extensor digitorum brevis muscle).

AMPS technique in patients with ALS

Data were collected from 22 patients with amyotrophic lateral sclerosis (ALS) (11 women and 11 men), whose age ranged from 36 to 76 years (mean 58 ± 11). On the first evaluation by AMPS (T0), none had received drug therapy; but all received riluzole after T0.

Reproducibility

In patients with ALS, when AMPS is performed twice in the same session with new electrode placements for the second trial, the coefficient of variation for both MUNE and average SMUP size was 4% between the two trials (Wang and Delwaide, 1998). In longitudinal studies, meticulous replication of electrode placement was sought by measuring in each patient the precise distance between the stigmatic electrode and tip of the thumb.

Ease of use

In our experience, MUNE is easier to obtain in patients with severe axonal loss than in healthy volunteers. In agreement with previous reports (Brown and Milner-Brown, 1976), there was less overlap of motor unit thresholds when denervation was severe and, therefore, alternation was less noticeable. Abundant fasciculation potentials, excessive spasticity or absence of relaxation could make the applications of AMPS somewhat trickier. Neuromuscular transmission defects, as frequently observed in patients with ALS (Mulder et al., 1959; Carleton and Brown, 1979; Bernstein and Antel, 1981), could induce changes of motor response size which could be interpreted as a different unit or activation of a new motor unit.

MUNE results in ALS subjects

Cross-sectional evaluation

Among 22 patients with ALS, 19 (86%) had initial thenar MUNE values less than the normal lower limit according to age (defined in a group of 70 healthy subjects). Figure 1 illustrates the statistically significant relationship between thenar MUNE values and time from symptom onset. As shown, MUNE data supports the finding that patients with a total disease duration (survival from time of disease onset) of less than 3 years ($n = 10$) had a greater rate of motor unit loss than in patients with a total disease duration of more than 3 years ($n = 12$).

The relationship between average SMUP size and the evolution time from the beginning of symptoms is shown in Fig. 2. In patients with a total disease duration of more than 3 years ($n = 12$) there was a progressive increase in average SMUP size. In patients with a survival of less than 3 years ($n = 10$) the increase in average SMUP size was less and followed by a secondary decrease in motor unit size. The initial motor unit size increase was mainly due to collateral reinnervation. The secondary decrease in average SMUP size might indicate less efficacious collateral sprouting, "disintegration" of motor units reinnervated at earlier stages (Emeryk-Szajewska et al., 1997) or the loss of particularly large motor units.

Longitudinal study

Figure 3 summarises longitudinal results of a 1-year follow-up in 17 patients with ALS who received riluzole after the first evaluation (T0). Thenar MUNE values every four months show a statistically significant decrease. The mean loss of

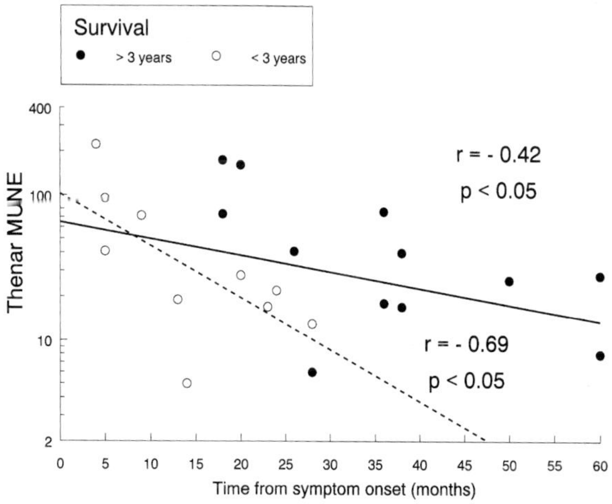

Fig. 1. Relationship between thenar MUNE and the duration between symptom onset and initial evaluation (T0) in 22 patients with ALS.

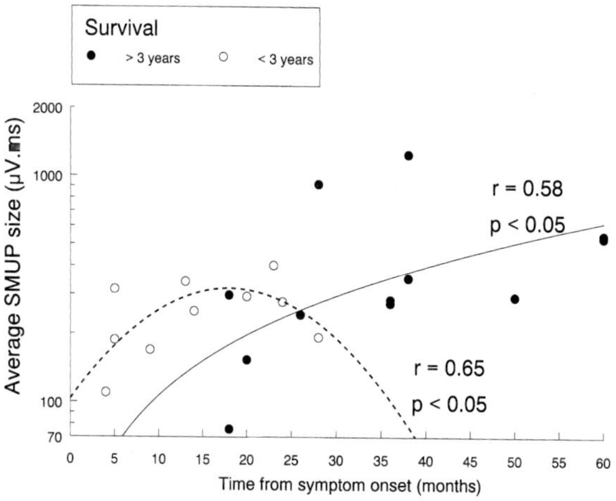

Fig. 2. Relationship between average SMUP size and the duration between symptom onset and initial evaluation (T0) in 22 patients with ALS.

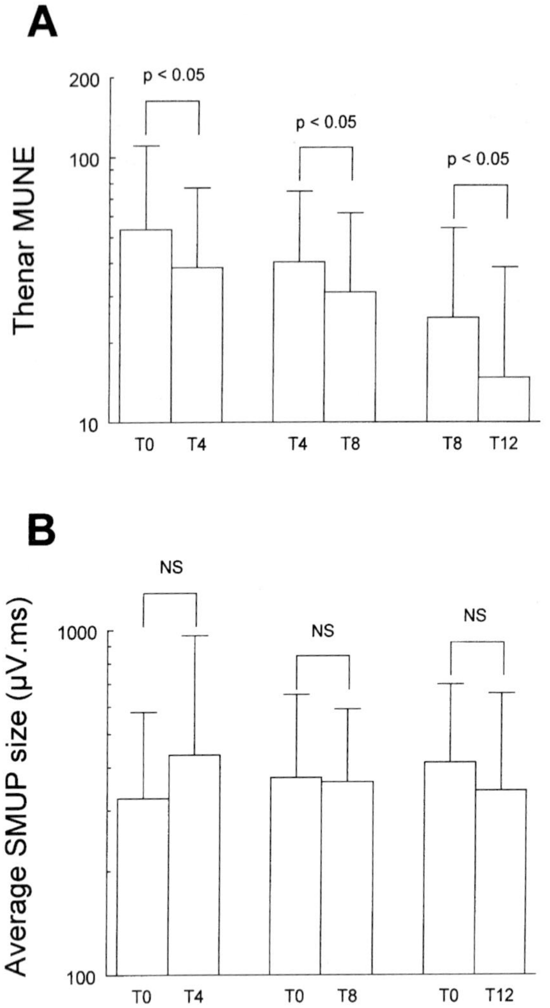

Fig. 3. Longitudinal results (mean + 1SD) of the AMPS method in 17 patients with ALS before (T0) and after 4 (T4, $n = 17$), 8 (T8, $n = 15$), and 12 (T12, $n = 13$) months of riluzole therapy. (A) Thenar MUNE. (B) Average SMUP size.

motor units over 12 months of treatment reached 72%, which contrasts with the 1.4% physiological loss of motor units with age (Wang and Delwaide, 1995) (Fig. 3A).

Conversely, the mean motor unit size did not significantly change even when results from T0 and T12 months were compared (Fig. 3B). These data probably reflect the fact that several parameters influence motor unit size in different ways and that patients were not at same stage of disease evolution. Collateral reinnervation, which was probably more efficacious in early stages, increased the size of some motor units. However, the disappearance of some large motor units and the "disintegration" phenomenon, which might occur in terminal stages, decreased the mean motor unit size.

Conclusion

We propose AMPS as a reliable MUNE technique that is comfortable for subjects and allows quantification of motor unit loss and changes in average SMUP size in ALS patients over time.

References

Bernstein, L.P. and Antel, J.P. Motor neuron disease: decremental responses to repetitive nerve stimulation. *Neurology*, 1981, 31: 204–207.

Brown, W.F. A method for estimating the number of motor units in thenar muscles and the changes in motor unit count with ageing. *J. Neurol. Neurosurg. Psychiatry*, 1972, 35: 845–852.

Brown, W.F. and Milner-Brown, H.S. Some electrical properties of motor units and their effects on the methods of estimating motor unit numbers. *J. Neurol. Neurosurg. Psychiatry*, 1976, 39: 249–257.

Carleton, S.A. and Brown, W.F. Changes in motor unit populations in motor neurone disease. *J. Neurol. Neurosurg. Psychiatry*, 1979, 42: 42–51.

Daube, J.R. Statistical estimates of number of motor units in thenar and foot muscles in patients with amyotrophic lateral sclerosis or the residual of poliomyelitis. *Muscle Nerve*, 1988, 11: 957 (Abstract).

Doherty, T.J. and Brown, W.F. The estimated numbers and relative sizes of thenar motor units as selected by multiple point stimulation in young and older adults. *Muscle Nerve*, 1993, 16: 355–366.

Emeryk-Szajewska, B., Kopec, J. and Karwanska, A. The reorganization of motor units in motor neuron disease. *Muscle Nerve*, 1997, 20: 306–315.

Kadrie, H.A., Yates, S.K., Milner-Brown, H.S. and Brown, W.F. Multiple point electrical stimulation of ulnar and median nerves. *J. Neurol. Neurosurg. Psychiatry*, 1976, 39: 973–985.

Lee, R.G., Ashby, P., White, D.G. and Aguayo, A.J. Analysis of motor conduction velocity in the human median nerve by computer simulation of compound muscle action potentials. *Electroencephalogr. Clin. Neurophysiol.*, 1975, 39: 225–237.

McComas, A.J., Fawcett, P.R.W., Campbell, M.J. and Sica, R.E.P. Electrophysiologic estimation of the number of motor units within a human muscle. *J. Neurol. Neurosurg. Psychiatry*, 1971, 34: 121–131.

Milner-Brown, H.S. and Brown, W.F. New methods of estimating the number of motor units in a muscle. *J. Neurol. Neurosurg. Psychiatry*, 1976, 39: 258–265.

Mulder, D.W., Lambert, E.H. and Eaton, L.M. Myasthenic syndrome in patients with amyotrophic lateral sclerosis. *Neurology*, 1959, 9: 627–631.

Sica, R.E.P., McComas, A.J., Upton, A.R.M. and Longmire, D. Motor unit estimations in small muscles of the hand. *J. Neurol. Neurosurg. Psychiatry*, 1974, 37: 55–67.

Stashuk, D.W., Doherty, T.J., Kassam, A. and Brown, W.F. Motor unit number estimates based on the automated analysis of F-responses. *Muscle Nerve*, 1994, 17: 881–890.

Wang, F.C. and Delwaide, P.J. Number and relative size of thenar motor units estimated by an adapted multiple point stimulation method. *Muscle Nerve*, 1995, 18: 969–979.

Wang, F.C. and Delwaide, P.J. Number and relative size of thenar motor units in ALS patients: application of the adapted multiple point stimulation method. *Electroencephalogr. Clin. Neurophysiol.*, 1998, 109: 36–43.

Motor Unit Number Estimation (Supplements to Clinical Neurophysiology Vol. 55)
Editor: M.B. Bromberg

Chapter 6

MUNE by intraneural microstimulation and the effects of averaging of unitary muscle action potentials

Keisuke Arasaki*

EMG/EEG Laboratory, Department of Neurology, NTT East Kanto Medical Center, 5-9-22 Higashi-Gotanda, Shinagawa-ku, Tokyo 141-0022, Japan

Introduction

A motor unit is a functional group of structures consisting of the spinal alpha motoneuron, its axon, and muscle fibers innervated by branches of the axon. Inasmuch as we cannot count the number of human motor units, we use as a substitute a motor unit number estimate (MUNE). Eight techniques, excluding the one presented here, have been described for obtaining a MUNE (McComas, 1998). Among them are five major techniques: increment stimulation, statistical, F-wave, spike-triggered averaging, and multiple point stimulation. The increment stimulation technique is associated with the problem of alternation (McComas, 1998), which leads to overestimation of the number of motor units. The statistical technique is based on the assumption that the variance of the submaximal compound muscle action potential (CMAP) amplitude follows the Poisson distribution (Daube, 1995), and the resulting MUNEs are dependent upon the intensity of the nerve stimulation. The F-wave technique requires that two identical F-responses be identified to be certain that they represent a unitary muscle action potential (MAP) and that there is no size bias (Stashuk et al., 1994).

Although spike-triggered averaging (Brown et al., 1988) and multiple point stimulation techniques (Doherty et al., 1993) are free from the pitfall of alternation, they involve another problem called phase cancellation (Stein et al., 1990). Phase cancellation occurs when a portion of the negative phase of a single unitary MAP is canceled by the positive phase of another unitary MAP. Because of phase cancellation, the area of the negative phase of the CMAP may be smaller than the sum of the areas of the negative phases of all unitary MAPs. Accordingly, when a MUNE is calculated by dividing the area of the negative phase of the maximal CMAP by the area of the negative phase of the average unitary MAP, the result may be an underestimation of the number of motor units.

Prior to our human studies, we performed animal studies to refine a new and reliable method to obtain MUNEs – a method unaffected by alternation or phase cancellation. Because MUNEs obtained by our new method were well correlated with anatomic estimates of the number of motoneurons (Arasaki et al., 1997), we applied this method to human subjects.

**Correspondence to*: Dr. Keisuke Arasaki, EMG/EEG Laboratory, Department of Neurology, NTT East Kanto Medical Center, Tokyo 141-0022, Japan.
Tel.: 81-3-3448-6455, Fax: 81-3-3448-6458.
e-mail: arasaki@rr.iij4u.or.jp

doi: 10.1016/S1567-424X(03)00006-0

Methods

We obtained MUNEs in 20 patients with headaches (age range 30–80 years) who had no spinal or peripheral nerve disorders. Before testing, we discussed the procedure and its possible adverse effects and obtained their consent. Our research project was reviewed and approved by the Committee for the Assurance of Clinical Study Quality in our institution.

Surface electrodes on the hypothenar and extensor digitorum brevis (EDB) muscles were used to record maximal CMAPs and unitary MAPs (Fig. 1). For microstimulation of motor axons, fine tungsten-needle electrodes with tip impedances of 9–13 MΩ at 1000 Hz and 10^{-8} A (Frederick Haer & Co., Brunswick, ME, USA) were inserted into the ulnar and peroneal nerves at the wrist and the ankle, respectively. Square wave current pulses (duration of 100 μs) were delivered to active single motor axon with the lowest threshold. While keeping the same insertion point, we manipulated the needle electrode manually so that its tip activated different axons in the nerve.

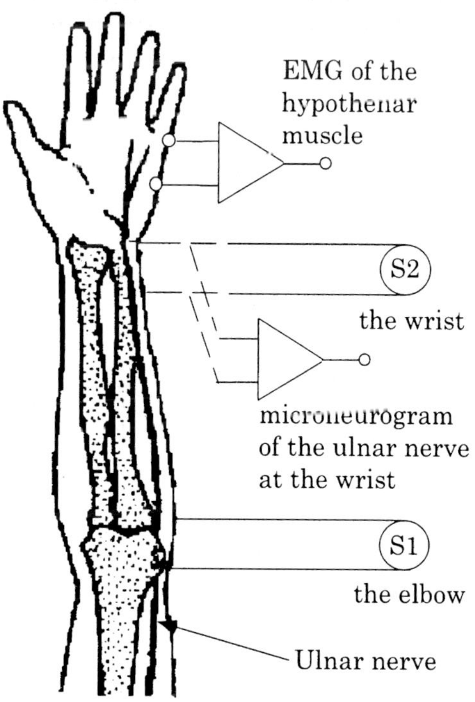

Fig. 1. Recording and stimulating arrangement for the intraneural microstimulation MUNE technique applied to the ulnar–hypothenar muscle.

The area of the negative portion of the maximal CMAP was measured by a computer with an integration algorithm installed (Fig. 1A). In our new method to obtain MUNEs, we recorded at least 10 unitary MAP waveforms (Fig. 1B) and then averaged them to obtain the mean unitary MAP waveform (Fig. 1C). A MUNE was calculated by dividing the area of the negative portion of the CMAP by that of the digitally averaged unitary MAP (Fig. 2).

Results

The negative CMAP areas of the CMAPs in the group of 20 patients with headaches at their first testing was 28.5 ± 6.9 mV*ms for the hypothenar and 24.7 ± 12.1 mV*ms for the EDB muscles. The negative areas of the unitary MAPs was 120 ± 98 μV*ms from hypothenar muscles and 290 ± 108 μV*ms from the EDB muscle. Corresponding MUNEs from hypothenar muscles at their first and second testings were 247 ± 94 and 259 ± 105, respectively, and from the EDB muscle were 107 ± 56 and 100 ± 47. The reproducibility of MUNEs thus obtained was tested by the test–retest plot (Fig. 3), and the correlation equations of the MUNEs of the hypothenar and EDB muscles were linear and had coefficients of 0.90 and 0.87, respectively.

Discussion

Our new technique of obtaining MUNEs in the present study has several advantages that other methods do not have. The validity of this technique has been tested and confirmed in past animal studies (Arasaki et al., 1997), and the animal data will be reviewed in another chapter of the proceedings. The only difference between the animal studies and the current human studies is that in the human studies, single MAPs with lowest thresholds to electrical stimulation by fine tungsten needles were recorded, while in the animal studies single muscle twitches

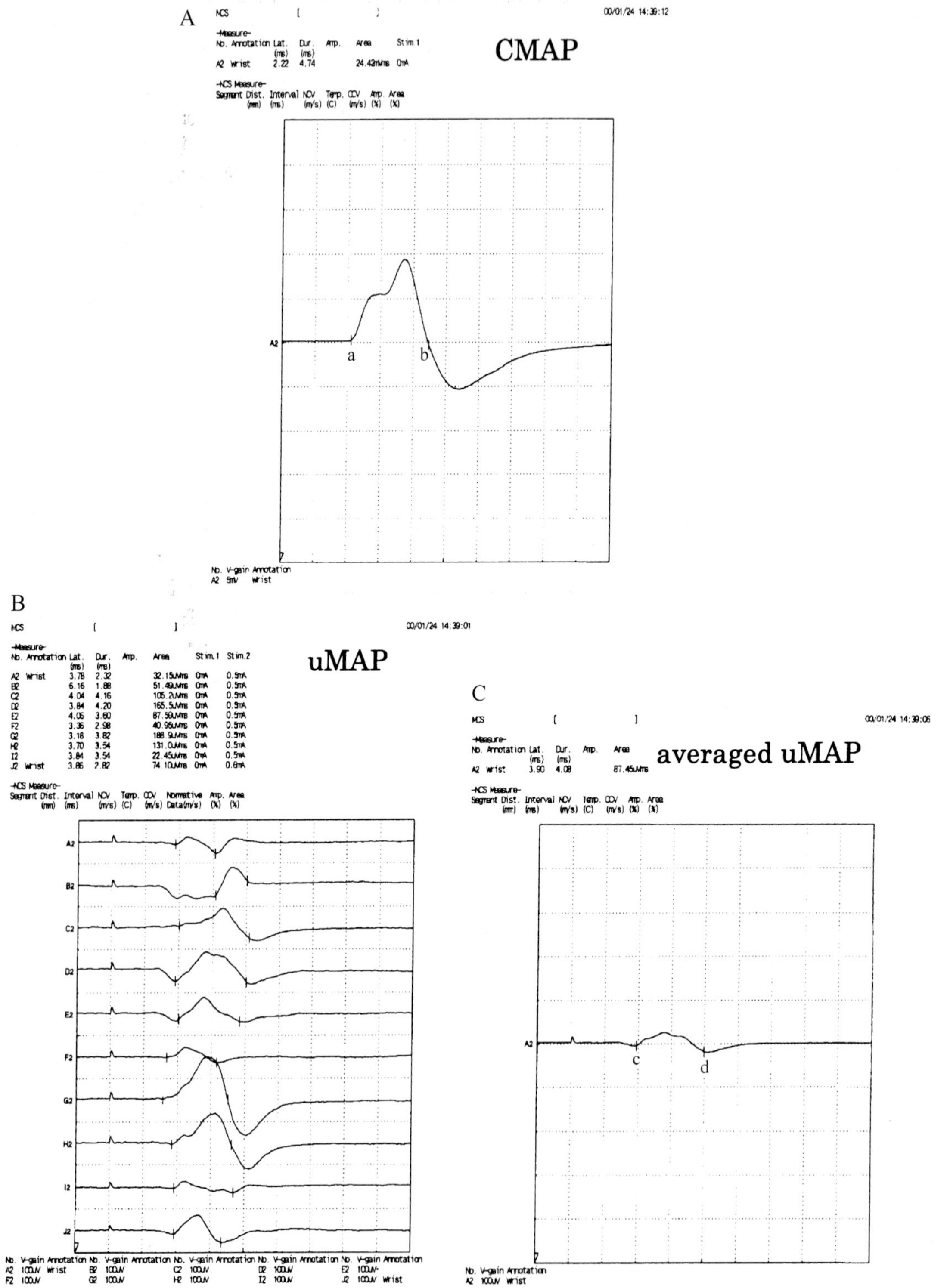

Fig. 2. Sample recording of maximal compound motor action potential (CMAP) and unitary motor unit action potentials (MAPs) and their integrated values used to calculate MUNE value. (A) Maximal CMAP with negative area marked by points a and b. (B) Ten unitary motor unit potentials. (C) The digitally averaged potential with negative area marked by points c and d.

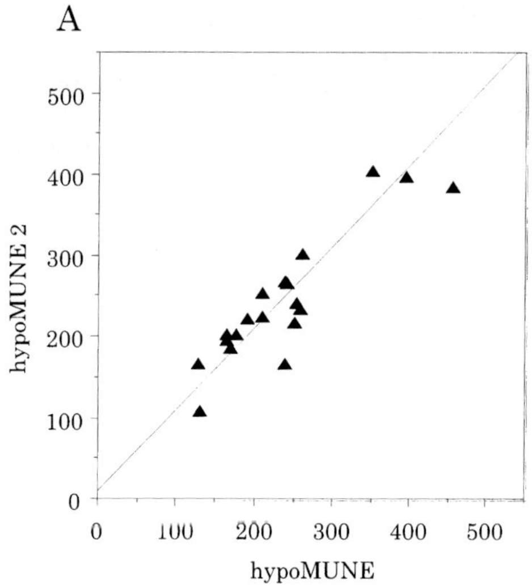

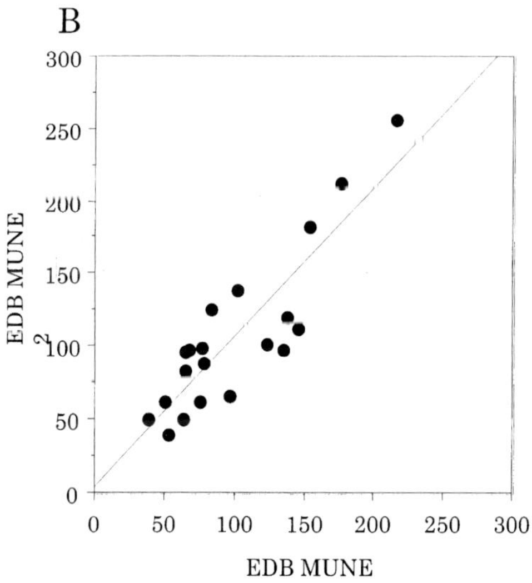

Fig. 3. Test–retest plot of intraneural microstimulation MUNE technique. (A) From ulnar nerve–hypothenar muscles (hypo). (B) From extensor digitorum muscle (EDB).

were recorded. Accordingly, MUNEs from the hypothenar and EDB muscles obtained by the techniques used in the present study are probably not significantly different from the number of functional spinal alpha motoneurons innervating these muscles.

Our technique might seem similar to multiple point stimulation because both utilize computer averaging of unitary MAPs. However, our method is different from the latter in that we do not move the stimulation electrode along the nerve in order to activate single MAPs. For this purpose we only need to manipulate the needle electrode in the nerve, which makes it possible to stimulate single motor axons at the same place as that for the maximal stimulation (Arasaki et al., 1998).

It is also noteworthy that we do not use the amplitudes of the negative peak of the CMAP and unitary MAPs, but measured the area of the negative part of these waveforms. When the CMAP is formed by unitary MAPs, the CMAP peak amplitude may not change significantly when unitary MAPs are added with significant latency differences. The CMAP area, however, will change even when unitary MAPs are not associated with phase cancellation. Accordingly, we expected that division of the CMAP area by the averaged unitary MAP area would reflect the number of motor units better than that of the CMAP peak amplitude by the average unitary MAP amplitude.

We are also aware of cons associated with our new technique to obtain MUNEs. It is invasive, using a fine tungsten needle electrode to insert into human nerves. It is significantly more time-consuming than other methods of obtaining MUNEs. It also requires well-trained examiners who can also perform microneurography. Accordingly, it is not readily available in many clinical research centers, which prevents us from adopting this method as a standard in obtaining MUNEs. It is, however, useful to ascertain the validity of MUNEs obtained by other routine methods because it is the only method proven to result in MUNEs consistent with the number of SA motor neurons anatomically determined (Arasaki et al., 1997).

Abbreviations

MUNE	motor unit number estimate
EDB	extensor digitorum brevis
CMAP	compound muscle action potential
MAP	muscle action potential

References

Arasaki, K. and Tamaki, M. A loss of functional spinal alpha motor neurons in amyotrophic lateral sclerosis. *Neurology*, 1998, 51: 603–605.

Arasaki, K., Tamaki, M., Hosoya, Y. and Kudo, N. Validity of electromyograms and tension as a means of motor unit number estimation. *Muscle Nerve*, 1997, 20: 552–560.

Brown, W.F., Strong, M.J. and Snow, R.S. Methods for estimating number of motor units in biceps-brachialis muscles and losses of motor units with aging. *Muscle Nerve*, 1988, 11: 423–432.

Daube, J. Estimating the number of motor units in a muscle. *J. Clin. Neurophys.*, 1995, 12: 585–594.

Doherty, T.J. and Brown, W.F. The estimated numbers and relative sizes of thenar motor units as selected by multiple point stimulation in young and older adults. *Muscle Nerve*, 1993, 16: 355–366.

McComas, A.J. Motor units: how many, how large, what kind? *J. Electromyogr. Kinesiol.*, 1998, 8: 391–402.

Stashuk, D.W., Doherty, T.J., Kaasam, A. and Brown, W.F. Motor unit number estimates based on the automated analysis of F-response. *Muscle Nerve*, 1994, 17: 881–890.

Stein, R.B. and Yang, J.F. Methods for estimating the number of motor units in human muscles. *Ann. Neurol.*, 1990, 28: 487–495.

Motor Unit Number Estimation (Supplements to Clinical Neurophysiology Vol. 55)
Editor: M.B. Bromberg

Chapter 7

MUNE by statistical analysis

Jasper R. Daube*

Department of Neurology – Mayo Clinic, 200 First Street SW, Rochester, MN 55905, USA

Introduction

Motor unit number estimate (MUNE) techniques record and directly measure samples of motor unit potentials obtained from the skin surface called "surface MUPs" (SMUPs). The size of the compound muscle action potential (CMAP) is divided by the average SMUP to obtain the MUNE. It is also possible to estimate the size of SMUPs indirectly from the statistical characteristics of a sequence of CMAPs. This "statistical" technique uses Poisson statistical assumptions that have been applied for many years in studies of the pathophysiology of neuromuscular junction disease (Katz and Miledi, 1972).

The Lambert–Eaton myasthenic syndrome (LEMS) and myasthenia gravis (MG) are diseases of the neuromusclar junction whose pathophysiology has been determined by analysis of electrical potentials recorded by microelectrodes at the junction (Elmqvist and Lambert, 1968). Stimulation of an axon in both LEMS and MG produces muscle fiber end plate potentials (EPPs). In MG, EPPs are of low amplitude due to a reduced post-synaptic receptor response to normal amounts of acetylcholine released from the nerve terminal. Miniature end plate potentials (MEPPs) are the electrical response to spontaneous release of single packets of acetylcholine, called quanta. In LEMS, MEPPs are readily recorded because the acetylcholine quantal size to spontaneous release is normal and the number of receptors is normal. With this knowledge of quantal size, the number of quanta released in LEMs by axonal stimulation can be readily calculated by dividing the size of the EPP by the size of an MEPP. The number is reduced. In MG, however, the size of MEPPs is too small to be recorded directly because of reduced numbers of receptors. This precludes a similar calculation of the number of quanta released with axonal stimulation in MG.

It is possible, however, to determine the size of an MEPP or a quantum by a Poisson statistical analysis of a series of EPPs (Hubbard and Quastel, 1969). An EPP can be considered to represent the sum of the number of quanta released with axon activation. The number of quanta in an EPP changes with each impulse, resulting in a measurable change in EPP amplitude. The change in amplitude represents additions and subtractions of quanta, and the size of a quantum can be estimated by analyzing the variation in EPP amplitude using Poisson statistics. A Poisson analysis can be applied to unitary data in which each sample is a multiple of a basic unit. In Poisson statistics the size of a single unit is equal to the variance of a series of responses made up of one or more units. Thus, the size of

**Correspondence to*: Dr. Jasper Daube, Department of Neurology – E8B, Mayo Clinic, Rochester, MN 55905, USA. e-mail: daube.jasper@mayo.edu

doi: 10.1016/S1567-424X(03)00007-2

the MEPP can be determined from the variance of the EPP. The number of quanta in an EPP is then the EPP divided by the estimated MEPP size. By this analysis, it was shown that the number of quanta released is normal in MG, but reduced in LEMS.

Poisson statistics assumes that samples are the same size, that the size of a single sample is the same each time it occurs, and that the histogram of all samples is skewed to the right. Modeling can help define the effect of these changes (Daube, unpublished). Modeling of differences in size of SMUPs of up to 100% showed no more than a 20% error in unit size using variance to determine unit size. Modeling variation in the size of a single unit up to 20% produced no more than a 10% error in unit size. Modeling of different distributions of data showed a 10% error for a normal distribution, with increasing error as the distributions becomes more skewed to the left. Quanta are not the same size in MG, but can be corrected to allow an accurate calculation of the number of quanta (Slawnych et al., 1996).

A critical component of all neurogenic diseases is the loss of functioning axons or anterior horn cells. MUNE is the only available direct and quantitative measure of this loss. There are a number of MUNE techniques, and most depend on the all-or-none activation of peripheral axons by electrical stimulation. Each axon has its own threshold of activation, and at any given stimulus intensity below supramaximal, some proportion of the axons will be activated while others will not. The threshold for activation of an individual axon is in fact a threshold region that follows a sigmoid curve, with low probability of activation at low intensity and higher probability at higher stimulus intensity (Fig. 1, bottom). When a fixed submaximal stimulus intensity is used, axons with a similar threshold will fire intermittently resulting in variations in the amplitude of the CMAP (Fig. 1, top). At a given stimulation intensity, different combinations of axons will be activated leading to varying size of the response, a term called "alternation". As a result, the size of sequential responses will be the actual number being activated factorial ($2f = 3$; $3f = 7$).

If the stimulus intensity is sufficiently low that only the lowest threshold axons are activated, some of the stimuli will activate no axons and the resulting CMAP will be zero. In that situation the variance of the response equals the SMUP size by Poisson assumptions. When the stimulus intensity is above the threshold for a number of axons, variations in the size of the CMAP will be superimposed on an unvarying baseline component of the CMAP. The calculation of variance then requires dividing the measured variance by the mean minus minimum CMAP. If we record "n" sequential, submaximal CMAP, "c"

$$c = [c_1, c_2, c_3, \ldots, c_n],$$

$$\mathrm{var}\, c = [\mathrm{Sum}\, c^2 - (\mathrm{Sum}\, c)^2/n]/(n-1),$$

$$S = \mathrm{var}\, c/[\mathrm{mean}\, c - \mathrm{minimum}\, c],$$

where S = single surface motor unit potential size.

MUNE is then be calculated from the maximal compound muscle action potential ($\mathrm{CMAP_m}$) divided by S, the calculated size of the SMUP.

$$\mathrm{MUNE} = \mathrm{CMAP_m}/\mathrm{S}.$$

These calculations assume that the threshold of an axon does not change over the period of testing. Our data suggest that this may not be the case (see normal findings below). This also may not be the case in amyotrophic lateral sclerosis (ALS) (Burke et al., 2001), however, the changes are minimal and not likely to have a measurable effect on the calculation of MUNE.

The use of Poisson statistics to calculate MUNE is still being improved, but the basic method has been well enough developed that it is being used in a number of laboratories. Other statistical approaches could be considered to determine if they provide better measures of the number of motor units.

Methods

Standard stimulation and recording methods are used for the statistical MUNE technique. A number of issues require special attention, as outlined below.

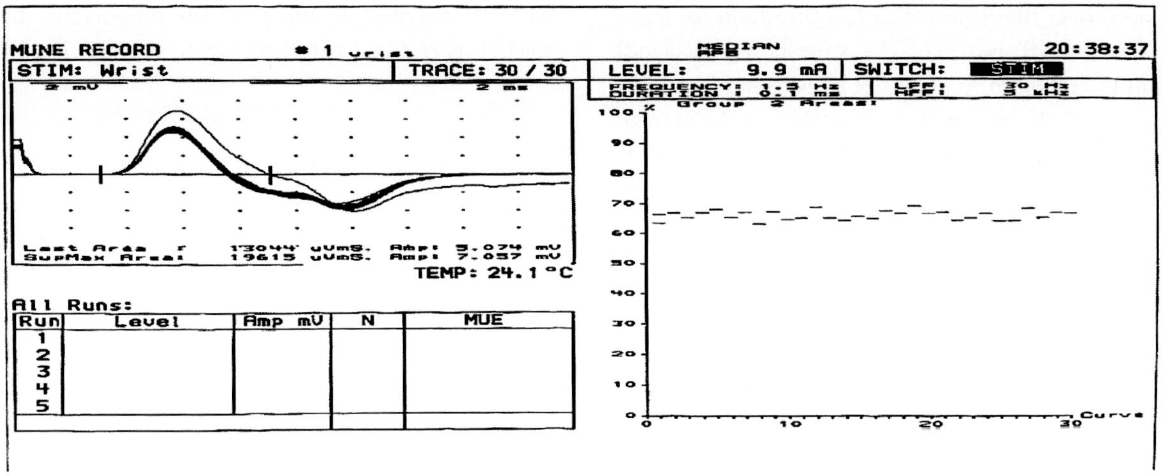

From Slawynch, '96

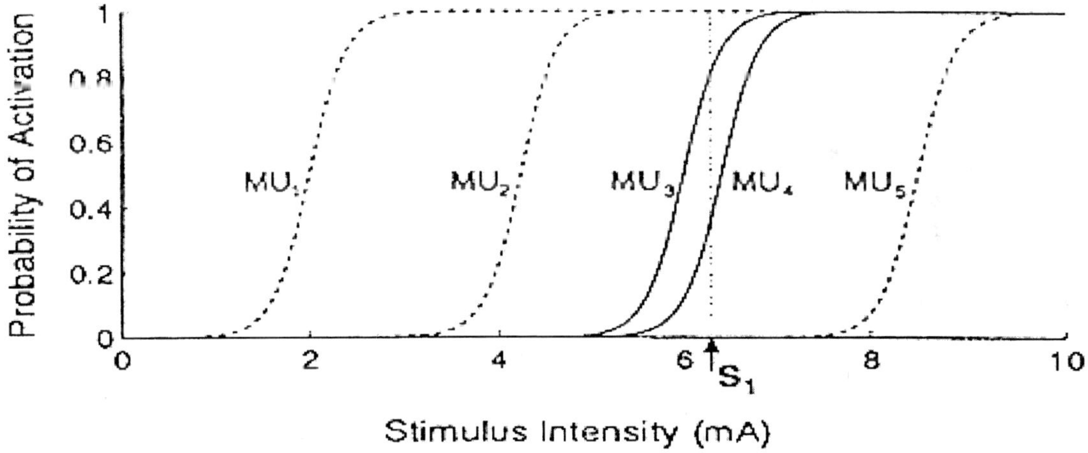

Fig. 1. *Top left:* Thirty sequential submaximal CMAP recordings and the maximal CMAP in a normal subject. Variation in thickness of the line of superimposed responses is due to CMAP size variation. *Top right:* measured variation in the size of the 30 CMAP that resulted from intermittent firing of seven axons. *Bottom:* schematic diagram of the mechanism of the variation in CMAP size due to differences in axon threshold that result from the percent likelihood of activation of an axon in a group of five axons. (From Henderson and Daube, 2003.)

Recording and stimulating

Recording electrodes are placed over the muscle and tendon. Different size and types of electrodes can be used as long as they maintain a reliable connection with the skin over the time taken to make the recording, which is often longer than standard nerve conduction studies. Recording artifacts induced by movement require that the extremity be immobilized, as in the fashion used for repetitive stimulation studies.

Stimulating electrodes must also be well fixed, since the slightest movement will shift the activation to a different group of axons. This is best accomplished with flat taped-on electrodes that do not depress the skin. The electrodes should be placed over the region of lowest threshold for nerve activation. If possible, the stimulating electrode should be placed to minimize activation of immediately underlying muscle that might cause electrode movement. They should also be moved away from nerves to extraneous muscles such as the lumbrical muscles. The maximal CMAP should be obtained with minimum stimulation duration and intensity. The rate of stimulation can be varied to enhance patient acceptance. Faster rates of stimulation, 1–2 Hz, may be helpful in reducing the variation due to a defect of neuromuscular transmission.

Display gain and sweep settings are determined by the size of the maximal CMAP. Filter settings of 30 Hz low and 5 kHz high minimizes baseline noise. Incomplete muscle relaxation causes background motor unit potential (MUP) activity will prevent a reliable recording. Immobilization will reduce MUP activity, but some patients will need manual manipulation of the hand or foot during the recording to eliminate MUP firing. Auditory monitoring of the MUP activity over the loudspeaker can assist both the patient and operator in assuring a quiet baseline.

Recording procedure

Stimulus parameters

The "setup" step determines the stimulation current levels for CMAP threshold and maximal responses. The "threshold" is the stimulus intensity at which a CMAP is first elicited. The "maximum response" is achieved by increasing the intensity until there is no further increase in CMAP size: the intensity is slowly decreased and increased to assure that the stimulus is eliciting a just maximal CMAP.

MUNE is most reliably measured from the negative portion of the CMAP. Automatic markers should be checked and reset to delimit the negative peak. Shock artifact and dispersed components of the CMAP are excluded. Accuracy of the marker placement is confirmed by reviewing the CMAP at a higher gain. Some diseases have positive CMAP components. When calculating the variance of the SMUP contributing the positive components, the CMAP is rectified before the analysis.

CMAP scan

A "scan" shows the series of CMAPs from minimum to maximum generated to graded stimuli. A series of CMAPs is recorded in response to stimuli automatically increased between the threshold and the maximum CMAP as determined in the setup step. A scan of 30 stimuli is standard, but more detailed search for large SMUP is facilitated by a larger number of stimulus increments in the scan. Fewer than 30 stimuli are inadequate. A reliable scan will have only a few responses at zero and only a few at maximal.

A normal scan is a sigmoid curve with larger steps in the mid-portion, but no sudden changes in the increment between stimuli ("steps") in the increment between threshold and maximum (Fig. 2). Sudden changes in step size or steps larger than 10–15% of the full CMAP may be due to single SMUPs. Large steps are tested to determine if they are due to a single SMUP (see below). The configuration of the scan is then reviewed to determine what stimulus intensities to test. Ideally, testing would include all axons. However, the number of stimuli and time required preclude this. Statistical MUNE values increase with the number of levels tested. Testing more levels of stimulus intensity increases reliability much less in normal subjects in whom SMUP sizes are nearly the same. Testing one level in the 5–25% range can provide a useable MUNE in a subject with a normal scan.

Data sampling

For most MUNE determinations, sampling 25–50% of all axons is satisfactory if large SMUPs have been identified and measured separately. Sampling is commonly done at stimulus intensities selected by the MUNE program from the scan to assess the largest steps and one small step; sampling is not performed at high intensities unless necessitated by large steps. Some operators prefer to test at preset levels such as 10–20%,

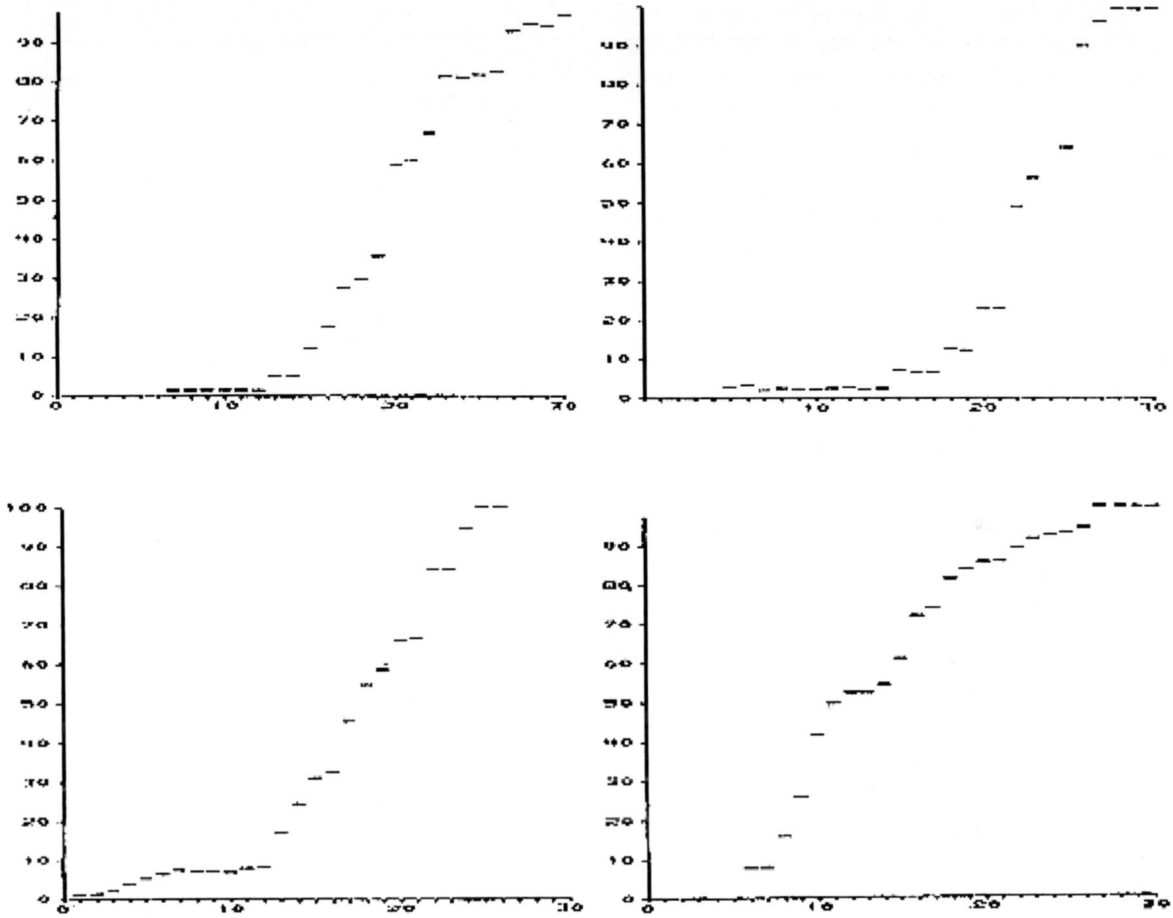

Fig. 2. Thirty sequential stimuli that were incremented in equal current steps between threshold and maximal at four points on the median nerve of a normal subject.

25–35%, 40–50% and 55–65%, unless large steps require altering these choices. No consistent differences have been shown with testing at low, intermediate or high levels of stimulus intensity. The effect of testing without a preset range has not been published.

Data analysis is typically performed multiple times on groups of 30 CMAPs (MUNE30), as shown in Fig. 3. This number provides a reasonable balance between larger numbers that would increase reproducibility, and smaller numbers that will allow more rapid completion of the study. MUNE30 studies enhance the reproducibility of the data by repeating groups of 30 CMAPs until the standard error is less than 10% with a minimum of four groups (120 responses). Reproducibility is increased to levels comparable with nerve conduction studies (< 10% error) by repeating the measurements twice (Lomen-Hoerth and Olney, 2000; Olney et al., 2000; Simmons et al., 2001).

Use of 500 data samples

Data to be reported here represent an expansion for the MUNE30 technique by using an automated program to collect 500 data samples. All CMAPs were evoked at a single stimulus intensity and were analyzed off line. Data was collected from normal subjects and from ALS patients.

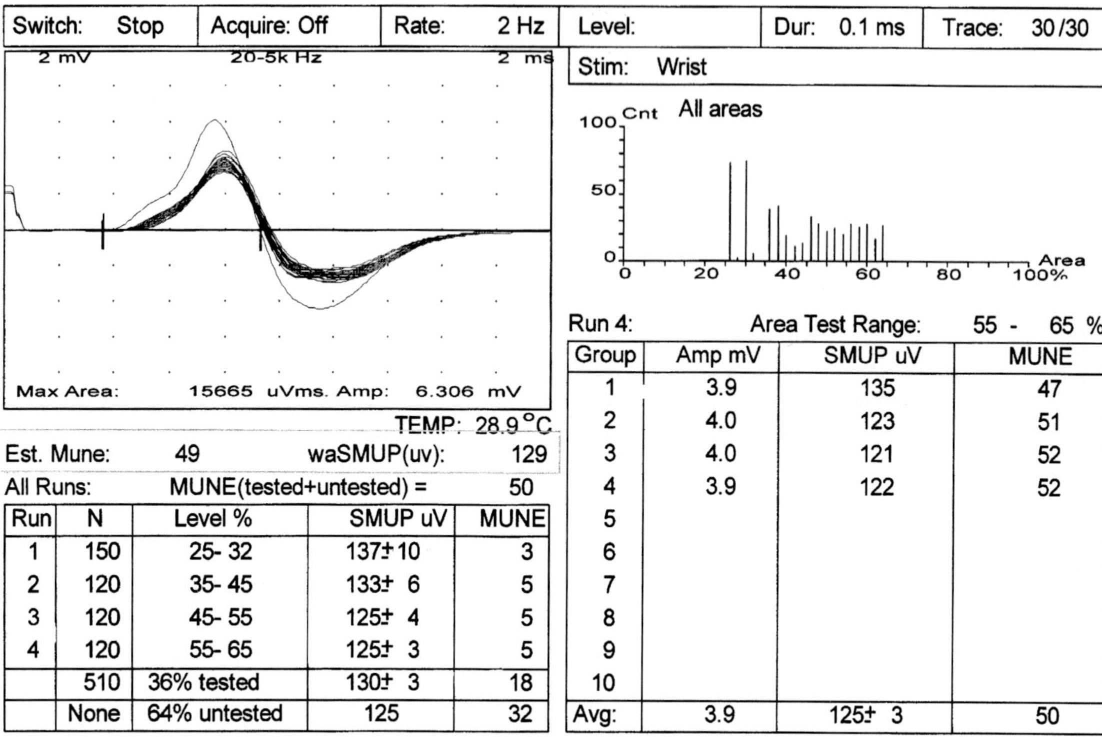

Fig. 3. Calculation of MUNE30 from a patient with moderate ALS with normal thenar muscle strength. *Top left:* last 30 superimposed CMAPs recorded at 55% stimulus intensity, and the maximal CMAP. *Top right:* histogram of all CMAPs recorded at four stimulus intensity levels between 20 and 60% of the CMAP. *Bottom right:* SMUP and MUNE calculation on four groups of 30 sequential CMAP between 55 and 60% of maximal. *Bottom left:* Results of the calculation of SMUP and MUNE at the four intensity levels. The number of stimuli, stimulus intensity, SMUP size and MUNE is give for each of these runs with the average for the measured segment of the CMAP and an estimate of the unmeasured segment. The box gives the weighted average (wa) SMUP size and the resulting MUNE. Normal MUNE is 100.

Objectives

Five specific questions will be addressed in this report, three that are pertinent for all methods of MUNE, and two focused specifically on statistical MUNE.

Questions for all MUNE methods:

1. What technical issues need to be considered?
2. What should be done with positive waveform responses?
3. What is the smallest acceptable SMUP?

Questions for statistical MUNE:

1. Should windows be a percent of maximum or an absolute microvolt/millisecond value?
2. What is the maximum effect of a decrement on statistical MUNE?

Technical issues

Examples of 500 CMAPs collected with no stimulus and at three stimulus intensities from three normal subjects and one ALS patient are shown in Fig. 4. The effects of poor relaxation are shown in the data set recorded at 0–10% with no stimulus (Fig. 4, “MUP”, left panel). If ongoing activity is present with stimulus intensities that evoke CMAP responses, this variability will be included with the CMAP variance to give spuriously high SMUP values leading to a low MUNE value. If the noise is continuous, the error can be

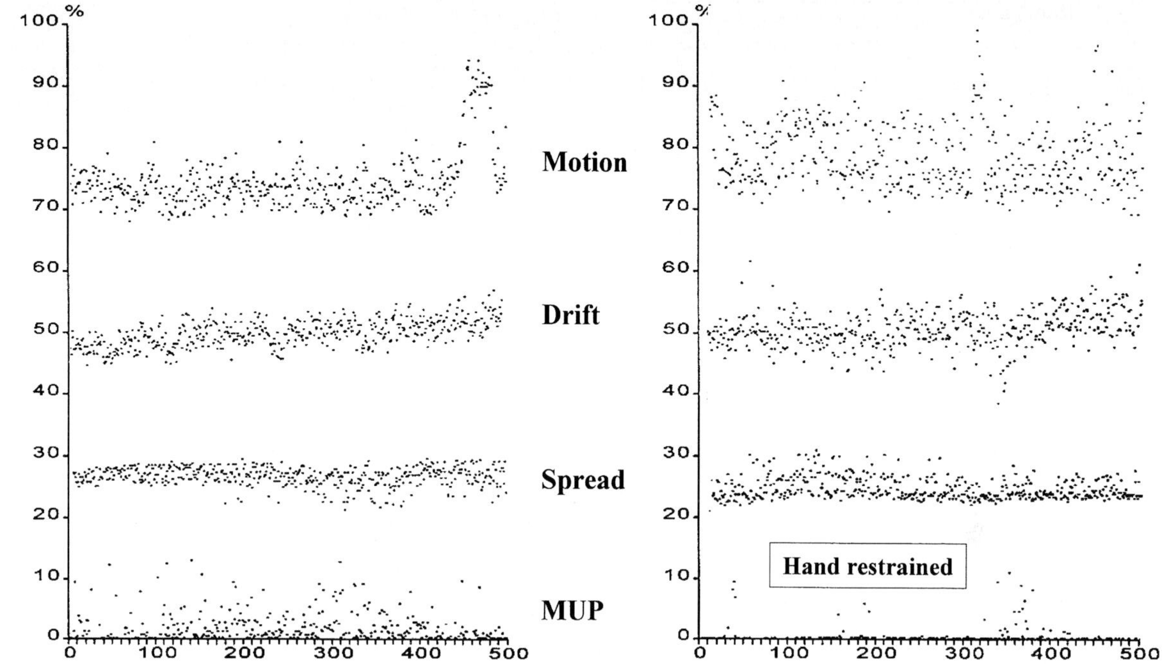

Fig. 4. Examples of technical problems identified during the recording of 500 sequential CMAP at a fixed stimulus intensity. The problems are described in the text. (From Henderson and Daube, 2003.)

corrected by subtracting this variance from the CMAP variance. However, it is more reliable to restrain the hand, and if necessary manipulate the fingers gently to reduce MUP firing (Fig. 4, "MUP", right panel).

Subjects may have movements that result in a burst of noise due to superimposed MUPs that are seen as a brief change in the CMAP size, as shown in the data set at 70–90% level (Fig. 4, "Motion"). These can be readily recognized visually, and are effectively eliminated without alteration of remaining data by selecting only the data within 2.5 standard deviations of the mean (Henderson and Daube, 2001).

There can be gradual increases or decreases in the average CMAP amplitude over the 500 stimuli, as shown in the data set at 40–50% levels (Fig. 4, "Drift"). Drift suggests a slow change in threshold for all axons, likely local changes in the nerve environment such as temperature, blood flow, local ion concentrations or local edema. If the drift is due to any of the latter, it will result in a gradual shift in the axons being tested, toward those with higher or lower thresholds. This would potentially cause a less accurate measure of SMUP size and of MUNE value. Applying a 2.5 SD data limit is not satisfactory in this case since it would eliminate different components at the beginning and end of the recording. Drifts are therefore best eliminated by minimal changes in the stimulus intensity to maintain activation of the same group of axons throughout the 500 stimuli. In standard MUNE30 testing that uses window limits of the data collected, such small stimulus adjustments are standard. Drift also might be corrected by using the mean consecutive difference (MCD) methods used in single fiber EMG.

A small number of subjects show a spread in the range of CMAP sizes occurring with a fixed stimulus (Fig. 4, "Spread"). Spread is not associated with increases or decreases in MUP firing or other noise, as monitored on the loudspeaker. It suggests that lesser or greater numbers of axons are being activated as the stimulus continues. This is most likely due to local factors of the type suggested above for drift.

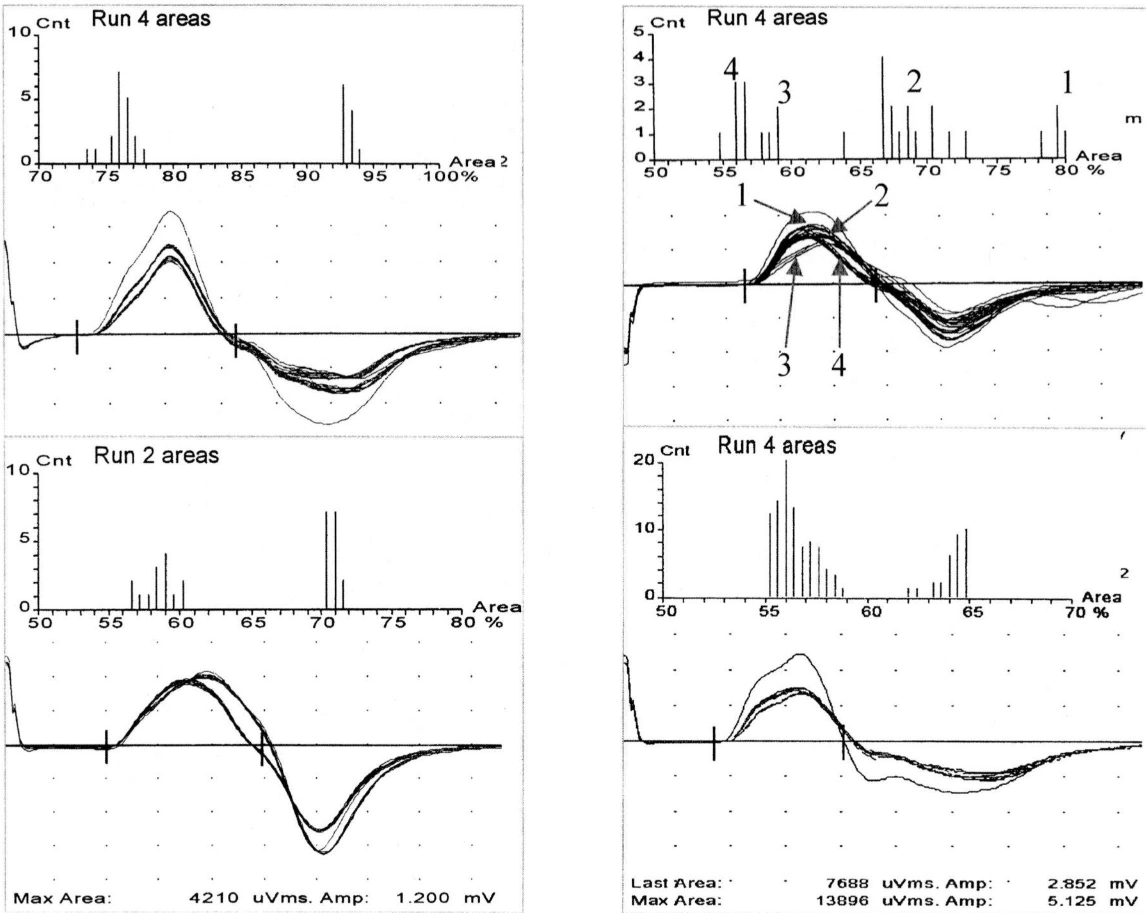

Fig. 5. Four sets of superimposed CMAP recorded during statistical MUNE to illustrate the variety of SMUP shapes. Each of the four examples includes the histogram of the areas of the CMAP. *Top left:* One SMUP that adds only amplitude to the CMAP. *Bottom left:* One SMUP that adds area due to a longer duration with little change in amplitude. *Top right:* Four SMUP that are distinguished by changes in shape and area with only a small change in amplitude. *Bottom right:* One SMUP that adds both area and amplitude.

CMAP amplitude has been the standard measure of size because of its ease of measurement. Amplitude is a reliable measure when the SMUPs contributing to a CMAP occur synchronously. However, if SMUPs are not synchronous, the addition of more SMUPs can increase the CMAP area with no change in amplitude (Fig. 5). In addition, the contribution to the CMAP of an SMUP with a different latency can increase the area without increasing the amplitude (Fig. 6). The capability of most EMG machines to measure area thus makes area a preferable measure of SMUP contribution to the CMAP.

Each of these technical problems must be considered for any MUNE technique. Drift and spread are less likely to cause errors in multiple point stimulation (MPS) and the adapted multiple point stimulation (AMPS) techniques since the stimulus intensity is altered at each new stimulation point, but they can affect the incremental stimulation (IS) technique. Noise from poor relaxation can impair the ability to isolate distinct SMUP in all techniques, especially AMPS and IS techniques. The measurement of SMUP size, amplitude or area, needs to be considered in any MUNE method.

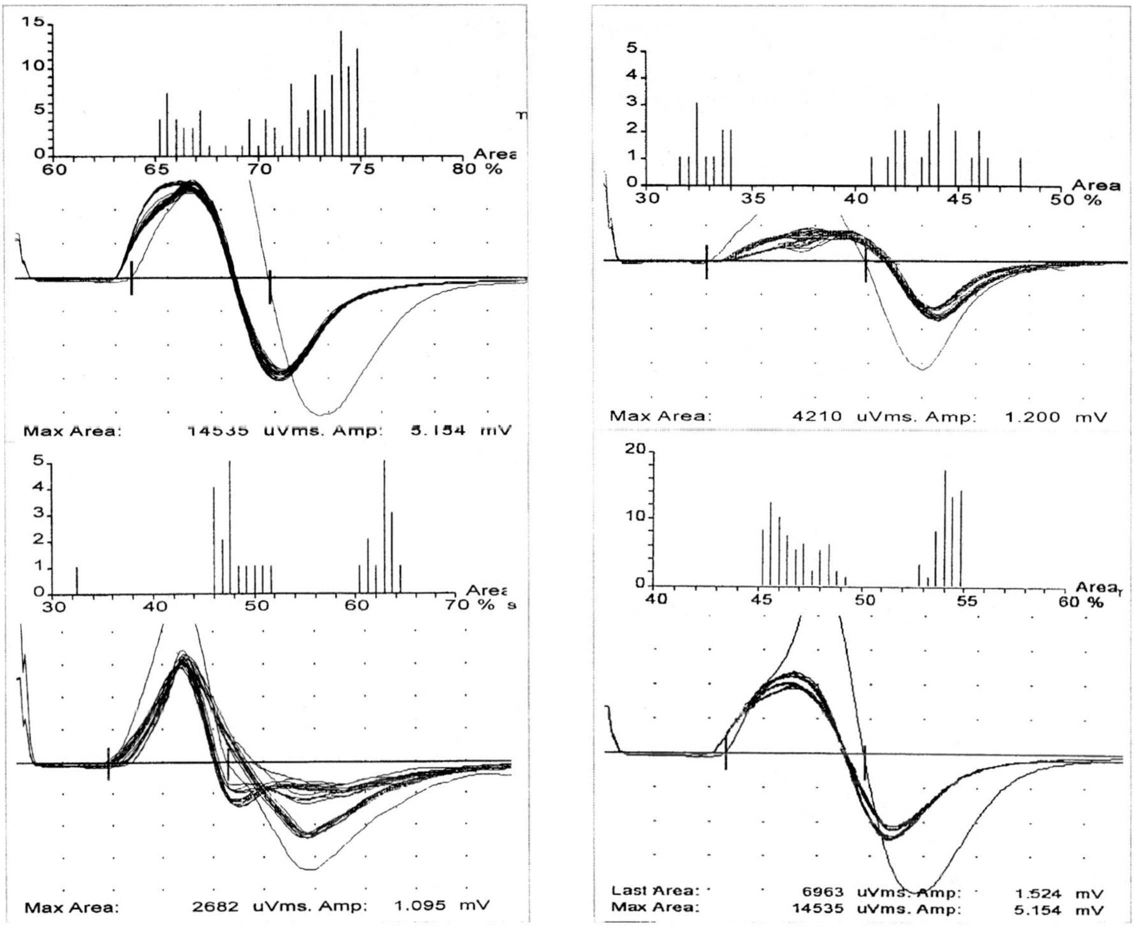

Fig. 6. Four examples of SMUP recorded during statistical MUNE in which the clear distinction between SMUP shown in the histograms is made solely on the basis of area and shape rather than amplitude. (From Henderson and Daube, 2003.)

Positive waveforms

CMAP waveforms recorded over the end plate region of a muscle are biphasic with an initially negative component. The negative component is usually measured for MUNE. MUNE analysis assumes that SMUPs are entirely or predominantly negative. If SMUPs from distant muscles contribute significantly, the CMAP may be predominantly positive. For example, positivity occurs when recording the CMAP from thenar muscles if the stimulating electrodes are positioned to selectively activate the nerve fascicle innervating the lumbrical muscles (Fig. 7). Note that there are multiple small steps in the positive lumbrical CMAP with an area of 20 μV ms (negative peak amplitude 8 μV). Such responses are smaller than most of those recorded over the thenar muscles because of their distance from the recording electrode. These small responses are best ignored in all MUNE techniques because of their minimal contribution to the CMAP.

Smallest measurable SMUP

The SMUP represents the surface potential generated by the activation of all muscle fibers in a motor unit in a nearby muscle. The physiologic determinants of SMUP size include the number of muscle fibers in the motor unit, the size of the muscle fibers, and their synchrony of firing.

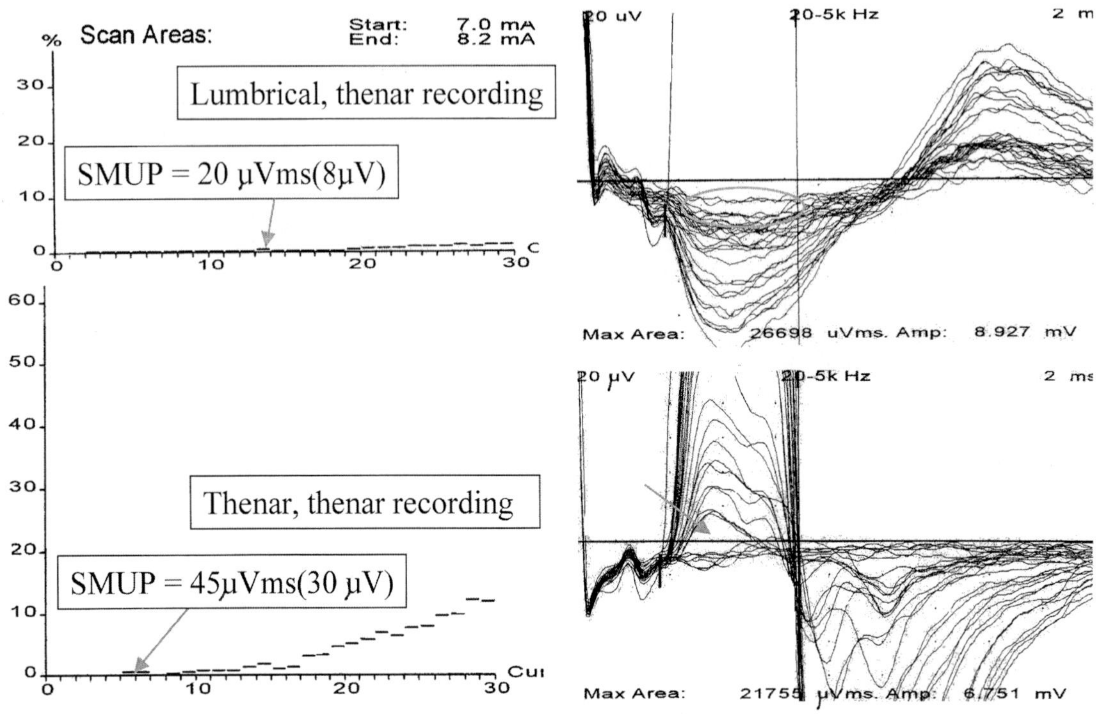

Fig. 7. Thirty sequential thenar CMAPs recorded in response to equal increment stimuli between threshold and slightly above threshold with two slightly different stimulating electrode locations. In the upper recording the stimulus elicited a visible lumbrical twitch alone; in the lower recording only a small thenar twitch was seen. The lumbrical recording shows very small SMUP increments (20 μV ms (8 μV)), while the thenar recording shows more typical size SMUP (45 μV ms (30 μV)). This illustrates the decreasing size of SMUP with distance of the recording electrode from the SMUP.

However, the location of the motor unit relative to the recording electrode has major influence on the size of the recorded SMUP because amplitude falls off exponentially with distance from the motor unit. Low amplitude SMUPs are seen in a number of settings.

Surface recordings from muscle during low level voluntary contraction and during recording of F-waves show low amplitude SMUPs recorded from distant MUPs in normal subjects and patients with ALS (Figs. 8 and 9). CMAP scans near threshold demonstrate small reproducible SMUPs in normal and ALS subjects (Figs. 10–14). These small SMUP are most readily recognized if there is a marked reduction in the number of remaining MUPs in a muscle (Fig. 13). The presence of small SMUPs can be confirmed on needle examination as arising from distant MUPs (Fig. 14). These findings confirm that there is no lower limit to the size of SMUP (Stålberg and Karlsson, 2001).

The amplitude of baseline noise with surface recordings are commonly in the range of 10 μV (Fig. 11). Identification of SMUP smaller than 10 μV (approximately 25 μV ms) is therefore not reliable in any of the MUNE techniques. A lower limit of 10 μV or 25 μV ms would be logical to consider for SMUPs. The corollary is that SMUP greater than this level can be recorded and should not be considered artifact. This permits measurements of SMUPs and determinations of MUNE values in myopathies in which all the SMUP remain greater than half the normal size. However, if some SMUP are smaller than this, MUNE becomes unreliable in myopathies, and may erroneously conclude that there is a reduction in MUNE.

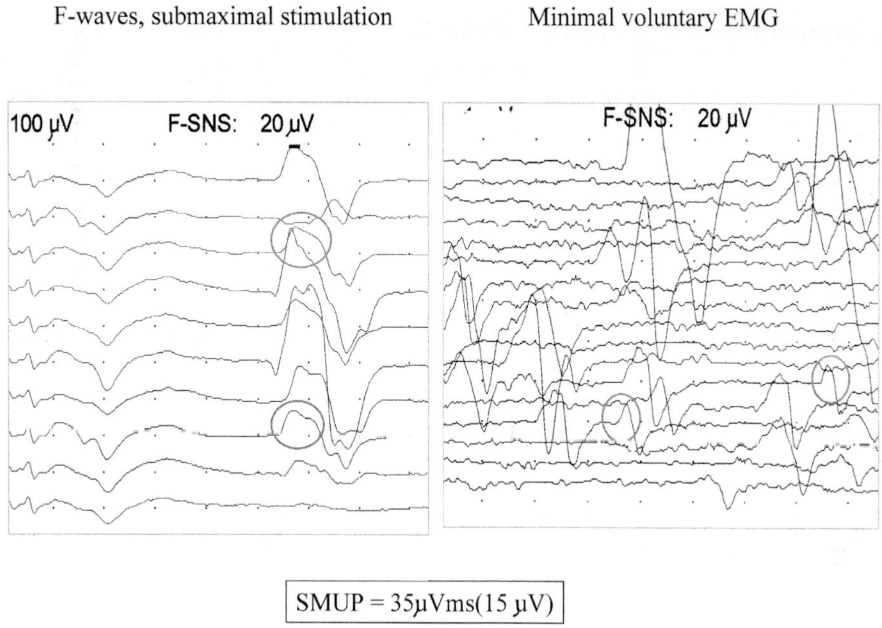

Fig. 8. Small SMUP recorded during F-wave testing and minimal voluntary EMG in a normal subject. *Left panel:* low intensity stimulus activated a small proportion of axons and a small CMAP. Multiple stimuli demonstrated reproducible, 15 µV SMUP (ovals). *Right panel:* Minimal voluntary EMG activity recorded on a raster display shows reproducible 15 µV SMUP (circles).

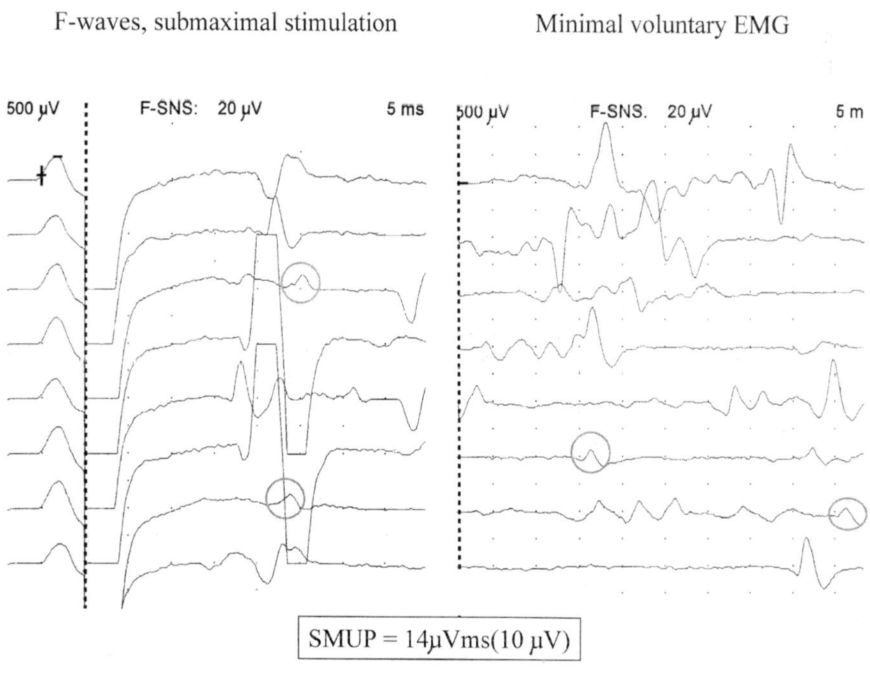

Fig. 9. Small SMUP recorded during F-wave testing and minimal voluntary EMG in a patient with ALS. *Left panel:* low intensity stimulus activated a small proportion of axons and a small CMAP. Multiple stimuli demonstrated reproducible, 10 µV SMUP (circles). *Right panel:* Minimal voluntary EMG activity recorded on a raster display shows reproducible 10 µV SMUP (circles).

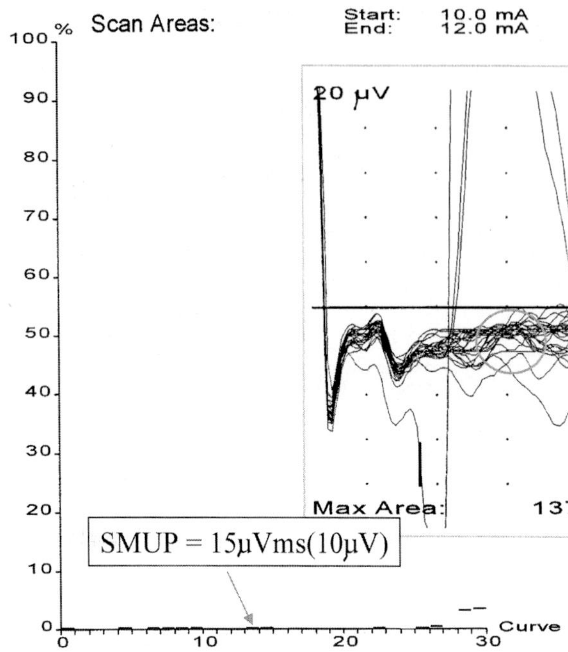

Fig. 10. Superimposed, small (10 μV) SMUP (circle) recorded from the thenar muscles in a normal subject with 30 sequential median nerve stimuli near threshold for a single axon. The area of each CMAP is plotted on the graph at the left.

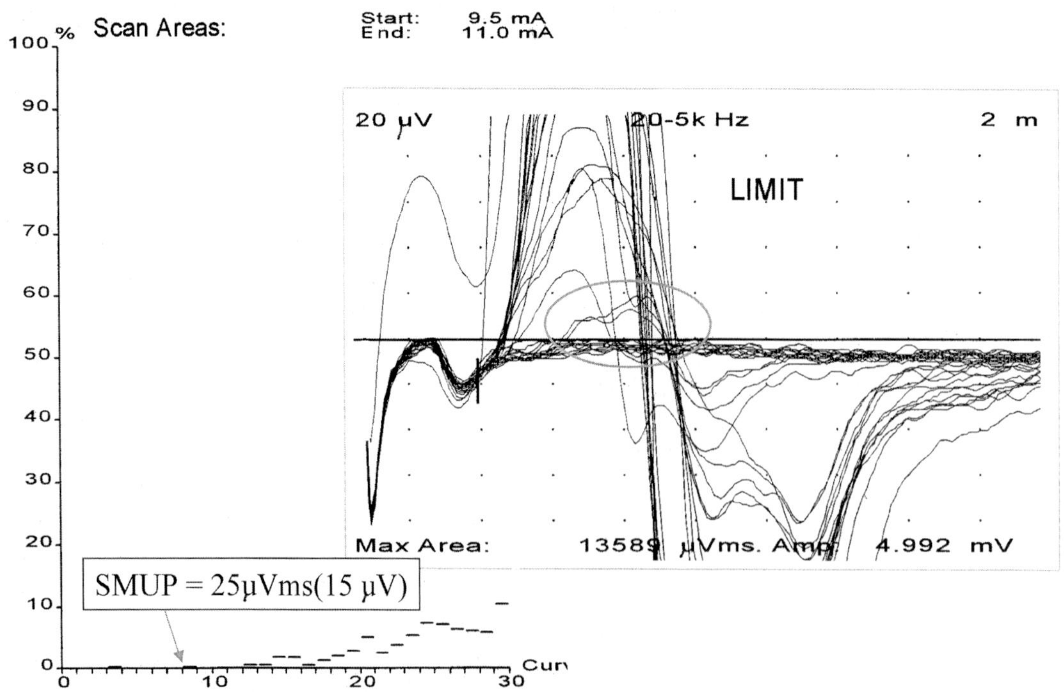

Fig. 11. Superimposed, small (15 μV) SMUP (circle) recorded from the thenar muscles in an ALS patient with 30 sequential median nerve stimuli near threshold for a single axon. The area of each CMAP is plotted on the graph at the left.

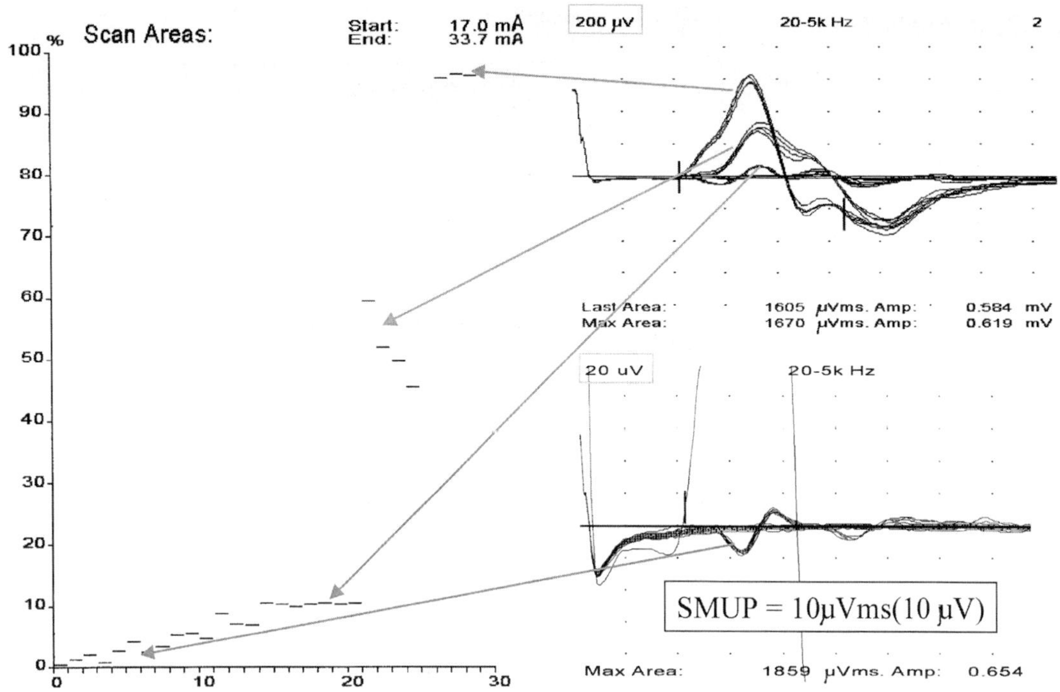

Fig. 12. Thirty sequential stimuli that were increased in equal current steps between threshold and maximal in a patient with ALS. Four distinct SMUP could be identified with the smallest (10 µV) seen only in the bottom right panel. The other three are seen in the top right panel. The areas of each CMAP are plotted in the graph on the left. The fourth SMUP shows a decrement in both the area plot, and the superimposed CMAP.

Window size

Figure 15 shows the spread of CMAP data over 10–25% of the CMAP amplitude range with 500 stimuli applied at three stimulus intensity levels in two normal subjects. This variation in CMAP amplitude with submaximal stimulation results mostly from alternations in the firing of axons with similar thresholds, as described above. However, other physiologic and technical factors are likely to contribute to the variation as well. These include temperature, blood flow, blood pressure, pulse, local metabolic changes, and variations in local current flow among the complex structures of the peripheral nerve. These factors will contribute to the variance, and thus to an over estimate of SMUP size in statistical MUNE. These variables are best recognized during baseline recordings with no stimulus.

Excess CMAP variation can be reduced by using a window and setting the stimulus intensity to elicit CMAPs in the lower 25% of the window. This results in CMAP responses with a skewed distribution, which better approximates the Poisson distribution (Fig. 16).

In the original MUNE30 method, windows were set to restrict or narrow the range of data analyzed. Data were accepted only if they lay within a defined set of ranges based an percentages of the maximal CMAP. The original MUNE30 program used two window sizes. One small window (5% of the CMAP amplitude) focused on the region of small steps in the scan to estimate the size of the small SMUP. Three additional windows were set to encompass the largest steps in a scan to estimate the size of large SMUPs. Steps due to single large SMUP (greater than 10% of the SMAP) were measured directly without using variance estimates. The variance calculation was applied to the remaining data. This sampling assured testing of regions in the scan (axons in a threshold range) likely to have both small and large SMUP.

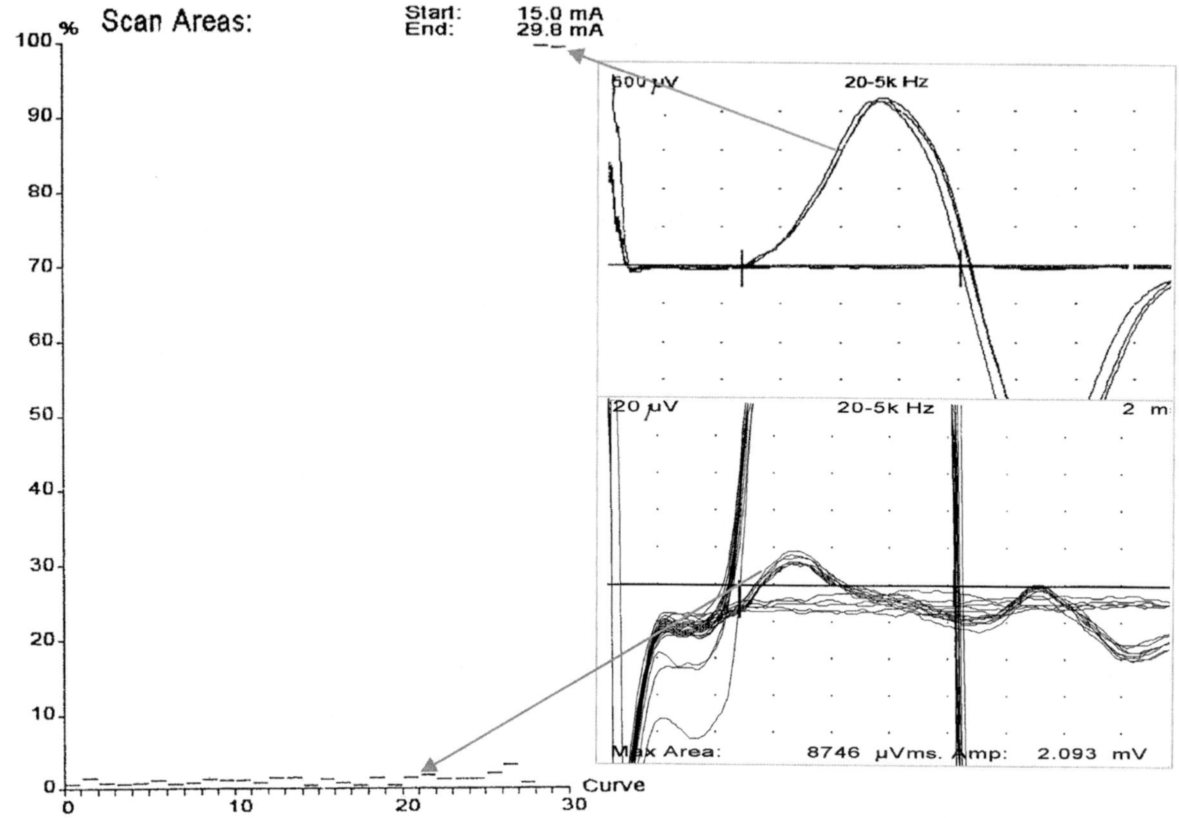

Fig. 13. Thirty sequential stimuli that were increased in equal current steps between threshold and maximal in a patient with ALS. Two distinct SMUP were recorded. The first was a 20 µV potential seen only in the bottom right panel. Most of the CMAP is made up of a single additional SMUP shown in the top right panel. The areas of each CMAP are plotted in the graph on the left. (From Henderson and Daube, 2003.)

However, window size defines the variance, and influences the estimates of SMUP size. Selection of window size can thereby limit the size of identified SMUPs. Recent statistical MUNE reports have used four standard sizes, each including 10% of the CMAP. Typical sizes are 10–20%, 25–35%, 40–50% and 55–65% of the CMAP (Lomen-Hoerth and Olney, 2001). Window ranges are modified if there are large steps within a window. This approach has the advantage of consistency, since no decisions need be made on window size and data range to test.

Using fixed, predefined window sizes defines the lower limit of SMUP size, as shown in Fig. 17 where a 1% window demonstrates much smaller SMUPs, on the order of 10–12 µV amplitude (28–36 µV ms area). In contrast, a 5% window identified larger SMUPs, on the order of 30–51 µV (94–151 µV ms). Ideally, at each stimulus intensity data should be tested with small and large windows to identify the range of SMUP sizes, but the time required makes this impractical. However, collection of a full set of 300–500 data points would allow multiple determinations of SMUP size with different window sizes to be calculated off line.

Use of a predetermined window size has another significant effect on SMUP measurement if defined as a percent of the CMAP. In most neurogenic processes there is a reduction in CMAP amplitude with disease progresses. A fixed percent window will therefore correspond to different absolute amplitudes. Thus as a CMAP decreases, the SMUP size calculated in statistical MUNE will decrease, resulting in an apparent

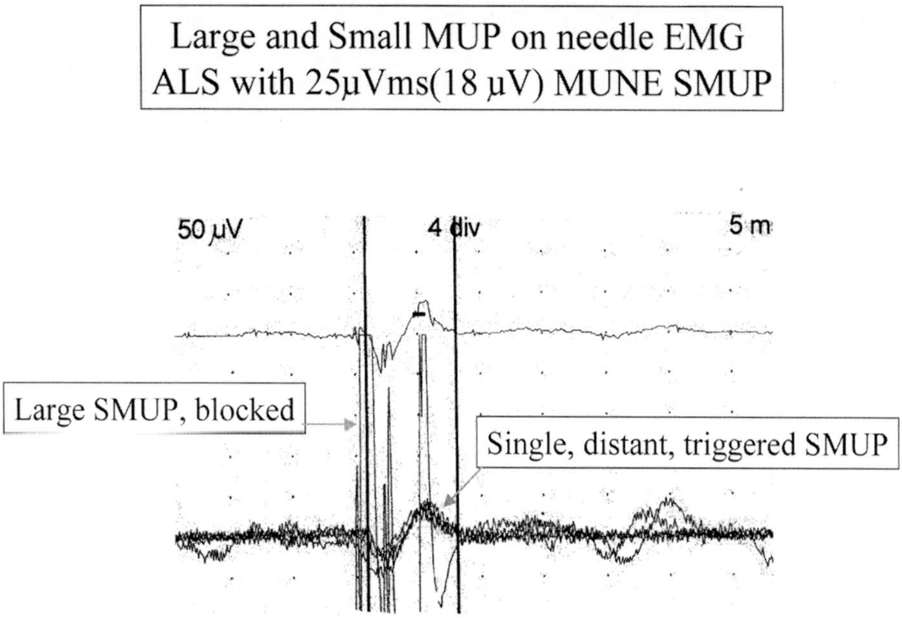

Fig. 14. Amplitude triggered needle EMG recording made from the same muscle from the ALS patient in Fig. 13 shows one small and one large MUP. A 1200 μV, polyphasic MUP is off the scale and seen as two vertical black lines and spikes between the lines. A 60 μV distant MUP (rise time 5 ms) is superimposed in the lower trace. (From Henderson and Daube, 2003.)

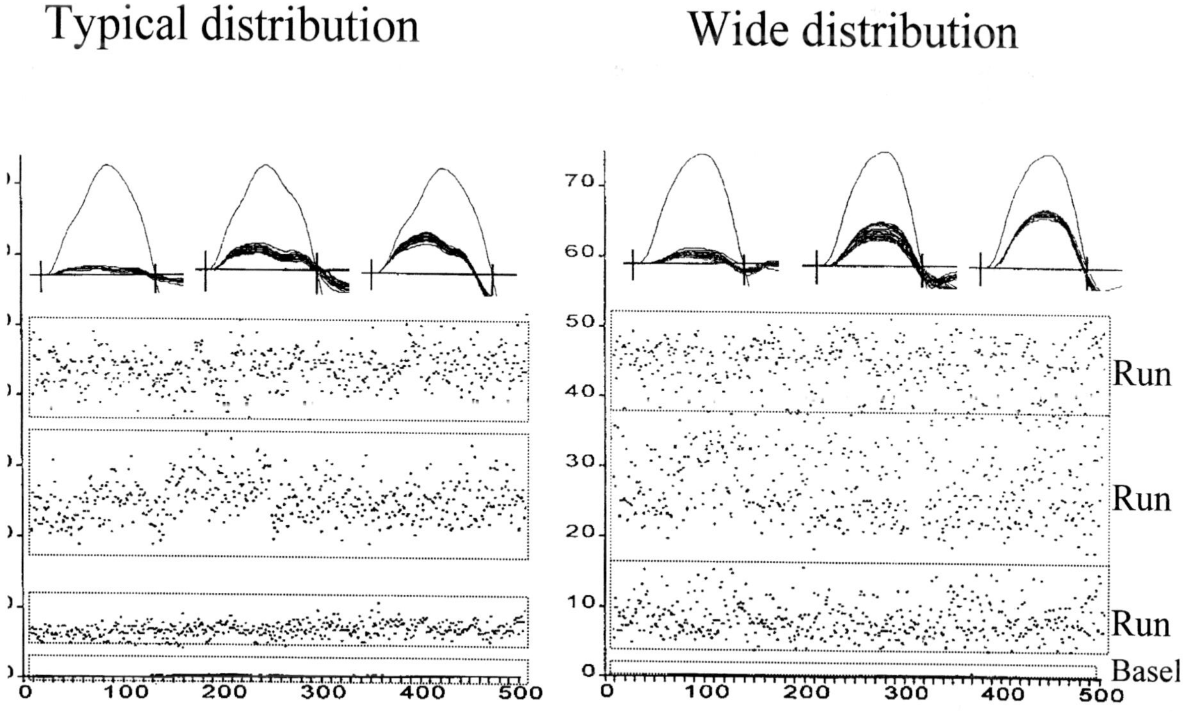

Fig. 15. Five hundred sequential stimuli applied to the nerve at four different and constant stimulus intensities show the variety of distributions of the CMAP in two normal subjects. The first 500 in each subject applied no stimulus to show the baseline noise. The scales at the left show the percent of the maximum CMAP for each response. The superimposed CMAP are shown at the top of each picture.

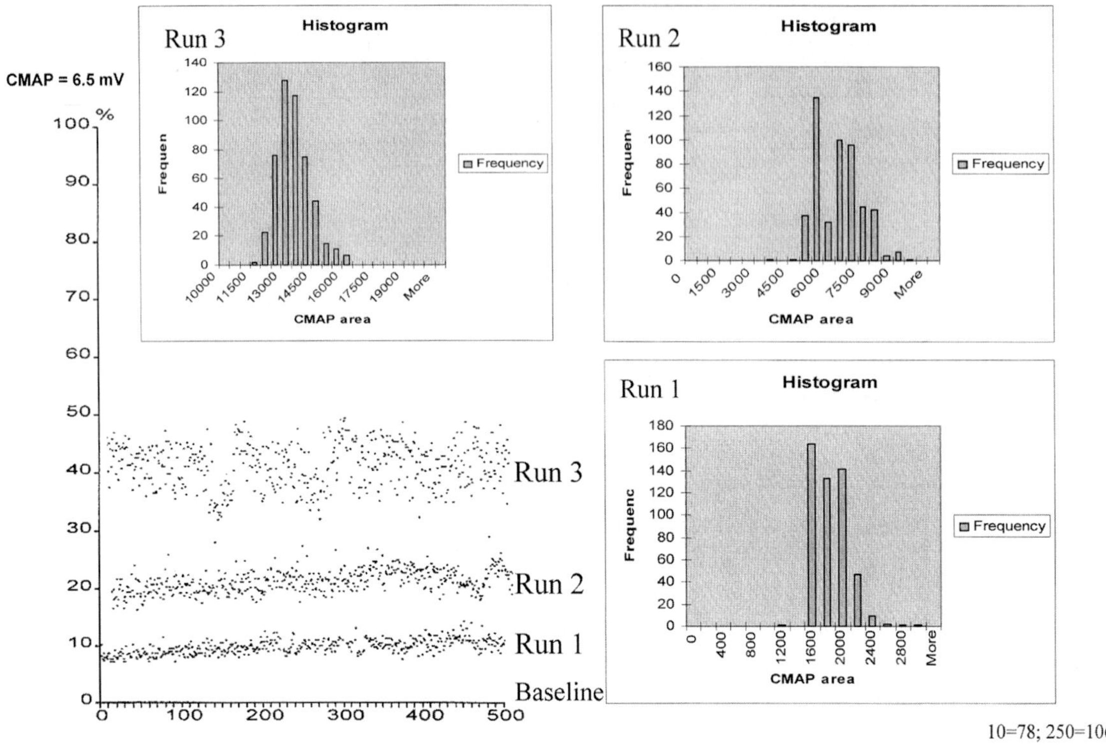

Fig. 16. Five hundred sequential CMAP areas evoked with stimuli at four different and constant stimulus intensities are shown in the bottom left panel. The first run applied no stimulus to provide a measure of baseline noise. The scales at the left show the percent of the maximal CMAP for each response. Histograms of the CMAP areas for each of the three runs are shown to the right and above the CMAP plots. (From Henderson and Daube, 2003.)

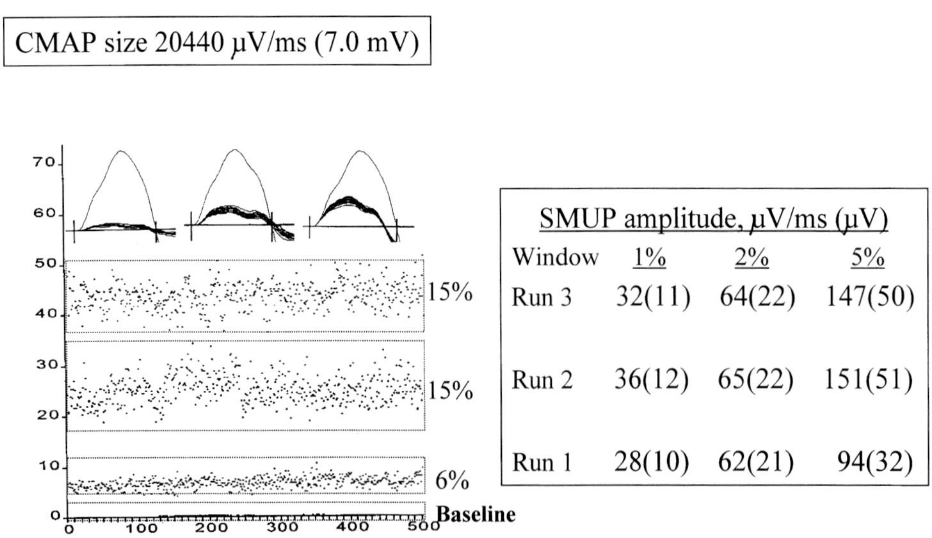

Fig. 17. Five hundred sequential CMAP areas evoked with stimuli at four different and constant stimulus intensities are shown in the bottom left panel. The first run applied no stimulus to provide a measure of baseline noise. The scale at the left shows the percent that each response is of the maximal CMAP. The superimposed CMAP are shown above the plots. The table at the right shows the effect of different window sizes on the calculated SMUP size for each of the three sets of 500. (From Henderson and Daube, 2003.)

TABLE 1

THE THEORETICAL EFFECTS OF DIFFERENT PERCENT AND AMPLITUDE WINDOWS ON THE SMUP SIZE THAT COULD BE MEASURED FOR DIFFERENT CMAP AND WINDOW SIZES

Effect of statistical window		
CMAP amplitude (mV)	Window amplitude (μV)	SMUP range[a] (μV)
Percent window, 10%		
10	1000	50–980
5	500	25–500
2	200	10–200
0.5	50	10– 50
CMAP amplitude (mV)	Window percent (%)	SMUP range[a] (μV)
Amplitude window, 250 μV		
10	2.5	10–230
5	5.0	10–230
2	12.5	10–230
0.5	50.0	10–230

[a] Theoretical with 10 μV baseline noise as lower SMUP limit.

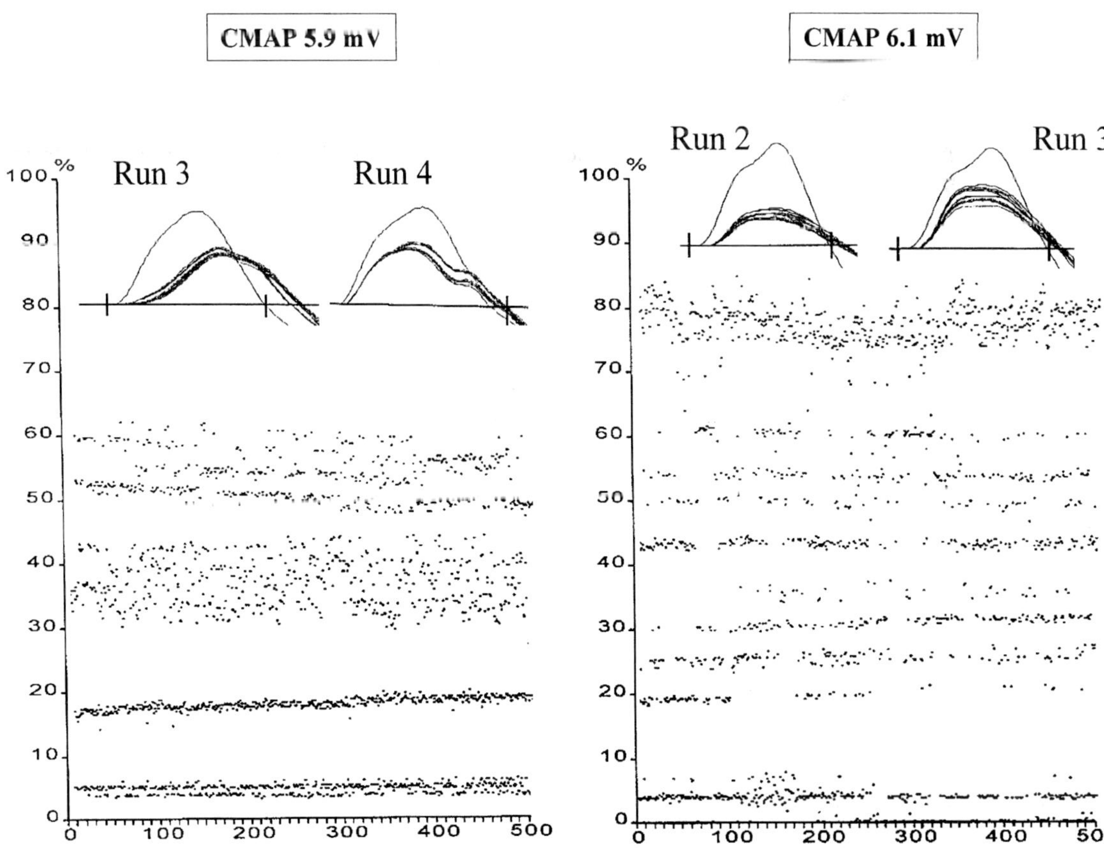

Fig. 18. Five hundred sequential CMAP areas recorded at four stimulus intensity levels in two patients with ALS. The corresponding CMAP for two of the sets of 500 are shown above the CMAP plots.

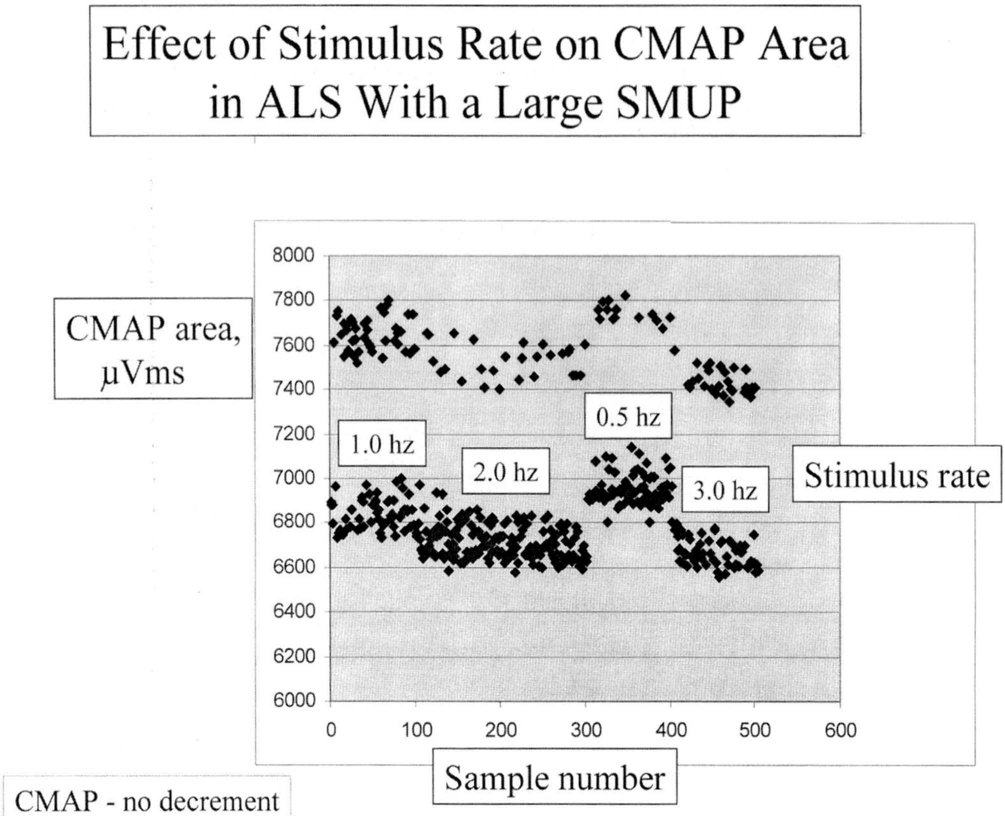

Fig. 19. Five hundred sequential CMAP areas recorded in a patient with ALS and no CMAP decrement with repetitive stimulation. The upper and lower limits of a single large SMUP range around 6800 and 7600 µV ms. The rate of stimulation is changed as shown after each 100 stimuli.

increase in MUNE, as shown in Fig. 17. This effect can be counteracted by using windows of fixed amplitude windows rather than windows of fixed CMAP percent (Table 1). A 250 µV (~600 µV ms) window allows the measurement of small SMUPs while not excluding larger SMUP up to 250 µV. SMUPs larger than that can be recognized as steps in a scan.

Fig. 18 shows examples of large steps in two ALS patients, and steps this large are not seen in normal subjects. Statistical MUNE calculation requires that the size of these single large SMUP be measured separately, with the variance calculation reserved for the remaining segments.

In the recordings in Fig. 18 from the patient on the left, run 1 (bottom) shows a single SMUP of approximately 120 µV. Run 2 appears to be a single SMUP peak with no defined lower limit. SMUP size from a run three variance calculation was three 85 µV responses. Run 4 (top) shows three SMUP of approximately 300 µV each. Calculated MUNE is 24. In the recordings from the patient on the right, there are only a few samples above and below, and most of the data in the run appear to show two SMUP of 150 µV. Run 3 shows three 300 µV, and one 100 µV SMUP. Run 3 has two 500 and one 300 µV responses. Variance calculation on run 4 shows three 110 µV SMUP. MUNE is 21.

Decrement

In some neurogenic disorders, such as ALS, newly formed nerve terminals from collateral sprouting causes a decrement with repetitive

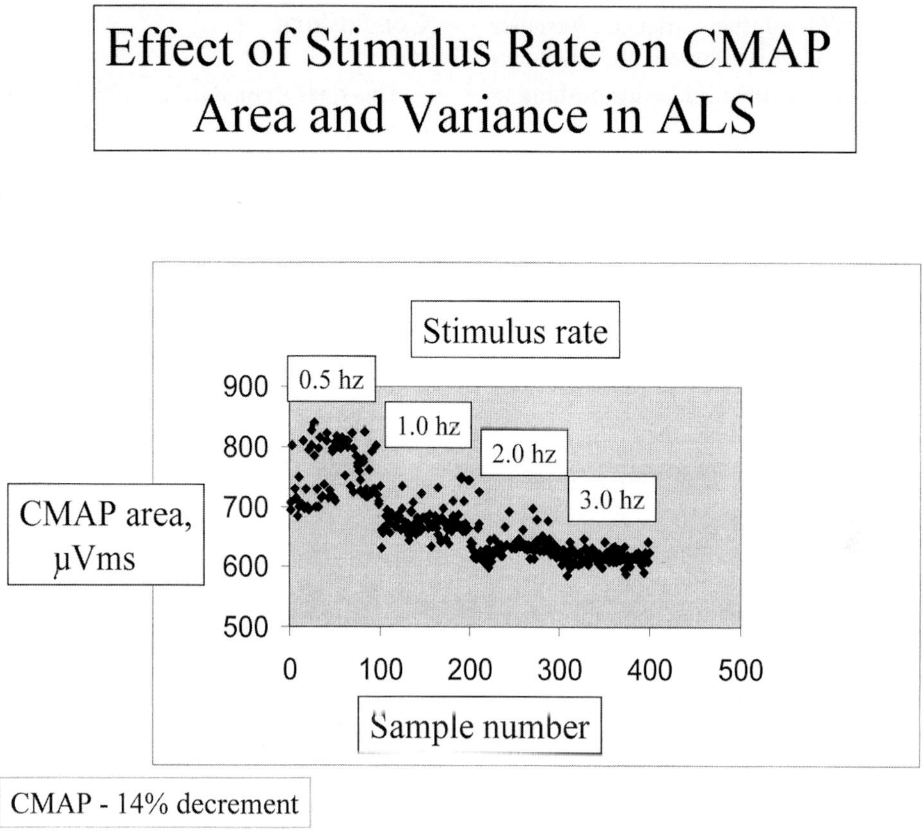

Fig. 20. Five hundred sequential CMAP areas recorded in a second patient with ALS who had a 14% CMAP decrement with repetitive stimulation at two per second. The rate of stimulation is changed as shown after each 100 stimuli.

stimulation and a variation of amplitude of single MUPs. This phenomenon introduces unwanted CMAP variation during statistical MUNE (Fig. 13). Estimates of the extent of this effect require study of a number of patients with different levels of decrement. Preliminary studies with 500 sequential stimuli suggest that this effect may be minimal.

The effect of different rates of stimulation on the sizes of two SMUP from two patients with ALS is shown in Figs. 19 and 20. The patient with no decrement (Fig. 19) showed no change in CMAP variance with different rates of stimulation, while a clear decrease in variance occurred in the patient with a 14% decrement (Fig. 20). Decrement occurs only with the initiation of stimulation, as shown in Fig. 13. During continuous stimulation the mobilization of acetylcholine stabilizes the amont released. The continuous stimulation in Figs. 19 and 20 began before the recording epoch, thereby eliminating the decrement. The reduction in variance with increased rate suggests that high rates will minimize the variance due to the neuromuscular junction instability to less than 10%.

SMUP size calculation

The considerations reviewed above suggest that the following be used in calculating the average SMUP size in statistical MUNE:

- The sizes of large steps in a scan that are due to a single, large SMUP are measured separately without calculation of the variance. Variance calculation with a large window that includes such steps would be correct, but adds nothing to a direct measurement.

- SMUP variance calculations are made with four levels of stimulus intensity that do not include the large SMUP measured directly.
- A fixed amplitude window is used to eliminate the effect of low amplitude CMAP on SMUP size calculations.
- The CMAP be recorded in the lower 25% of the window if the variation is less than the full window.
- Window size is expanded if necessary to incorporate well-defined steps.
- Variance due to baseline noise is subtracted from the CMAP variance to provide a more accurate measure of the variance from all or none activation of the MUP.
- The average SMUP size be calculated from the four levels of stimulation by a weighted average (Shefner et al., 1999) that takes into account the number of SMUP of a given size as well as their size.

Practical issues of the statistical MUNE technique

The advantages and disadvantages of the statistical MUNE methods are listed.

Advantages:

- Testing at multiple stimulus intensity levels.
- Limited operator dependence.
- Rapid and efficient.
- Reproducible.
- Includes entire waveform with latency and positivity summation.
- Eliminates issue of alternation.

Disadvantages:

- Patient cooperation.
- Number of stimuli needed.
- Time required with poor patient cooperation.
- Unable to test proximal muscles (anterior compartment).

Conclusions

This review considered a number of issues related to MUNE. Some are applicable to all MUNE techniques while others are pertinent to the statistical technique.

Considerations for all techniques:

- Technical problems must be recognized and minimized.
- Measure SMUAP area rather than amplitude.
- Eliminate positive SMUAP responses from calculations.
- Consider 25 μV ms (10 μV) to be the smallest acceptable SMUP.

Considerations for the statistical technique:

- Consider using a 250 μV window.
- Consider collecting 300 or more CMAPs at each stimulus level without windows to be analyzed at multiple window sizes off-line.
- Determine the maximum effect of decrement on calculation of SMUP variance.

References

Burke, D., Kiernan, M.C. and Bostock, H. Excitability of human axons. *Clin. Neurophysiol.*, 2001, 112(9): 1575–1585.

Daube, Unpublished data.

Elmqvist, D. and Lambert, E.H. Detailed analysis of neuromuscular transmission in a patient with the myasthenic syndrome sometimes associated with bronchogenic carcinoma. *Mayo. Clin. Proc.*, 1968, 43(10): 689–713.

Henderson, R.H. and Daube, J.R. Assessment of statistical MUNE data collection. *Muscle Nerve*, 2001, 24(3): 455 (abstract).

Henderson, R.H. and Daube, J.R. Effect of changing data collection parameters on statistical motor unit number estimates. *Muscle Nerve*, 2003, in press, permission requested.

Hubbard, L.R. and Quastel, D.M. *Electrophysiological Analysis of Synaptic Transmission*. E. Arnold, London, .

Katz, B. and Miledi, R. The statistical nature of the acetycholine potential and its molecular components. *J. Physiol.*, 1969, 224(3): 665–699.

Lomen-Hoerth, C. and Olney, R.K. Comparison of multiple point and statistical motor unit number estimation. *Muscle Nerve*, 1972, 23(10): 1525–1533.

Lomen-Hoerth, C. and Olney, R.K. Effect of recording window and stimulation variables on the statistical technique of motor unit number estimation. *Muscle Nerve*, 2000, 24: 1659–1664.

Olney, R.K., Yuen, E.C. and Engstrom, J.W. Statistical motor unit number estimation: reproducibility and sources of error in patients with amyotrophic lateral sclerosis. *Muscle Nerve*, 2001, 23(2): 193–197.

Shefner, J.M., Jillapali, D. and Bradshaw, D.Y. Reducing intersubject variability in motor unit number estimation. *Muscle Nerve*, 2000, 22(10): 1457–1460.

Simmons, Z., Epstein, D.K., Borg, B., Mauger, D.T., Kothari, M.J. and Shefner, J.M. Reproducibility of motor unit number estimation in individual subjects. *Muscle Nerve*, 1999, 24(4): 467–473.

Slawnych, M., Laszlo, C. and Herschler, C. Motor unit estimates obtained using the new "MUESA" method. *Muscle Nerve*, 2001, 19(5): 626–636.

Stålberg, E. and Karlsson, L. Simulation of the normal concentric needle electromyogram by using a muscle model. *Clin. Neurophysiol.*, 1996, 112(3): 464–471.

Motor Unit Number Estimation (Supplements to Clinical Neurophysiology Vol. 55)
Editor: M.B. Bromberg

Chapter 8

Multiple point stimulation MUNE with integrated single motor unit tracking

Clifton L. Gooch* and Petra Kaufmann

Department of Neurology, Columbia Presbyterian Medical Center, 710 West 168th Street, New York, NY 10032, USA

Introduction

Motor unit number estimation (MUNE) tech niques provide unique insights into the pathophysiology of motor unit survival and loss in human subject and have assumed increasing importance in the quantitative assessment of neuromuscular disease. MUNE is being used in natural history studies and as outcome measures in therapeutic trials, particularly those involving amyotrophic lateral sclerosis (ALS) (McComas et al., 1971; Daube, 1988; Dantes and McComas, 1991; Bromberg et al., 1993; Doherty and Brown, 1993; Stashuk et al., 1994; Felice, 1995; Gooch and Harati, 1997; Yuen and Olney, 1997; Armon and Brandstader, 1999; Shefner et al., 1999). In concert with estimates of functional motor unit numbers, complementary information about individual single motor unit action potential (S-MUAP) size and changes over time is also important, and enables a more full assessment of the extent of reinnervation during progressive motor unit loss. The multiple point stimulation (MPS) is a well-established and reproducible MUNE technique in which percutaneous stimulation of the nerve is used to elicit a number of S-MUAP waveforms (Doherty and Brown, 1993). The principles of the MPS technique can also be used to track the same individual S-MUAPs over time (Gooch and Harati, 1997). In this chapter, we discuss our experience with a modified MPS MUNE method which integrates S-MUAP tracking (MPS MUNE-T).

MUNE with integrated single motor unit tracking

A combined method of performing both MPS MUNE and S-MUAP tracking in the same patient over several sessions would have obvious advantages, but S-MUAP sampling bias introduced by such an approach might artifactually influence the MUNE value. We developed a MPS MUNE technique that includes S-MUAP tracking (MPS MUNE-T), and compared it to traditional MPS MUNE without S-MUAP tracking (MPS MUNE) in normal controls to assess the feasibility, efficiency and reproducibility.

Methods

Our recording and stimulating techniques have been previously reported (Gooch and Harati, 1997). Recording electrodes were disposable 8×30 mm

**Correspondence to*: Dr. Clifton L. Gooch, Department of Neurology, Columbia Presbyterian Medical Center, 710 West 168th Street, New York, NY 10032, USA. e-mail: CLG33@columbia.edu

doi: 10.1016/S1567-424X(03)00008-4

adhesive strips (TECA Co., Pleasantville, NY) placed transversely over the thenar eminence in close approximation to the end-plate zone of the abductor and flexor pollicis muscles. Reference electrodes were placed over the distal interphalangeal joint of the thumb, and ground electrodes were placed over the ulnar surface of the palm. The recording electrode position was noted using anatomical surface landmarks for future reference. Median nerve stimulation was performed with a hand-held bipolar electrode (Nicolet Biomedical, Madison, WI) through saline-soaked felt pads (5 mm diameter, 30 mm apart, cathode distal). S-MUAPs and compound motor action potentials (CMAPs) were recorded from the thenar musculature on an Advantage EMG system (Advantage Medical, London, Canada) with a bandpass of 2 Hz–2 kHz (12 bit resolution). S-MUAPs were activated by 0.05 ms square wave pulses at various intensities, from 5 to 50 mA. A surface map of the median nerve was made noting anodal and cathodal positions and current levels that produced a given S-MUAP.

Single motor units were identified using previously published criteria (Doherty and Brown 1994). (1) Each S-MUAP demonstrated an "all-or-nothing" response with no fractionation. Specifically, stimuli near threshold produced either a MUAP with consistent morphology and latency, or no response. (2) The threshold for eliciting a given S-MUAP was distinctly different from that eliciting the next highest motor axon at a specific stimulation site. Repeat excitation of the same baseline S-MUAP during sequential sessions was assumed when the potential fulfilled the above criteria, more closely resembled its predecessor than any other potential elicited from other stimulation sites, and was activated from the same anodal

TABLE 1

DATA FOR THREE S-MUAP TRACKED OVER TWO SESSIONS IN EACH OF FIVE SUBJECTS

	S-MUAP A		S-MUAP B		S-MUAP C		Mean ± SD	
	Session 1	Session 2	Session 1	Session 2	Session 1	Session 2	Session 1	Session 2
Subject A								
Latency (ms)	2.9	3.2	3.7	3.7	2.5	2.7	3.0 ± 2.6	3.2 ± 0.5
Amplitude (μV)	79	65	39	35	102	95	73 ± 32	65 ± 30
Duration (ms)	3.9	3.3	4.1	5.0	6.1	5.6	4.7 ± 1.2	4.8 ± 1.3
Subject B								
Latency (ms)	4.4	4.1	5.4	5.1	4.1	4.1	4.6 ± 0.7	4.4 ± 0.8
Amplitude (μV)	111	140	65	70	163	177	113 ± 49	125 ± 54
Duration (ms)	4.7	4.4	2.5	2.9	5.1	4.9	4.1 ± 1.4	4.1 ± 1.0
Subject C								
Latency (ms)	2.9	2.7	4.5	4.5	8.7	8.7	5.4 ± 3.0	5.3 ± 3.1
Amplitude (μV)	159	141	55	60	38	47	84 ± 66	82 ± 50
Duration (ms)	5.4	5.4	4.1	3.6	3.5	2.9	4.3 ± 1.0	4.0 ± 1.3
Subject D								
Latency (ms)	3.6	3.5	2.9	2.9	5.2	5.0	3.9 ± 0.8	3.8 ± 1.1
Amplitude (μV)	25	30	179	181	100	110	101 ± 77	107 ± 76
Duration (ms)	3.7	3.5	4.8	4.1	3.2	2.9	3.9 ± 0.8	3.5 ± 0.5
Subject E								
Latency (ms)	2.9	2.7	4.7	5.0	3.2	3.5	36.0 ± 1.0	3.8 ± 1.2
Amplitude (μV)	95	79	48	35	71	52	61 ± 31	55 ± 22
Duration (ms)	6.8	7.1	5.2	5.2	5.5	4.5	5.5 ± 1.2	5.6 ± 1.4

Individual values are listed, as well as mean values (and standard deviations). S-MUAP, single motor unit action potential.

TABLE 2

AVERAGED DATA FOR COMPOUND MUSCLE ACTION POTENTIAL (CMAP) AND S-MUAP AND RESULTANT MUNE VALUES CALCULATED WITH AND WITHOUT TRACKING IN EACH OF FIVE SUBJECTS OVER TWO SESSIONS

	CMAP		Average single MUAP (groups of 10)				MUAP			
	Session 1	Session 2	Session 1 without tracking	Session 2 with tracking	Session 1 without tracking	Session 2 with tracking	Session 1 without tracking	Session 2 with tracking	Session 1 without tracking	Session 2 with tracking
Subject A										
Latency (ms)	2.3	2.4	NA	NA	NA	NA	304	284	284	260
Amplitude (μV)	15.6	15.5	59	65	64	63				
Duration (ms)	5.6	5.8	4.8	4.2	4.9	5.0				
Subject B										
Latency (ms)	3.8	3.4	NA	NA	NA	NA	263	273	236	235
Amplitude (μV)	10.3	11.7	52	49	58	62				
Duration (ms)	8.0	8.2	3.5	3.5	3.9	4.0				
Subject C										
Latency (ms)	3.2	2.5	NA	NA	NA	NA	238	253	262	274
Amplitude (μV)	12.7	13.3	61	64	61	69				
Duration (ms)	5.4	5.3	4.7	4.4	4.9	4.8				
Subject D										
Latency (ms)	3.3	3.1	NA	NA	NA	NA	390	350	348	319
Amplitude (μV)	17.4	17.1	48	52	58	64				
Duration (ms)	5.4	5.4	3.5	5.8	4.1	4.2				
Subject E										
Latency (ms)	2.9	3.0	NA	NA	NA	NA	342	371	312	335
Amplitude (μV)	15.5	14.3	51	43	59	51				
Duration (ms)	6.9	7.0	5.1	4.5	5.0	4.8				

Without tracking: data from 10 S-MUAPs. With tracking: data from 3 to 10 S-MUAPs. CMAP, compound muscle action potential. S-MUAP, single motor unit action potential. MUNE, motor unit number estimation. NA, not applicable.

and cathodal coordinates with similar stimulus strengths as at baseline.

Results: data and feasibility

We performed traditional MPS MUNE using previously described methods (Doherty and Brown 1993) to randomly sample ten S-MUAPs in five normal control subjects. In the same subjects, we also performed the modified MPS MUNE-T technique combining three tracked and seven randomly sampled S-MUAPs. Each technique was repeated at a follow-up session from 1 h to 5 days later. Electrodes were removed and replaced between sessions 1 and 2.

Three S-MUAPs (labeled A, B and C) fulfilling the above criteria were tracked in each patient (Table 1). The latency of each S-MUAP remained relatively constant throughout the study, with no more than a 0.3 ms variation, attributed to minor temperature changes over the course of each session. The negative peak amplitudes of each S-MUAP also remained relatively constant from session to session, with most variations less than 15% and none greater than 30%. The mean and standard deviation of each of these parameters for each group of the three tracked S-MUAPs demonstrated minimal change, with coefficients of variance ranging from 0.98 to 1.00 for most parameters. For each of the tracked CMAPs, mean amplitudes varied less than 15%, with most varying less than 5%.

Mean S-MUAP amplitudes derived from all 10 sampled units, with and without tracking, also varied less than 15% (Table 2). MUNE values from the traditional MPS technique ranged from 238 to 371, and reproducibility between sessions 1 and 2 was high (correlation coefficient $r = 0.88$). MUNE values from the modified technique were similar (236–348), and had good reproducibility between sessions 1 and 2 ($r = 0.86$). MUNE values obtained during the same recording sessions without tracking and with tracking were highly correlated ($r = 0.94$ in session 1 and $r = 0.88$ in session 2), with minimal variation between the two techniques. Performing MPS MUNE-T was reasonably time efficient, averaging only 30–35 min, compared to 20–25 min to perform traditional MPS MUNE.

Summary

MPS MUNE-T is both feasible and reproducible. When compared to traditional MPS MUNE, values are similar, and the range of values among normal subjects matches those reported previously (Doherty and Brown 1993, 1994). MPS MUNE-T had high reproducibility and was also efficient in time, adding only 5–10 min to each study. The ability to track both S-MUAP parameters and derive MUNE values longitudinally provides data regarding the relationship between reinnervation and subsequent denervation in a variety of patient populations. This may be especially promising for detecting the preservation and/or resuscitation of injured motor neurons in patients with neuromuscular disease undergoing experimental therapies.

References

Armon, C. and Brandstader, M.E. Motor unit number estimate-based rates of progression of ALS predict patient survival. *Muscle Nerve*, 1999, 11: 1571–1575.

Bromberg, M.B., Forshew, D.A., Nan, K.L., Bromberg, J., Simmons, Z. and Fries, T.J. Motor unit number estimation, isometric strength and electromyographic measures in amyotrophic lateral sclerosis. *Muscle Nerve*, 1993, 12: 1218–1219.

Dantes, A. and McComas, A. The extent and time course of motor neuron involvement in ALS. *Muscle Nerve*, 1991, 14: 416–421.

Daube, J.R. Statistical estimates of number of motor units in thenar and foot muscles in patients with amyotrophic lateral sclerosis or the residue of poliomyelitis. *Muscle Nerve*, 1988, 11: 957-A.

Doherty, T.J. and Brown, W.F. The estimated numbers and relative sizes of thenar motor units as selected by multiple point stimulation in young and older adults. *Muscle Nerve*, 1993, 16: 355–366.

Doherty, T.J. and Brown, W.F. A method for the longitudinal study of human thenar motor units. *Muscle Nerve*, 1994, 17: 1029–1036.

Felice, K.J. Thenar motor unit number estimates using the multiple point stimulation technique: reproducibility studies in ALS patient and normal subjects. *Muscle Nerve*, 1995, 18: 1412–1416.

Gooch, C.L. and Harati, Y. Longitudinal tracking of the same single motor unit in amyotrophic lateral sclerosis. *Muscle Nerve*, 1997, 20: 511–513.

McComas, A.J., Fawcett, P.R.W., Campbell, M.J. and Sica, R. E.P. Electrophysiological estimation of the number of motor units within a human muscle. *J. Neurol. Neurosurg. Psychiatry.*, 1971, 34: 121–131.

Shefner, J.M., Reaume, A.G., Flood, D.G., Scott, R.W., Kowall, N.W., Ferrante, R.J., Siwek, D.F., Upton-Rice, M. and Brown, R.H. Mice lacking cytosolic Cu/ZN SOD display a distinctive motor axonopathy. *Neurology*, 1999, 53: 1239–1246.

Stashuk, D.W., Doherty, T.J., Kassam, A. and Brown, W.F. Motor unit number estimates based on the automated analysis of F-responses. *Muscle Nerve*, 1994, 17: 881–890.

Yuen, E.C. and Olney, R.K. Longitudinal study of fiber density and motor unit number estimate in patients with amyotrophic lateral sclerosis. *Neurology*, 1997, 49: 573–578.

Motor Unit Number Estimation (Supplements to Clinical Neurophysiology Vol. 55)
Editor: M.B. Bromberg

Chapter 9

Statistical MUNE in larger muscles

Clifton L. Gooch* and Werner Trojaborg

Department of Neurology, Columbia Presbyterian Medical Center, 710 West 168th Street, New York, NY 10032, USA

Introduction

Most motor unit number estimation (MUNE) techniques derive motor unit numbers by dividing the compound muscle action potential (CMAP) area or amplitude of a given muscle by that muscle's average, surface-recorded single motor unit action potential (S-MUAP) (McComas et al., 1971). MUNE techniques differ principally in the way in which this average S-MUAP is obtained and calculated. The statistical MUNE technique utilizes computerized Poisson analysis of CMAP variation with repetitive nerve stimulation at a given stimulus intensity to derive this data (Daube, 1995). The software for this method is proprietary and available only a single EMG system, but that EMG system is widely utilized. The statistical technique continues to undergo further refinement as it is increasingly employed in research and, more recently, clinical trials (Daube, 1995; Slawnych et al., 1996; Shefner et al., 1999). This technique has been previously studied only in small, distal muscle groups, but MUNE in proximal and larger distal muscles is also important for the assessment of a number of neuromuscular diseases. In this chapter, we review our techniques for, and the reproducibility of statistical MUNE in the elbow flexor and anterior tibialis muscles of normal subjects (Trojaborg et al., 2000a,b).

**Correspondence to*: Dr. Clifton L. Gooch, Department of Neurology, Columbia Presbyterian Medical Center, 710 West 168th Street, New York, NY 10032, USA.
e-mail: CLG33@columbia.edu

doi: 10.1016/S1567-424X(03)00009-6

Statistical MUNE in elbow flexor muscles

Assessment of MUNE in the elbow flexor muscles by other methods has proven challenging. Variable results have been obtained due to both the nature of stimulated and volitional activation in this region and to issues specific to each technique (McComas et al., 1971; Brown et al., 1988; Bromberg, 1993; Bromberg and Abrams, 1995). We assessed the feasibility of statistical MUNE in this muscle group (Trojaborg et al., 2000a).

Methods

The musculocutaneous nerve was stimulated in the axilla, between the axillary artery and the median nerve. Depending on body habitus, stimulation was with either a bipolar bar electrode (placed longitudinally over the nerve) or a superficial disc cathode and a large anode placed on the lateral aspect of the arm at the same level. Stimulus pulses were 0.1–0.1 ms in duration with intensities up to 40–60 mA and delivered at a frequency of 1 Hz. The CMAP was recorded with a self-adhesive strip electrode placed transversely over the endplate zone of the biceps muscle (between the upper two and the lower one-third of the muscle) referred to a second self adhesive disc electrode over the distal tendon. The arm was fixed to a board to minimize elbow flexion, and care was taken during stimulation to avoid simultaneous activation of forearm flexor muscles.

The statistical MUNE technique was performed using the Viking IV EMG System and the MUNE software package (Nicolet Biomedical, Madison, WI). Each session included two complete statistical MUNE studies, each of which included 3–4 tested ranges chosen according to the original software acquisition parameters (Daube, 1995). MUNE values were calculated by two methods, the original method proposed by Daube (MUNE-D) and a weighted averages method proposed by Shefner (MUNE-S), and comparisons were made (Daube, 1995; Shefner et al., 1999). The two studies during each session included both MUNE-D and MUNE-S calculations, and the paired studies were averaged to give average MUNE-D and average MUNE-S values. In addition, one normal elderly subject was studied over 11 sessions on separate days, and each session included two statistical MUNE studies (with both MUNE-D and MUNE-S calculations), averaged to derive the MUNE for that session.

Results: data and reproducibility

Seven normal subjects ranging from 21 to 76 years old were studied in two separate sessions on subsequent days to assess reproducibility. The mean, standard deviation and range for MUNE values was 176 ± 28 (140–230.5) by the MUNE-D method and 137 ± 17 (114.5–165.5) by the MUNE-S method (Table 1). Reproducibility was low regardless of which calculation method was used, with correlation coefficients of 0.15 for MUNE-D and 0.30 for MUNE-S. The mean MUNE-D value in a longitudinal study of one subject over 11 sessions was 190 ± 36 (127–212), and the mean MUNE-S value was 140 ± 1 (121–166) (Table 2). There was a decrease of MUNE with increasing age, but poor correlation overall ($r = -0.07$ for MUNE-D and $r = -0.2$ for MUNE-S), likely due to the limited number of elderly subjects, one of whom was unusually athletic.

TABLE 1

DEMOGRAPHIC AND MUNE VALUES FROM ELBOW FLEXOR MUSCLES FROM SEVEN SUBJECTS

Age	MUNE-D	MUNE-S
26	177	156
30	186	132.5
31	140	129
34	230.5	114.5
36	165.5	165.5
37	163	132.5
76	171.5	130.5
Mean: 42	180	145
SD: 17	27	26

MUNE-D refers to MUNE values calculated by the original software acquisition parameters (Daube, 1995), and MUNE-S refers to values calculated by a weighted averages method (Shefner, 1990). See text for details.

TABLE 2

AVERAGE AND MUNE VALUES FROM ELBOW FLEXOR MUSCLES RECORDED FROM ONE SUBJECT OVER 11 SESSIONS

Session	MUNE-D	MUNE-S
1	176	136
2	167	125
3	174	125
4	250	166
5	209	159
6	190	153
7	144	129
8	222	163
9	127	121
10	218	128
11	212	138
Mean	190	140
SD	36	16

MUNE-D refers to MUNE values calculated by the original software acquisition parameters (Daube, 1995), and MUNE-S refers to values calculated by a weighted averages method (Shefner, 1990).

Summary and comparisons with other methods

Mean MUNE values for the elbow flexor muscles have varied among studies, likely attributed to different techniques. The automated incremental method (Galea et al., 1991) yielded a mean MUNE of 113 ± 40 (60–250) for the elbow flexors in a group of 40 healthy subjects (age range 21–56 years). This method was also applied in another group of 79 healthy young and elderly volunteers (age range 20–98 years) and yielded mean MUNEs of 111 ± 32 in patients aged 20–29, and 93 ± 37 in those over 80 (Galea, 1996). These values are lower than those obtained by us using the statistical technique, but in other muscles MUNE values obtained from the incremental stimulation technique are generally lower than those obtained by the statistical technique (particularly when calculated by the MUNE-D algorithm). Differences in stimulation methods may also partially account for lower MUNE values. For example, Galea et al. stimulated the biceps brachii over the middle of the muscle, at or near the motor point with the stimulating electrodes oriented in the long axis of the muscle, whereas we stimulated the musculocutaneous nerve. Another issue is the phenomenon of alternation, which automation of the incremental method was designed to minimize, but does not entirely eliminate. Our study demonstrated no significant correlation between MUNE values and advanced age, but included few elderly subjects, and one 70-year-old subject was exceptionally athletic and cycled several miles each day.

Biceps brachii MUNE values obtained from the spike triggered averaging (STA) technique (Brown et al., 1988) yield considerably higher and more variable MUNE values in normal subjects, ranging from 400 to 1300. Similar results were reported in another study in which STA reproducibility was assessed, and showed a high test–retest difference (45.3%) and low correlation coefficient ($r = 0.07$) (Bromberg, 1993). The STA technique has yielded the highest MUNE values recorded, perhaps because this technique samples S-MUAPs at low levels of voluntary contraction, causing disproportionate sampling of smaller motor units, resulting in lowerer average S-MUAPs and larger MUNEs. Volume conduction from remote muscles activated during initial stimulation may also resulting in spuriously large CMAPs, further increasing MUNE values. The low reproducibility of STA may be due to a sampling effect, as the sample size of 5–20 recorded units is a much smaller proportion of the total MUNE, and the possibility of sampling variation from session to session correspondingly greater (Bromberg and Abrams, 1995). In our study with the statistical MUNE technique, there was also a relatively wide variance and low reproducibility with both calculation methods, though lower standard deviations were seen with MUNE-S calculations.

Statistical MUNE in the anterior tibialis muscle

MUNE techniques have been extensively applied to the smallest, distal muscle groups (Kadrie et al., 1976; Stein and Yang, 1990; Daube, 1994; Gooch and Harati, 1997), but larger muscles such as the anterior tibialis muscle have not extensively studied. The anterior tibialis muscle has the potential to provide information about how neuromuscular diseases progress in the lower extremities. We have assessed the feasibility of the statistical MUNE in the anterior tibialis muscle.

Methods

The leg was placed in a brace to minimize ankle dorsiflexion. The maximal CMAP was recorded by stimulating the deep peroneal nerve below the fibular head, with care to avoid simultaneous activation of branches to the peroneus muscle (Devi et al., 1977). Stimuli at 1 Hz were delivered at a duration of 0.1–0.2 ms and an intensity of 35–55 mA utilizing a standard bar electrode, which was fixed once the correct position was determined. The active (recording) electrodes was a 45 × 15 mm self-adhesive strip placed at the junction of the upper and lower two-thirds of a line drawn vertically between the tibial tuberosity and the tip of the lateral malleolus. The reference electrode was a round 1 cm self-adhesive electrode placed over the distal tendon or along the medial aspect of the tibia (passive electrode) (Fig. 1). Following CMAP acquisition, statistical MUNE was performed using the Viking IV EMG System and a resident software package (Nicolet Biomedical, Madison, WI). Motor unit numbers were calculated by both the Daube method (MUNE-D) and Shefner's method of weighted averages (MUNE-S) and compared (Daube, 1995, Shefner et al., 1999). Each session included two complete statistical MUNE studies, each included 3–4 tested ranges chosen according to the original software acquisition parameters (Daube, 1995). The two studies during each session included both MUNE-D and MUNE-S calculations, and like MUNEs were averaged to provide both average MUNE-D and average MUNE-S for a given session. In addition, one normal elderly subject was studied during separate sessions on 13 separate days. Each session included two statistical MUNE studies (with both MUNE-D and MUNE-S calculations) averaged to derive the MUNE for that session.

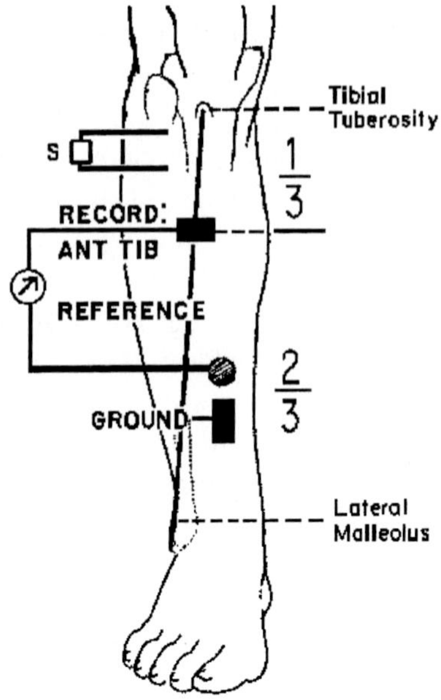

Fig. 1. Setup for statistical MUNE in the anterior tibialis muscle. The deep peroneal nerve is stimulated immediately below the fibular head by a standard bar electrode. A self-adhesive active strip recording electrode is placed at the junction of the upper and lower two-thirds of a line drawn vertically between the tibial tuberosity and the tip of the lateral malleolus. The reference round is a self-adhesive electrode placed over the distal tendon or at the medial aspect of the tibia.

Results: data and reproducibility

Eleven healthy control subjects, aged 21–76 years, were studied during two separate sessions on subsequent days to assess reproducibility. The mean and standard deviation for MUNE in the 11 normal subjects was 176 (± 42) by the MUNE-D method and 129 (± 21) by the MUNE-S method (Table 3). The range for all studies was 104–318. Correlation coefficients were significantly higher than those for the technique applied to the elbow flexor muscles, with a reproducibility of 0.64 for MUNE-D and 0.79 for MUNE-S. The mean MUNE-D in a longitudinal study of one subject over 13 sessions was 182 ± 42 (range 127–256) and the mean MUNE-S was 132 ± 20 (range 104–169) (Table 4). The correlation coefficients between first and second study MUNE results for all 13 sessions were 0.65 for MUNE-D and 0.72 for MUNE-S. MUNE decreased with increasing age for both MUNE-D ($r = -0.42$) and MUNE-S ($r = -0.56$),

TABLE 3

DEMOGRAPHIC AND MUNE VALUES FROM ANTERIOR TIBIALIS MUSCLES FROM 11 SUBJECTS

Age	MUNE-D	MUNE-S
21	190	151
26	151	147
27	238	209
33	194	159
37	189	182
38	204	196
46	198	147
47	177	145
61	206	156
64	97	123
76	166	133
Mean	182	159
SD	36	26

MUNE-D refers to MUNE values calculated by the original software acquisition parameters (Daube, 1995), and MUNE-S refers to values calculated by a weighted averages method (Shefner, 1999).

TABLE 4

AVERAGE AND MUNE VALUES FROM ANTERIOR TIBIALIS MUSCLES RECORDED FROM ONE SUBJECT OVER 13 SESSIONS

Session	MUNE-D	MUNE-S
1	156	111
2	143	115
3	146	119
4	183	131
5	256	157
6	155	128
7	127	118
8	230	169
9	145	104
10	220	125
11	151	132
12	226	159
13	233	153
Mean	182	132
SD	44	20

MUNE-D refers to MUNE values calculated by the original software acquisition parameters (Daube, 1995), and MUNE-S refers to values calculated by a weighted averages method (Shefner, 1999).

with better correlations than those observed for statistical MUNE in the elbow flexor muscles.

Summary and comparison with other methods

Statistical MUNE in the anterior tibial muscle has not been previously reported. This technique results in limited intra- and inter-subject variability that is similar to that reported in previous studies investigating smaller muscles. The MUNE-S method of calculation yielded lower values for the abductor digiti minimi in normal controls and improved reproducibility when compared to MUNE-D calculations ($r=0.57$ vs. $r=0.44$) (Shefner, 1990). Consistent with previous studies, we noted lower values for MUNE-S than MUNE-D in our study (129 vs. 176) with remarkably similar correlation coefficients ($r=0.54$ for MUNE-S vs. $r=0.49$ for MUNE-D). Even better intra-individual reproducibility was noted during longitudinal study of one subject over 13 sessions ($r=0.72$ for MUNE-S and $r=0.65$ for MUNE-D). This relatively high reproducibility despite the relatively large size of the anterior tibialis may be due to a number of factors, including the stability and easy localization of the stimulation and recording sites. Decreasing MUNE with advancing age is also consistent with prior studies of other muscle groups (Brown et al., 1988). This technique appears promising for future application and may have similar reliability compared to statistical MUNE in smaller, more distal muscle groups.

References

Brown, W.F., Strong, M.J. and Snow, R. Methods of estimating numbers of motor units in biceps-brachialis muscles and losses of motor units with aging. *Muscle Nerve*, 1988, 11: 423–432.

Bromberg, M.B. Motor unit estimation: reproducibility of the spike-triggered averaging technique in normal and ALS subjects. *Muscle Nerve*, 1993, 16: 466–471.

Bromberg, M.B. and Abrams, J.L. Sources of error in the spike-triggered averaging method of motor unit number estimation. *Muscle Nerve*, 1995, 18: 1139–1146.

Daube, J.R. Statistical estimates of number of motor units in thenar and foot muscles in patients with amyotrophic lateral sclerosis or the residue of poliomyelitis. *Muscle Nerve*, 1994, 17: 1029–1036.

Daube, J.R. Estimating the number of motor units in a muscle. *J. Clin. Neurophysiol*, 1995, 12: 585–594.

Devi, S., Lovelace, R.L. and Duarte, N. Proximal peroneal nerve conduction velocity: recording from anterior tibial and peroneus brevis muscles. *Ann. Neurol.*, 1977, 2: 116–119.

Galea, V. Changes in motor unit estimates with aging. *J. Clin. Neurophysiol.*, 1996, 13: 253–260.

Galea, V., De Bruin, H., Cavasin, R. and McComas, A.J. The number and relative sizes of motor units estimated by computer. *Muscle Nerve*, 1991, 14: 1123–1130.

Gooch, C.L. and Harati, Y. Longitudinal tracking of the same single motor unit in amyotrophic lateral sclerosis. *Muscle Nerve*, 1997, 20: 511–513.

Kadrie, H.A., Yates, S.K., Milner-Brown, H.S. and Brown, W. F. Multiple point electrical stimulation of ulnar and median nerves. *J. Neurol. Neurosurg. Psychiatry.*, 1976, 39: 973–985.

McComas, A.J., Fawcett, P.R.W., Campbell, M.J. and Sica, R. E.P. Electrophysiological estimation of the number of motor units within a human muscle. *J. Neurol. Neurosurg. Psychiatry.*, 1971, 34: 121–131.

Shefner, J.M., Jillapalli, D. and Bradshaw, D.Y. Reducing intersubject variability in motor unit number estimation. *Muscle Nerve*, 1999, 10: 1457–1460.

Slawnych, M., Laszlo, C. and Herschler, C. Motor unit number estimates obtained using the new MUESA method. *Muscle Nerve*, 1996, 19: 626–636.

Stein, R.B. and Yang, J.F. Methods for estimating the number of motor units in human muscles. *Ann. Neurol.*, 1990, 28: 487–495.

Trojaborg, W., Kaufman, P. and Gooch, C.L. MUNE in a larger muscle: normative data and reproducibility studies. *Muscle Nerve*, 2000a, 23: 1635.

Trojaborg, W., Kaufman, P. and Gooch, C.L. Statistical MUNE in the elbow flexor muscles: techniques and normative data. *Muscle Nerve*, 2000b, 23: 1635.

Motor Unit Number Estimation (Supplements to Clinical Neurophysiology Vol. 55)
Editor: M.B. Bromberg

Chapter 10

Comparison of statistical and multiple point stimulation MUNE techniques

Catherine Lomen-Hoerth* and Richard K. Olney

Department of Neurology, University of California, San Francisco, School of Medicine, 505 Parnassus Avenue, Box 0114, San Francisco, CA 94143-0114, USA

Introduction

Motor unit number estimation (MUNE) refers to a group of techniques to estimate the number of lower motor neurons innervating a muscle (McComas, 1995). This number must be estimated, since there is no method to count the number of functioning motor neurons innervating a given muscle. Techniques vary in the way they obtain samples of surface-recorded motor unit potentials (SMUPs), but all calculate MUNE by dividing the size of the maximal CMAP by the size of the mean SMUP.

Multiple point stimulation and the statistical MUNE represent two techniques used in studies of amyotrophic lateral sclerosis (ALS) patients to quantify the rate of motor unit loss over time (Bromberg, 1998; Daube, 1995). Multiple point stimulation was first described by Kadrie, and Doherty later applied the technique to MUNE (Kadre and Milner Brown, 1976; Doherty et al., 1993b). Multiple point stimulation involves setting the stimulation intensity low enough to activate only one motor axon, and different motor axons are activated by moving the stimulating electrode up or down the motor nerve. Superficial nerves with long segments are required, and it is not painful for the patient. Typically, 10–20 SMUPs are measured to calculate the MUNE value (McComas, 1995). A longitudinal study over 1 year showed that change in MUNE was a more sensitive measure of ALS progression compared with changes in CMAP amplitude, isometric hand grip, manual muscle testing, Appel ALS functional rating scale, and forced vital capacity (Felice, 1997).

The statistical technique was developed based on the observation that when a nerve is stimulated at a given current level, the responses naturally tend to form a Poisson distribution, as is typical of other natural phenomena such as quanta release at the neuromuscular junction (Daube, 1988). A Poisson distribution has a right skew, with decreased numbers at higher values (named for the direction of the long tail). Analysis of the variance of submaximal CMAP responses that have a Poisson distribution is used to determine the mean SMUP size at that stimulus intensity (Daube, 1988). The technique is useful to determine SMUP size at stimulus intensities where many SMUPs are activated. Similar to

**Correspondence to*: Dr. Catherine Lomen-Hoerth, Department of Neurology, University of California, San Francisco, School of Medicine, 505 Parnassus Avenue, Box 0114, San Francisco, CA 94143-0114, USA. e-mail: cathylh@itsa.ucsf.edu

doi: 10.1016/S1567-424X(03)00010-2

multiple point stimulation, statistical MUNE has been found to be more sensitive to change over time in ALS patients than change in strength or CMAP amplitude (Yuen and Olney, 1997). The statistical technique is quick to perform, but is more complicated than multiple point stimulation due to the number of operator-determined variables, such as stimulation current, recording window levels, recording window size, and recording window number.

Methods

Subjects

Ten ALS patients and 20 healthy control subjects gave written informed consent for these studies, which were approved by the University of California San Francisco (UCSF) Institutional Review Board. The ALS patients were diagnosed with probable or definite ALS based on the World Federation of Neurology criteria (Brooks et al., 2000). The control subjects were volunteers with no neurological symptoms or findings on examination All subjects were screened for ulnar neuropathies, and one ALS patient was thus excluded.

Multiple point stimulation technique

Recording electrodes were set up as for a typical motor nerve conduction study with the active electrode over the motor point of the hypothenar muscle group and the reference placed on the tendon. A maximum CMAP was generated. The stimulating electrode was then moved up and down the nerve to obtain different SMUPs at different sites along the nerve. The current was gradually increased and decreased to ensure all-or-none responses. Ten responses were recorded from different stimulation sites and averaged together to determine the mean SMUP. The MUNE was calculated by dividing the maximum CMAP by the mean SMUP value. The multiple point stimulation procedure was performed twice (tests 1a, 1b), the electrodes were then removed and replaced, and performed two more times (tests 2a, 2b).

Statistical technique

Recording electrodes were set up as for a typical motor nerve conduction study with the active electrode over the motor point of the hypothenar muscle group and the reference placed on the tendon. Stimulating electrodes were taped over the nerve and a maximum CMAP was generated. The stimulating electrodes remained in this position. The upper and lower stimulus intensity–CMAP response relationships were determined; the stimulus intensity that evoked a 0% CMAP response was just below the initial threshold for generating a SMUP, and the stimulus intensity that evoked a 100% CMAP response was the stimulus intensity that just activated all motor units. Using this 0–100% stimulus intensity–CMAP response range, a "scan" of CMAP responses was obtained using 30 stimuli within this range. The 0–100% stimulus intensity–CMAP response range was divided into "windows" covering 10–20, 25–35, 40–50, and 55–65% of the CMAP response. Within each recording range or window, a series of 30 submaximal CMAPs were recorded until the standard error was less than 10% of the mean. To ensure a Poisson distribution of CMAP responses within a window, the stimulation current small adjustments were made during the 30 stimuli to ensure that CMAP responses occurred in the entire range of the window. For ALS patients, the standardized recording window levels were not used if there was a large step, making up greater than 15% of the scan. The recording windows were also enlarged if there was no CMAP variation within the 10% recording window due to loss of motor units or if more than 50% of the responses fell outside of the recording window. The statistical procedure was performed twice (tests 1a, 1b), the electrodes were then removed and replaced, and performed two more times (tests 2a, 2b).

The MUNE value was calculated by the number-weighted statistical method, where the mean SMUP amplitude was multiplied by the number of motor units estimated at each level, the products added, and the result divided by the sum of the number of motor units determined at each level (Shefner et al., 2001). The maximal CMAP was divided by this modified mean SMUP to calculate the MUNE. For ALS patients where a single SMUP accounted for greater than or equal to 15% of the entire CMAP range by itself, the calculations were modified. The size of the large SMUP was measured as a percent of the CMAP range, and it was counted as one (1) toward the MUNE. The corresponding percentage was subtracted from 100% before calculating the remaining number of motor units (Lomen-Hoerth and Olney, 2000).

Optimization of the statistical technique

In a subset of 15 control subjects and 10 additional ALS patients with intermediate motor unit loss, further modifications of the statistical method were explored (Lomen-Hoerth and Olney, 2001). In addition to the 10% recording windows mentioned above, 5% recording windows set at 10–15, 25–30, 40–45, and 55–60% of the CMAP response were used in control subjects. Before recording began in each window, the stimulation current was set in the lower quarter of the window in test 1, in the middle half of the window in test 2, and in the upper quarter of the window in test 3 (Fig. 1). Submaximal CMAPs were recorded without adjusting the current. For the 5% windows only the lower quarter and middle half settings were used, since there were no differences in MUNE or reproducibility between the stimulation current set in the middle half or upper quarter of these small recording windows. Lastly, results were compared with the method described above where current was adjusted to fill out the window ("current forced" method). The standardized windows were not used in ALS patients if there was a greater than 15% gap as described above. All testing was performed twice to obtain reproducibility information for a single test.

Results

Primary results

Recordings from a typical multiple point stimulation recording in a control subject and ALS subject are illustrated in Fig. 2. Recordings for the statistical method are illustrated in Fig. 3.

Reproducibility

Reproducibility results are shown in Fig. 4. Paired test results of mean SMUP and MUNE are very reproducible for both methods, as demonstrated by the scatter plots. Test–retest correlation coefficients (r) for mean SMUP are 0.83–0.86 for multiple point stimulation, and 0.91–0.99 for the statistical method (all $P < 0.001$). Test–retest correlation coefficients for MUNE are 0.82–0.90 for multiple point stimulation and 0.94–0.98 for the statistical method. Paired t-tests do not detect a significant difference for test–retest comparisons of tests 1a and 1b for each method without electrode movement or of tests 1a and 2a for each method with electrode movement, showing that electrode movement does not have a significant effect on reproducibility.

The MUNE results for both methods correlated well with each other, $r = 0.55$ ($P < 0.001$), however the reproducibility was significantly different from each other ($P < 0.05$), as shown in Fig. 5. Additionally, the mean of paired tests was compared with single tests to determine if an increased number of tests improved reproducibility. Reproducibility was improved with the paired tests ($P < 0.05$), increasing from a MUNE coefficient of variation of 11–7% for the statistical method and from 18 to 12% for multiple point stimulation. The statistical method was somewhat faster to perform than multiple point stimulation, taking 15–20 min per test for multiple point and 6–10 min for one four-level statistical method test in control subjects.

Comparison of current level and window size

The effect of changing the current level and window size in a sample control subject is shown in Fig. 1. When the stimulation current is set in the lower quarter of the recording window, a right skewed distribution results (Poisson distribution) (Fig. 1b). When the stimulation current is set in the middle of the recording window, a normal

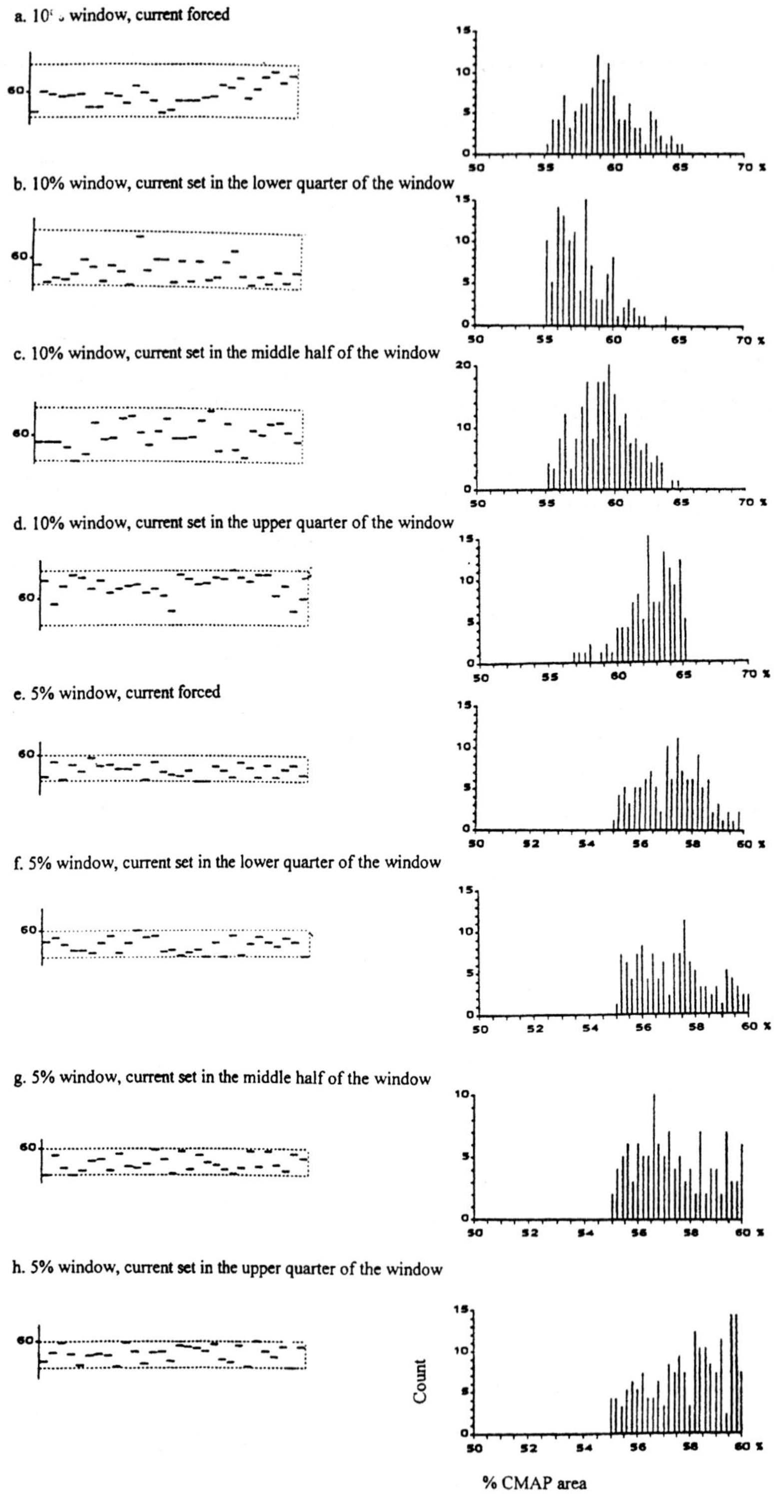

Fig. 1. The left-hand portion of the figure shows representative samples of submaximal CMAP areas generated with 30 stimuli in the 55–65% of the maximum CMAP amplitude range for 10% windows and 55–60% for 5% windows. The right-hand portion of the figure is a histogram of the results. For the histogram, the vertical axis is the number of responses to individual stimuli and the horizontal axis is the stimulus intensity recorded.

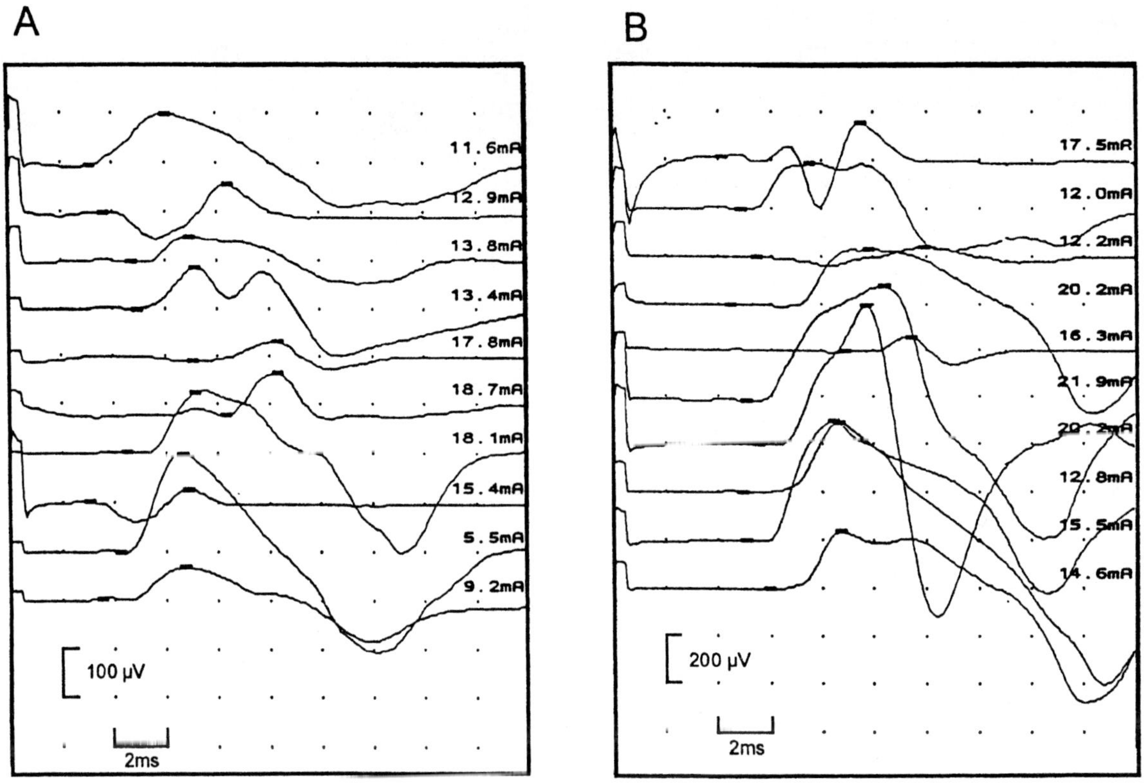

Fig. 2. Samples of hypothenar SMUPs collected by multiple point method in a control subject (**A**) and in an ALS patient (**B**). Recordings were initially made using a gain of 100–200 μV per division; however, if individual SMUPs blocked the amplifier, then lower gains (e.g. 500 mμV per division) were used. Notice the differences in gain between the control and ALS patient.

distribution typically results (Fig. 1c). When the stimulation current is set in the upper portion of the recording window, a left skewed distribution results, which is the opposite of a Poisson distribution (Fig. 1d). For the 5% recording windows, the stimulation current was set in the lower (Fig. 1f) and middle portions (Fig. 1g) of the recording window. Since the recording windows were narrow, it was difficult to detect differences with these two recordings, and the stimulation current was not set in the upper quarter of the recording window for the remaining subjects (Fig. 1h). Lastly, we compared these results to our previous "current forced" method, where the current was slightly changed at the end of each recording to completely fill out the window (Fig. 1a and e). Table 1 shows the primary results for all subjects demonstrating that MUNE tends to be lower when 10% recording windows are used and when the current is set in the lower portion of the windows. However, setting the stimulation current in the lower portion of the window contributes to better reproducibility (Table 2). Increasing the number of recording windows also improved MUNE reproducibility (Table 3). Testing three and four recording windows significantly improved reproducibility compared with one and two windows ($P < 0.03$).

Application in ALS

Applying the most reproducible technique in ALS, setting the stimulation current in the lower quarter of the recording window and using 10% windows resulted in excellent reproducibility. Patients were chosen who had an intermediate motor unit loss, since these patients are often the most difficult to test with MUNE methods reproducibly. The recording window was expanded when

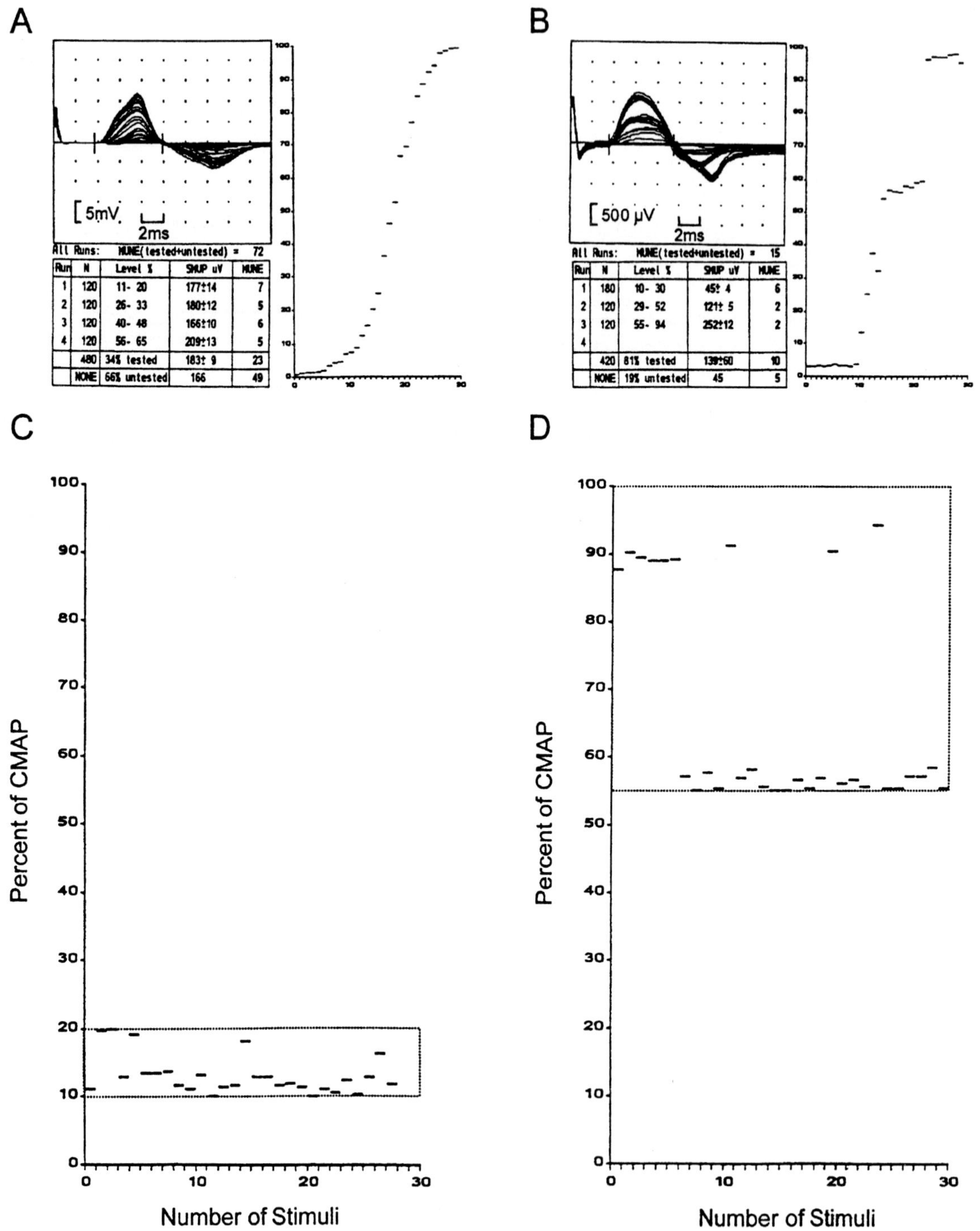

Fig. 3. Samples of scans spanning from 0 to 100% stimulus (**A**,**B**) and recording windows spanning an individual testing range (**C**,**D**) performed by the statistical method in a control subject (A,C) and in an ALS patient (B,D). For controls, 30 submaximal stimulations at 2–3 Hz were recorded (one group demonstrated in C) and the process repeated at each of the above stimulus ranges until the standard error of the mean SMUP was < 10% or 10 trials were completed (one run). For controls, the four standard levels were chosen for all four runs. For the ALS patient, D demonstrates a single large SMUP that was counted visually and manually calculated in to the total MUNE using the modified statistical method. This resulted in a value nearly identical to the program determined value and higher than the weighted statistical values.

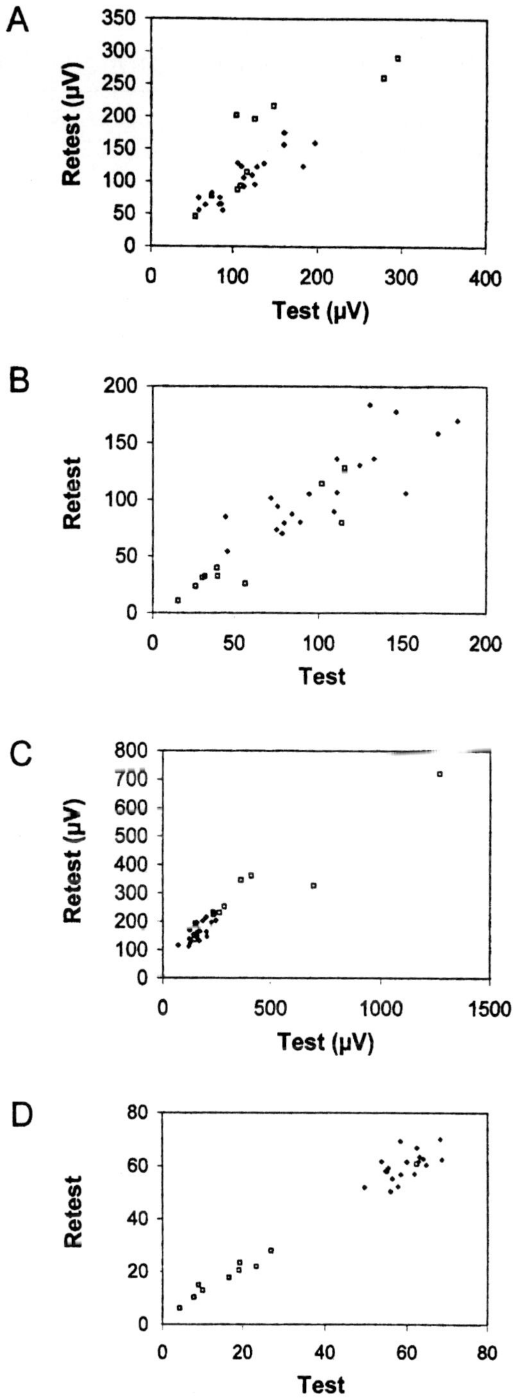

Fig. 4. Scatter-plots of the weighted statistical and multiple point methods paired mean SMUP and MUNE results for ALS patients (open squares) and controls (diamonds). (**A**,**C**) Mean SMUP results for the multiple point and weighted statistical methods, respectively. (**B**,**D**) MUNE results for the multiple point and weighted statistical methods, respectively.

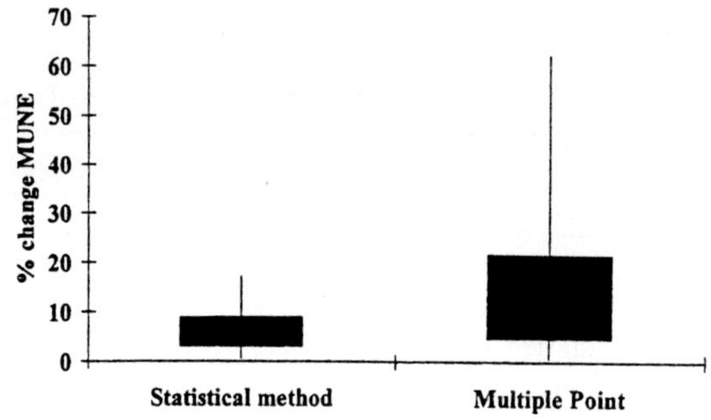

Fig. 5. Reproducibility of multiple point and weighted statistical methods in control subjects. The % change in MUNE was calculated by taking the absolute value of the difference of the average of tests 1a and 1b from the average of 2a and 2b and dividing by the mean of 1a, b, 2a, b. The lines show the range of values and the dark box includes the 25th to the 75th quartiles. The results are plotted here for the size weighted statistical method where the 25% quartile was 2.8% and the 75% quartile was 8.9%. Results were similar for the number weighted method. For multiple point, the 25% quartile was 4.4% and the 75% quartile was 21.8%.

necessary, as described in Section 2. Results showed an average SMUP of 144 µV (range 64–258) and an average MUNE of 42 (range 24–59). The coefficient of variation was 10% for SMUP and 7% for MUNE. Thus, even with a single determination of MUNE value, the coefficient of variation was excellent in ALS patients with intermediate motor unit loss.

Discussion

Comparison of multiple point stimulation and statistical techniques

These studies compare the multiple point stimulation and statistical techniques in the same subject population. The MUNE values were twice as large with the multiple point stimulation technique than the statistical technique in our hands. There are limited data for the statistical technique on the hypothenar muscle group, but in one study of 30 control subjects MUNE values ranged from 70 to 285 (Daube, 1995). These data were based on using the smallest SMUP to account for the SMUPs in the untested CMAP range. This approach produces

TABLE 1

PRIMARY RESULTS FOR ULNAR NERVE-ABDUCTOR DIGITI MINI MUSCLE FOR CONTROL SUBJECTS

	SMUP (μV)	Change in SMUP (μV)	MUNE	Change in MUNE[a]
10% *Recording window size*				
Stimulation current set at				
Lower quarter	130 ± 33 (60–197)	17 ± 12 (1–41)	81 ± 14 (62–103)	8 ± 6 (0.2–18)
Middle half	117 ± 34 (61–174)	13 ± 11 (1–37)	91 ± 19 (61–123)	15 ± 14 (0.4–51)
Upper quarter	92 ± 35 (49–149)	15 ± 11 (1–43)	119 ± 23 (83–153)	15 ± 12 (0.1–40)
5% *Recording window size*				
Stimulation current set at				
Lower quarter	91 ± 25 (40–147)	9 ± 8 (0.2–26)	120 ± 15 (108–135)	11 ± 13 (1.0–25)
Middle half	83 ± 17 (54–97)	10 ± 11 (0.2–20)	133 ± 17 (120–154)	15 ± 18 (0.5–73)

Values are means and ± standard deviation (range) for the paired mean of tests 1 and 2. SMUP, surface motor unit potential. MUNE, motor unit number estimation.

[a] Test–retest absolute difference.

TABLE 2

REPRODUCIBILITY OF MUNE IN CONTROL SUBJECTS

Current set in window	Coefficient of variation (%)	
	5% Windows	10% Windows
Lower quarter	6	7
Middle half	8	11
Upper quarter	NT	9
Forced	7	5

NT, not tested.

TABLE 3

REPRODUCIBILITY CHANGE IN MUNE WITH INCREASING NUMBER OF RECORDING WINDOWS TESTED IN CONTROL SUBJECTS

Number of recording windows tested	Coefficient of variation (%)	
	5% Windows	10% Windows
1	9–14	11–14
2	6–10	6–11
3	7–8	6–9
4	6	7

a higher MUNE value than the newer, weighted approaches (Shefner, 1999; Lomen-Hoerth and Olney, 2000). For the multiple point stimulation technique, MUNE values of 115–256 have been reported for the hypothenar muscle group, which are also higher than the MUNE values in our study (Daube, 1995).

It is not possible to determine the true number of functioning motor units in a muscle in order to make comparisons between MUNE techniques. Santo Neto et al. (1998) used histological methods to estimate the number and size of human flexor digiti minimi muscle motor units from ten fresh cadavers aged 33–74 years. Assuming that 60% of all large-sized myelinated nerve fibers were alpha motor neurons, they showed an average number of 130 motor units ± 15. Thus, the multiple point stimulation results correlate better with the number found anatomically, however the statistical technique is more reproducible. For following patients longitudinally, reproducibility is likely to be more important than how well the absolute number correlates with anatomic numbers. There was also better separation between patients and controls with the statistical as compared with multiple point stimulation technique, which may be important for early diagnosis or detection of a sub-clinical phenotype.

The only other published comparison of MUNE techniques in the same patient population compared multiple point stimulation with spike triggered averaging in control subjects (Doherty and Brown, 1993a). These techniques gave similar

MUNE values for the thenar muscles and showed excellent test–retest correlation in 23 subjects $r=0.88$ ($P<0.001$). Felice reported multiple point stimulation reproducibility in 20 ALS patients and 16 control subjects for the thenar muscle. His results were similar to Doherty and Brown, with $r=0.85$ ($P<0.001$) in control subjects and $r=0.99$ ($P<0.001$) in ALS subjects for test–retest (Felice, 1997). In our study $r=0.90$ ($P<0.001$) for test–retest with multiple point stimulation for ALS and control subjects, fitting with the above previously reported values.

Limited data are available on the reproducibility of the statistical technique. Daube reported a standard deviation of < 10% for SMUPs with repeated measurement of groups of 30 stimuli in control subjects (Daube, 1995). Reproducibility studies in ALS patients showed excellent test–retest reproducibility in the hypothenar muscle group $r=0.86$ ($P<0.001$) (Olney et al., 2000). In our study $r=0.96$ ($P<0.001$) for test–retest with the statistical method for ALS and control subjects.

The statistical technique is, therefore, a more reproducible method than multiple point stimulation in our hands, with median percent test–retest differences of 6% for statistical and 11% for multiple point stimulation technique. The reproducibility of MUNE techniques determines their sensitivity in detecting rate of change over time in patients with ALS or other progressive neurogenic diseases.

Optimization of the statistical technique

The statistical technique was developed based on the observation that when a nerve is stimulated at a given current level, the responses naturally tend to form a Poisson distribution. The Poisson equation models several natural phenomena such as quanta release at the neuromuscular function and tree ring growth. The fall in MUNE value with increasing recording window size is expected because the equation is based on the variance of the response, which is inversely proportional to the MUNE value. Variance increases as recording window size increases, and the MUNE value is lowered. Setting the current in the lower quarter of the window is best, since a Poisson distribution results almost every time. However, a normal distribution, such as occurs when the current is set in the middle of the window, also results in a similar MUNE value. Reproducibility is improved when the current is set in the lower portion of the window rather than in the middle of the window. This may be due to more variability in the distribution when the stimulation current is set in the middle as opposed to the lower quarter of the recording window.

Increasing the window size from 5 to 10% in control subjects reduces the MUNE value, which means that the operator can influence the MUNE results by expanding or shrinking the recording windows. In a subject with suspected ALS, expansion of the recording window may result in a MUNE value suggesting motor unit loss. This could be real or artifact. Operators have different criteria for expanding recording windows, including the presence of gaps on the scan and the number of responses falling outside of the recording window.

Based on our data, we suggest using 10% recording windows with the current set in the lower portion of the window. With 10% recording windows, there is no need to expand the window in control subjects or in ALS patients with a very mild loss of motor units, because the majority of the responses fall within this window. By contrast, with 5% recording windows, more than 50% of the responses fall outside of the recording window in a number of control subjects and many ALS patients with mild motor unit loss. As motor unit loss increases, more responses fall outside of the recording window, necessitating an increase in the window size. Early in ALS, it is important to ensure that an artificially low motor unit number estimate is not produced by opening the window prematurely. Guidelines need to be developed to decide when to expand recording windows in ALS patients for consistent results following patients longitudinally.

Conclusions

In summary, we suggest the use of the statistical technique above the multiple point stimulation technique, based on better reproducibility in our hands. We suggest 10% recording windows with the stimulation current set in the lower quarter of the window for optimal reproducibility with the statistical method. This maximizes response collection, consistently results in a Poisson or normal distribution, and has excellent reproducibility. The decision to expand the recording window in the setting of a neurogenic process must be made carefully, since the decision to expand the recording window does produce a lower MUNE value even in normal subjects. The high reproducibility of the statistical method for MUNE supports its use in measuring rate of motor unit loss in clinical trials for treatment of ALS or in research that utilizes rate of change to study disease mechanisms.

References

Bromberg, M. Electrodiagnostic studies in clinical trials for motor neuron disease. *J. Clin. Neurophys.*, 1998, 15: 117–128.

Brooks, B.R., Miller, R.G., Swash, M. and Munsat, T.L. for the World Federation of Neurology Research Group on Motor Neuron Diseases. El Escorial revisited: revised criteria for the diagnosis of amyotrophic lateral sclerosis. *Amyotroph Lateral Scler. Other Motor Neuron Disord.*, 2000, Suppl. 2: S293–S298.

Daube, J.R. Statistical estimates of number of motor units in thenar and foot muscles in patients with amytrophic lateral sclerosis or the residual of polymyelitis. [abstr]. *Muscle Nerve*, 1988, 3: 957.

Daube, J.R. Estimating the number of motor units in a muscle. *J. Clin. Neurophysiol.*, 1995, 12: 585–594.

Doherty, J. and Brown, W.F. Estimated numbers and relative sizes of thenar motor units as selected by multiple point stimulation by young and older adults. *Muscle Nerve*, 1993a, 16: 355–366.

Doherty, T.J., Stashuk, D.W. and Brown, W.F. Determinants of mean motor unit size: impact on estimates of motor unit number. *Muscle Nerve*, 1993b, 16: 1326–1331.

Felice, K.J. A longitudinal study comparing thenar motor unit number estimates to other quantitative tests in patients with amyotrophic lateral sclerosis. *Muscle Nerve*, 1997, 20: 179–185.

Kadre, H.Y.S. and Milner Brown, W.F. Multiple point electrical stimuation of ulnar and median nerves. *J. Neurol. Neurosurg. Psychiatry*, 1976, 39: 973–985.

Lomen-Hoerth, C. and Olney, R.K. Comparison of multiple point and statistical motor unit number estimation. *Muscle Nerve*, 2000, 23: 1525–1533.

Lomen-Hoerth, C. and Olney, R.K. Effect of recording window and stimulation variables on the statistical technique of motor unit number estimation. *Muscle Nerve*, 2001, 24: 1659–1664.

McComas, A.J. Motor unit estimation: anxieties and achievements. *Muscle Nerve*, 1995, 18: 369–379.

Olney, R.K., Yuen, E.C. and Engstrom, J.W. Statistical motor unit number estimation: reproducibility and sources of error in patients with amyotrophic lateral sclerosis. *Muscle Nerve*, 2000, 23: 193–197.

Santo Neto, H, De Carvalho, V.C. and Marques, M.J. Estimation of the number and size of human flexor digiti minimi muscle motor units using histological methods. *Muscle Nerve*, 1998, 21: 112–114.

Shefner, J.M., Jillapalli, D. and Bradshaw, D.Y. Reducing intersubject variability in motor unit number estimation. *Muscle Nerve*, 2001, 24: 467–473.

Yuen, E.C. and Olney, R.K. Longitudinal study of fiber density and motor unit number estimate in patients with amyotrophic lateral sclerosis. *Neurology*, 1997, 49: 573–578.

Discussion after Section III

Alan McComas, London, Ontario

I would like to ask Ken Arasaki a question about his technique. Do you think that you are actually impaling the nerve fiber in order to stimulate it, or do you think that the tip of the electrode is against a node of Ranvier? Are there clues to this from the stimulus intensities used? I thought possibly if you were just at threshold stimulus intensity, and you were to see the latency jump by say 50 μs, that it would be suggestive evidence that you were actually stimulating at a node of Ranvier. If the latency changed by a smaller amount, then perhaps you had been stimulating in between nodes.

Ken Arasaki, Tokyo, Japan

You can tell whether the tip of the microelectrode is in the fascicle itself or outside of it by the stimulation threshold. If the tip is at a perifascicular position, the threshold current is about 3–9 A with a pulse duration of 200 μs, whereas if it is in the fascicle the threshold is 0.1–2 mA. I have not looked carefully into the issue you raised.

Mark Bromberg, Salt Lake City, Utah

I have a question with regard to positive waves that you see with low-intensity scans in the statistical technique. Have you tried placing an electrode in lumbrical muscles to determine if in fact the wave forms come from these muscles?

Jasper Daube, Rochester, Minnesota

In the example I showed you, the only twitch is from a lumbar muscle. We have placed surface recording electrodes over the lumbrical muscle, and you see a well-defined compound muscle action potential.

Richard Olney, San Francisco, California

I think that the issue of whether to exclude small SMUPs should be discussed in regard to both the statistical and multiple point stimulation techniques. With regard to the statistical technique, it seems clear that small motor units are real, and I do not know if it is fair to arbitrarily exclude small, primarily negative SMUPs. It might be reasonable to count the very small ones individually, as we do the very large ones. They can have a major influence and skews the average SMUP value if we include them in the calculation for the average value. With regard to the multiple point stimulation technique, later today we will present reproducibility data comparing the statistical and multiple point stimulation techniques. It is not clear whether those who use the multiple point technique also exclude small SMUPs. I think it is the small potentials that may largely account for the lower reproducibility of the multiple point stimulation technique in our hands. If we excluded arbitrarily all SMUPs less than 25 μV, probably the multiple point technique would have had similar reproducibility to the statistical technique.

Jeremy Shefner, Syracuse, New York

I am going to be talking more about my concern with small units later, but I do not want to support the contention that there are no small units in ALS or in normal subjects. When one encounters small units in the multiple point stimulation technique, the importance of a single unit will take up no more than whatever percentage of units are sampled. For example, if you sample 15 units, the importance of a single small unit can never be more than 6 or 7% of the total estimate. However, small units have been a problem with the statistical technique, and can affect our ability to evaluate changes with time and progression in ALS. Even with the modification that weights the total average SMUP according to the number of fibers that have been estimated, a single very small unit has a very large influence on the total MUNE. There has to be some method to account for this factor, and such a method has to apply to the way we are calculating MUNE in our clinical trials and the way the computer-generated algorithm calculates the MUNE. With the computer algorithm, you never get more than four individual estimates of SMUP size, and a single very small unit can contribute much more than 25%, in fact it can contribute up to 60–70%.

Richard Olney, San Francisco, California

Let me briefly comment that I think the magnified effect of small units is particularly true with the statistical technique, whether using the computer algorithm or the number-weighted method. I do not think that the size-weighting method is the answer.

Timothy Doherty, London, Ontario

I agreed with much of what Jasper said about the difficulty of dealing with small units. I want to make a comment about our experience with the multiple point stimulation technique. Despite trying to locate the active electrode as close as possible over the endplate zone, you can see positive onset units that are clearly coming from median innervated thenar muscles and not lumbrical muscles. Our observations are based on both our longitudinal tracking and force data. We observed this by looking for dimpling of the skin over the thenar eminence in association with positive onset units. When we collected simultaneous force measurements, the associated twitches produce a force vector from the thumb. I think it is not strictly correct to throw out positive onset units because we assume they do not come from the appropriate muscle group. That being said, we may still may agree to exclude them.

We have observed very few units smaller than 10 μV with the multiple point stimulation technique in control subjects. I think there are two issues; inclusion of very small units may not be absolutely important because small motor units (10, 15, or 20 μV contribute little to the maximum CMAP potential.

Jasper Daube, Rochester, Minnesota

I do not suggest that the small potentials with a significant negative component from thenar muscles should be discarded.

My issue is with potentials that are entirely positive. Where do they come from and how should we deal with them?

Jeremy Shefner, Syracuse, New York

I want to address an issue in the data presented by Ken Arasaki and Tim Doherty regarding the difference in the amplitude of a single motor unit based on whether it was generated by an average single motor unit or averages of multiple single motor unit areas. Using the analysis of the computer-assisted multiple point stimulation technique, Tim presented data suggesting that there was only a 4% difference between the two methods. However, Ken's data showed more like a 20% difference, which is greater than the variability when amplitude measures are used. And given that the location of the stimulus is not changing, the situations would seem to me to be very similar, and I am wondering whether either of you have any thoughts on why that difference exists.

Ken Arasaki, Tokyo, Japan

Well, the point is when you measure the mean single motor unit potential area, you get phase cancellation that normally occurs with the maximal CMAP waveform. What I suggested was that you get the 20% difference in the area because of phase cancellation. By averaging the arithmetic means of each motor unit amplitude area is 20% more than the averaged area because of a computerized averaging technique.

Sanjeev Nandedkar, Hawthorne, New York

I am going to go back to our discussion on amplitude. We have to keep in mind that all EMG amplifiers have a peak-to-peak noise of about 5 μV. Thus, individual responses less than the noise level are not acceptable. Perhaps responses less than 15–20 μV should be excluded to ensure a sufficiently high signal to noise ratio. Smaller signals can be extracted reliably using multiple trials to demonstrate reproducibility and with averaging. By averaging about 100 sweeps the noise level could be reduced by a factor or 10, to about 0.5 μV. Without stating it explicitly, we use this rule in sensory nerve conduction studies, and unless the signal has an amplitude greater than 10–15 μV, I find it hard to accept the value without averaging or showing two superimposing trials. In the multi channel decomposition methods, the noise includes background motor units that may have amplitudes in excess of 100 μV. If these signals are treated as noise, averaging 100 discharges would reduce the noise to only 10 μV. Therefore, I hesitate to accept motor units with an amplitude of less than 15–20 μV.

Richard Olney, San Francisco, California

My question is to Jasper; your suggestion of focusing on an amplitude for the data acquisition windows in the statistical technique is interesting. In referring to the 500 responses from ALS patients where you could see the different motor units separating from one another, there are obviously some gaps in the motor units. How are you going to account for them? I have concerns about a 10% window and a 0.5-mV response in ALS patients who have so few motor units; we always open up the window if there are more than 50% falling outside the window. There needs to be some way to account for different gaps in those recordings, and just having a 250-μV window is not always going to encompass that data.

Jasper Daube, Rochester, Minnesota

I agree. What I wanted to do is to raise the issue of using amplitude rather than percent as the criteria for our windows. You may have to look back at the initial scan for large steps that you can readily define. Those patients who had clear steps had surprisingly high amplitude, but that is a bit unusual and I selected those on purpose. I would like us to discuss first whether we should think about using amplitude rather than the percent that we are currently using.

Richard Olney, San Francisco, California

It seems like using amplitude could be very reasonable, but I would like to see more data before changing procedures.

Jasper Daube, Rochester, Minnesota

We are currently collecting more data on our patients, and we will need to make comparisons. It seems that there is an interest in this procedure.

Jeremy Shefner, Syracuse, New York

The whole issue of window size when you record multiple repetitions is an interesting one. If you recorded 5000 instead of 500 stimulus repetitions, you could go down to 0.5% window and get enough units to calculate a standard deviation. An important issue is the fact that you can get some variability and derive an estimate of an average SMUP amplitude, but that does not mean that the amplitude is a physiological truth. There are so many other things that happen. One question is, what would happen if you went the other way, if you did not use windows at all?

Jasper Daube, Rochester, Minnesota

In fact, that is exactly what we have done with 10 patients and 10 normal subjects. We have used no windows and we have used 5, 10, 15, and 20% windows. We have used cutoffs for standard deviation and tried to get rid of the noise. The data are preliminary and will be presented at a later time. For those people who are doing the statistical methods, the software for delivering 500 stimuli is available.

I hope we can agree that we should reject motor units below 10 μV amplitude or 25 μV ms area. Theoretically, there may be smaller units, but we have to decide where to stop, and I suggest 10 μV or 25 μV ms as the lower limit. Therefore, windows 0.5 or 0.25% make no sense. There probably are some in that window, but it is not worth looking at them.

Alan McComas, Hamilton, Ontario

I have two questions about the statistical technique. First, for those who use it, have you any explanation for the fact that MUNE values you obtain from control subjects for the thenar and hypothenar muscles are considerably lower than those from other MUNE techniques, and also lower than the anatomical data. Second, I had thought that in order for a Poisson analysis to be valid, that the unitary events had to be approximately the same size. That is the case if you are looking at packets of acetylcholine, but it is not the case if you are looking at motor unit potentials. If I am right, how are you dealing with this?

Jasper Daube, Rochester, Minnesota

That is correct. Poisson statistics is based on units that are the same size, but even acetylcholine quanta are not all the same size, and miniature endplate potentials in somebody who has the myasthenic syndrome are of different sizes. We have performed simulation studies, and if the values of the individual units have large differences in size, the Poisson distribution breaks down. That is why a number of people have talked about the skewness of the distribution of the data. If you get a skew to the wrong side or get a normal distribution, the mean values are less likely to be correct. This is an important question that has been addressed. Maybe Cathy should answer the question why their statistical technique MUNE values are low.

Catherine Lomen-Hoerth, San Francisco, California

In one study with the statistical technique, towards the end of the data acquisition run we turned up slightly the current to completely fill the 10% window, and our average MUNE value was approximately 60. When we left the current unchanged and filled only the lower quarter of the window our average value was 84. This is close to the anatomic report of 100 units innervating the abductor pollicis brevis muscle. We have achieved good separation between control and ALS subjects. In practical terms, since MUNE is an estimate, the important questions are how reproducible is the technique, how well does it separate normal from abnormal subjects, and can it be used to follow subjects over time.

Jasper Daube, Rochester, Minnesota

When we first selected our windows we used a smaller window in normal subjects and had MUNE values similar to those obtained by others. Other investigators have taken steps, that make sense, to address issues of the reproducibility, and may have different values.

Richard Olney, San Francisco, California

Let me supplement what Cathy said. We were successful with some of the variations we used to reduce the variance and improve reproducibility. These variations included minor adjustments of the stimulation current or "current forcing", studying multiple data acquisition levels, and not using the built-in calculation algorithm. I agree that current forcing is not technically preferable, and we have gotten away from it. The MUNE values from the statistical technique are still a bit lower than from other techniques. The weighting average method that Jeremy has introduced (Muscle Nerve, 1999, 22: 1457–1460) improves reproducibility and raises the MUNE values, but they still are not as high as those from the built-in calculation algorithm. I am not sure if I know all the factors. I do not know if the variability in the size of motor units within a recording window contributes to the lower number.

Mike, I recall you have data that estimate how much of an error is introduced by violating the assumption that all motor units are similar in size.

Michael Slawnych, Calgary, Alberta

Unfortunately, I cannot recall the data you mentioned. However, if you go back to the original papers of Katz and Meledi in 1954, there is a correction factor that can be used to help with this issue, at least to a first approximation. Cathy and I are currently writing a paper on the theory and practice of the statistical technique that will hopefully be a guide to help deal with these issues.

Richard Lewis, Detroit, Michigan

When I have tried the statistical technique, I do not get a feel for what the single motor unit potential is that ends up on the screen. It can be manipulated by the size of the window, which windows you use, and how many windows. So my question is, when you train people, did you ever have two or three different people do the same patient and see if they came up with the same numbers?

Jeremy Shefner, Syracuse, New York

In the creatine clinical trial several sites had more than one investigator certified to participate. When two investigators investigated the same patient twice, the values were very close. From my own experience, if you use the windows that are predefined, I think it is remarkable how reproducible the statistical technique is.

Richard Lewis, Detroit, Michigan

Is that opposite to what Rick is saying? That when they do not use the predefined windows, they get more reproducibility, or am I missing the point?

Richard Olney, San Francisco, California

For hypothenar muscles, we looked at reproducibility of the statistical technique, including taking electrodes off and reapplying them (Muscle Nerve, 2000, 23: 1525–1533). We found that what introduced the most variability was when the scan varied.

Richard Lewis, Detroit, Michigan

In the method that Rick and Cathy use, there are defined window sizes and percentages. If you use those in a normal subject, will you get very similar results with repeated testing?

Jeremy Shefner, Syracuse, New York

There are defined procedures for a normal subject, and you deviate only when certain assumptions are not met.

Jasper Daube, Rochester, Minnesota

I would like to just confirm that we have our technicians performing MUNE, and when they perform it in a fixed way, it is quite reproducible.

Let me shift the topic. Several people have talked about the importance of electrode placement, electrode orientation, and electrode size. Yet as I recall, Ken said it does not make any difference. Our experience has also been that it does not make any difference because whatever electrode you use to record the CMAP will be the same for the SMUP. We have seen no differences in motor unit number estimates with electrodes of different sizes and shapes and even shifting them off a little bit. If this is the case, why do we keep talking about the importance of the type and location of the electrode?

Ken Arasaki, Tokyo, Japan

You remembered what I said correctly, that the types or the widths or the placement of electrodes really did not matter. I did a reproducibility study using three different kinds of electrodes and two different systems, and only the system made a difference. The older system based on Mac Lab did not pick up the smaller single motor unit potentials, and MUNE values are heavily dependent upon the systems rather than on the recording electrodes.

Timothy Doherty, London, Ontario

I agree that theoretically it really should not matter if you have a wide-strip or small circular electrode. However, there may be a technical issue with MUNE techniques where you have lost the temporal relationship, such as the multiple point stimulation and the spike triggered averaging techniques. If you focus on negative peak areas as opposed to amplitudes and there is a poor signal to noise ratio, being able to find the onset of the potential is important. Positioning the electrode as close to the innervation or endplate zone of as many of the potentials as possible allows for a nicer takeoff to position the onset marker.

Joleen, Blok, Nijmegen, Netherlands

I agree that if the electrode is in about the same position, its size or shape does not really matter. Electrode positioning might make a difference when it is shifted to the side or towards or away from the tendons. For larger muscles, position should have a larger affect because the electrode can be further away from the endpoint region, while for smaller muscles, like the thenar muscles, electrode position is less of a factor.

Jasper Daube, Rochester, Minnesota

I would like to ask a different question. I have heard a variety of different approaches on how to define the term "reproducibility". It is difficult to compare reproducibility when different methods of calculation are used.

Carmel Armon, Loma Linda, California

I agree that using different methods to calculate reproducibility limits comparability. I would suggest that at least one method to calculate reproducibility be used in common. Then if people want to use additional methods, they should feel free to do so. I propose the following when you are comparing two MUNE estimates: measure 1 minus measure 2, divided by the mean of the measures, and take the absolute value. You can call it a variance if you want to translate to percentages, or you can call it percent variability. Taking the mean is the best estimate of the true value. Taking as the denominator the lower of the two measures would perhaps more conservative because it would set you up to show a greater degree of variance. Taking the larger of the two measures would tend to be more liberal in the sense that it would make you look a little better than what I think the mean would show.

I would also emphasize the need to clarify exactly the methodology used. Are you making two measures leaving the electrodes on or taking them off? Are you testing the same or different subjects? Even though data do not seem to show that electrode position matters, I still feel in general that it makes sense to standardize how things are done. Are you going to use an anatomic location that is going to be fixed no matter what happens to the muscle if it atrophies? Are you going to hunt for a maximal surface negativity over the maximal area? I think that does need to be standardized basically because I do not know whether it would make a difference or not.

Jasper Daube, Rochester, Minnesota

I wonder if we should try to put forward a consensus at the end of the weekend to define reproducibility.

Section IV

Voluntary MUNE Techniques

Motor Unit Number Estimation (Supplements to Clinical Neurophysiology Vol. 55)
Editor: M.B. Bromberg

Chapter 11

Spike triggered averaging MUNE technique

Mark B. Bromberg*

Department of Neurology, University of Utah, 50 North Medical Drive, Salt Lake City, UT 84132, USA

Introduction

The spike triggered averaging (STA) technique of motor unit estimation (MUNE) was initially described in a brief report by Nandedkar and Barkhaus (1987). It was more fully described, including applications to the study of amyotrophic lateral sclerosis (ALS) subjects, by Brown and colleagues in 1988 (Brown et al., 1988; Strong et al., 1988). Bromberg and colleagues explored the technique and its relationship to other electrophysiologic and strength measurements in normal and ALS subjects (Bromberg, 1993; Bromberg et al., 1993), and used STA as a secondary endpoint measure (Bromberg et al., 2001) in a small multicenter ALS drug trial (Tandan et al., 1996). STA has features and limitations that make it unique among MUNE techniques. This chapter will review the STA technique in detail, including technical issues and applications.

Methods

The STA technique is similar to other MUNE techniques in that it is based on the ratio of the maximal compound muscle action potential (CMAP) amplitude (or area) divided by the mean surface single motor unit potential (SMUP) amplitude (or area). It is also similar in that the CMAP is recorded using routine techniques with surface electrodes in a belly-tendon arrangement following electrical stimulation of the nerve supplying the muscle or group of muscles under study. STA differs operationally from other MUNE techniques in that SMUPs are obtained by identifying single motor units with an intramuscular needle electrode and recording their surface potential using STA. Another difference is that single motor units are activated by weak voluntary muscle contraction.

In practice, two amplifiers and several display channels are used (Fig. 1). The intramuscular electrode, through the first amplifier, records single motor units during weak voluntary activation (Fig. 2). Motor units are isolated, as in routine quantitative needle EMG studies, by adjusting the intramuscular electrode to record a short rise time. A voltage or window trigger level is set to capture the isolated motor unit potential. One display channel is set to continuous sweeps (free run mode) and the second display channel is used to observe the isolated single unit potential. The belly-tendon electrodes, through the second amplifier, record the surface signal. The surface signal undergoes triggered averaging using the single motor unit spike potential as the trigger. Another display

**Correspondence to*: Dr. M. Bromberg, Department of Neurology, University of Utah. Tel.: 801-581-6873. Fax: 801-585-2054.
e-mail: Mark.Bromberg@hsc.utah.edu

doi:10.1016/S1567-424X(03)00011-4

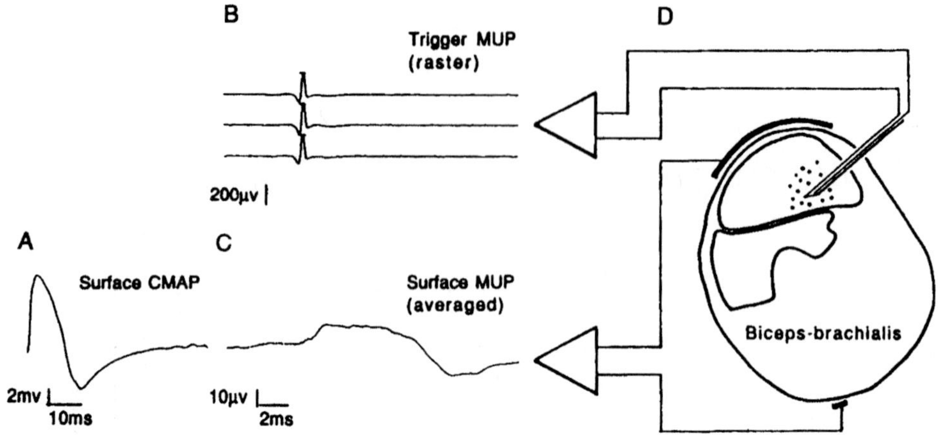

Fig. 1. Recording arrangement for spike triggered averaging MUNE in biceps-brachialis muscles. (A) CMAP following supramaximal stimulation of the musculocutaneous nerve. (B) Triggering motor unit action potentials shown in raster mode. (C) Averaged S-MUAP. (D) Cross section of muscles showing intramuscular trigger electrode, surface strip electrode, and reference electrode.

channel is used to observe the averaged surface potential. Approximately 100–200 surface potentials are averaged to achieve a clean SMUP.

Alternation

Most MUNE techniques activate SMUPs by electrical stimulation of the motor nerve. Overlap between axonal excitability curves leads to alternation between combinations of activated axons. Alternation can be a major issue in the identification of SMUPs in certain MUNE techniques (McComas et al., 1971; Brown and Milner-Brown, 1976). The STA technique, by activating motor units through voluntary contraction, avoids alternation.

Proximal and distal muscles

The STA technique can be readily applied to any muscle where a CMAP can be obtained, including many proximal muscles. Most MUNE techniques require a stable segment or suitable length of motor nerve for placement of stimulating electrodes to obtain SMUPs, which can be problematic for proximal muscles.

Intramuscular motor unit information

SMUPs are recorded from the surface of the muscle in all MUNE techniques, but surface recordings do not provide specific information about collateral reinnervation. A variety of intramuscular electrodes can be used in the STA technique, including concentric, monopolar, single fiber or macroEMG types. Accordingly, additional information about the pathophysiology of reinnervation can be obtained from the trigger potentials, including quantitative motor unit analysis, fiber density and macroEMG amplitude. With special software that can decompose a complex discharge pattern into several trigger potentials, the recruitment pattern and discharge rates of the different trigger potentials can be obtained.

Hardware and software availability

Several MUNE techniques require special software, or are facilitated by special software, that is frequently proprietary and available only on specific EMG machines. STA software and two amplifiers are relatively common features of EMG machines, making the STA technique widely available.

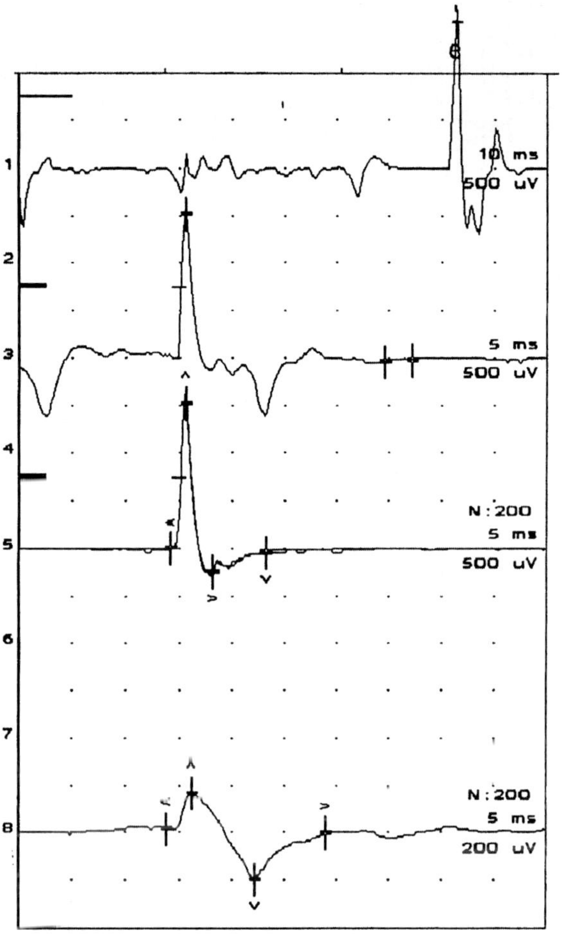

Fig. 2. EMG machine recording arrangement for displaying waveforms for spike triggered averaging MUNE technique. *First trace:* continuous run (free run) mode of intramuscular electrode data. *Second trace:* triggered intramuscular electrode data showing motor unit potential used to trigger averaging of surface potential. *Third trace:* averaged intramuscular motor unit potential. *Fourth trace:* averaged surface motor unit potential.

Motor unit sampling bias

All MUNE techniques have inherent SMUP sampling bias. The STA technique relies on voluntary muscle activation at low levels of contraction. This favors early recruited motor units and a bias toward small SMUPs based on the size principle of motor unit recruitment (Henneman et al., 1965; Milner-Brown et al., 1973). Bias towards small motor units can be reduced by two methods. A window discriminator for selecting the triggering motor unit allows for sampling a greater variety of recruited motor units (Brown et al., 1988). Software has been developed that decomposes a moderately full interference pattern into four to eight individual motor units can be used as triggers to extract corresponding SMUPs activated at higher recruitment efforts (see other chapters) (Stashuk, 1999). Bias towards small motor units will be less in denervating diseases such as ALS, because the order of motor neuron death is not based on size (Strong et al., 1988).

SMUP bias among different MUNE technique has been investigated. It is likely that for all MUNE techniques, bias may be less problematic than basic biophysics and physiology might suggest. Most other MUNE techniques rely on electrical stimulation of the motor nerve to activate SMUPs. Axon excitability is proportional to axon diameter, leading to possible bias toward large diameter axons in stimulation-based MUNE techniques. However, a bias toward larger axons has not been reported, and local factors that affect current flow, such as the geometry of the nerve and regional impedance, are more influential (McComas, 1991; Doherty and Brown, 1993). Direct comparisons of SMUPs obtained by STA, percutaneous nerve stimulation and microstimulation of intramuscular nerves in the same subjects were not significantly different (Stein and Yang, 1990). Another comparison of SMUPs from the STA and multiple point stimulation techniques showed high correlations between averaged SMUP values (Doherty and Brown, 1993).

Samples of 10–20 SMUPs represent 5–10% of the motor units in a normal muscle, and a greater percentage in denervated muscle. Efforts have been made to determine the distribution of SMUPs in normal and ALS subjects. In both normal and ALS subjects, the range of SMUP values is skewed toward smaller sized units (Bromberg and Abrams, 1995). The range is narrow for each group (within one order of magnitude), and median and mean values are similar (Fig. 3). Occasional outlying values are observed in normal and ALS subjects.

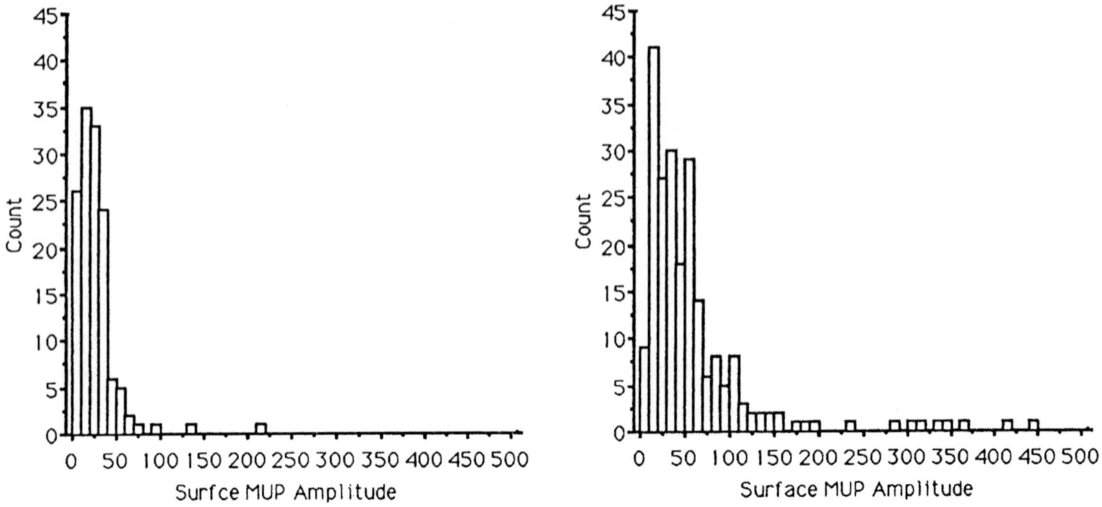

Fig. 3. Distributions of single surface motor unit potentials from normal subjects (left histogram) and subjects with ALS (right histogram). Motor unit potential amplitude in microvolts.

Subject cooperation

Active cooperation by the subject is not required with electrical stimulation MUNE techniques, although subjects must remain physically quiet. The STA technique requires subject cooperation for voluntary muscle contraction and motor unit isolation and concentration to keep a steady discharge rate during the averaging procedure.

Proximal CMAP waveforms

The accurate recording of CMAP waveforms from proximal muscles can be challenging. MUNE studies in proximal muscles may include one or more muscles, and the position of the stimulating electrode can influence how many muscles contribute to the CMAP (Galea et al., 2001). An example is stimulation of the musculocutaneous nerve in the axilla will activate the biceps brachii and brachialis muscles, while stimulation of the motor branch over the biceps brachii muscle is more selective and activates only the biceps brachii.

Current spread to other motor nerves in proximal segments of the arm can be problematic (Brown et al., 1988). This can lead to contamination of the CMAP by volume conduction from neighboring muscles (Fig. 4). Palpation of neighboring muscles and reports of paresthesias are helpful in identifying current spread to other nerves. Volume conducted components tend to occur later in the CMAP

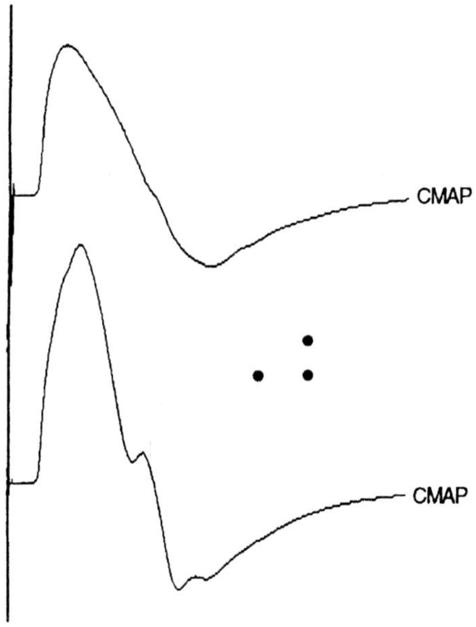

Fig. 4. Effects of volume conduction on biceps-brachialis CMAP amplitude and area. *Upper trace:* normal CMAP. *Lower trace:* inflated CMAP due to volume conduction, which will inflate negative area more than peak-to-peak values. Time: 5 ms/div, voltage: 5 mV/div (from Bromberg and Abrams, 1995).

TABLE 1

PERCENTAGE CHANGE IN AVERAGED SMUP AMPLITUDE WHEN DIFFERENT NUMBERS OF SPURIOUS POTENTIALS OF DIFFERENT RELATIVE AMPLITUDES ARE ADDED TO A RUNNING AVERAGE OF 200 POTENTIALS (FROM BROMBERG AND ABRAMS, 1995)

Relative amplitude of spurious signals	Number of spurious potentials added to the average		
	0.5% (1/200)	2.5% (5/200)	5% (10/200)
0.5	99.8	99	98
1	100	100	100
2	100.5	102	105
5	102	110	119
10	104	122	143
20	109	143	
30	114		

waveform and inflate the negative peak area and negative peak amplitude values more than peak-to-peak amplitude values. A consensus was reached during the Symposium in favor or using negative peak areas for MUNE calculations (see chapter on Consensus), but calculations based on peak-to-peak amplitude may be more accurate for MUNE determinations from proximal muscles.

Trigger potentials

STA relies on a consistent trigger potential. There are a number of situations where unwanted trigger potentials or changes in trigger potentials could affect the averaging process.

Spurious triggers

The occurrence of spurious trigger potentials leads to contamination of the averaged surface SMUP by waveforms from other motor units. Fasciculation potentials are examples of spurious trigger sources that may occur frequently in ALS subjects. Another example is inadvertent recruitment of other motor units that cross the trigger threshold and are included in the average.

The effect of a spurious trigger on the averaged surface waveform depends upon the frequency of occurrence and size of spurious motor units. The true size cannot be determined because there is no relationship between the size of the spurious trigger potential and the size of the whole motor unit. The effects of spurious potentials can be assessed in modeling studies (Bromberg and Abrams, 1995). In a model where 200 potentials were averaged, the effects of different numbers of smaller and larger spurious motor unit potentials has been determined (Table 1). Spurious potentials smaller than the primary potential have little effect on the average. However, spurious potentials larger than the primary potential can have an effect, and two to five potentials twice the size of the primary potential can artificially inflate the averaged SMUP value by 5–10%.

Although the true size of a spurious motor unit cannot be known, the range of spurious motor unit amplitudes can be assessed from the distribution of motor units within normal and ALS subjects (Fig. 3). The practical impact is likely to be low because the distributions of SMUP sizes in normal and ALS subjects largely overlap, with rare outlying values exceeding an order of magnitude above the mean value. However, during the acquisition of trigger potentials it is important to be vigilant, and the data acquisition run should be repeated if more than 5% of potentials are spurious.

Time shifts within the trigger potential

In subjects with denervation and reinnervation, motor unit potentials with long durations and

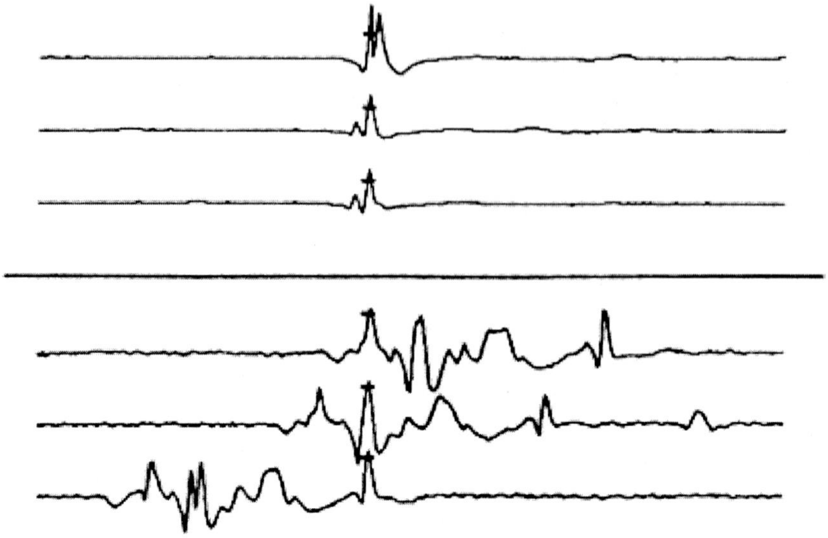

	Number of spurious potentials added to the average		
Trigger time shift	5% (10/200)	10% (20/200)	20% (40/200)
2 ms	99	97	95
4 ms	95	97	82

Fig. 5. Time shifts of the trigger point within the trigger potential due to amplitude changes of spike components within the trigger potential. *Top raster:* example of small temporal shift. *Bottom raster:* example of large temporal shift. Time: 2 ms/div, voltage: 20 μV/div. *Table:* Percent change in averaged SMUP amplitude when various numbers of trigger potentials with shifting trigger points are added to a simple running average of 200 potentials (from Bromberg and Abrams, 1995).

multiple phases may be used as the trigger. Small inadvertent movements of the intramuscular recording electrode may change the relative amplitudes of the phases used for triggering. When different motor unit components cross the trigger threshold the trigger potential may jump ahead or behind the trigger point (Fig. 5). When complex motor units are of long duration the jumps can exceed 5 ms, and these jumps will be associated with shifts of the surface potentials during the averaging process. Modeling of the effects of shifts indicates that occasional shifts less than 2 ms are acceptable (Bromberg and Abrams, 1995).

Component blocking

Another factor associated with ongoing denervation and reinnervation that may affect MUNE is neuromuscular blockade at newly reinnervated neuromuscular junctions (Stålberg, 1982). This process can be identified in the triggering potential as an unstable motor unit. Tenuous neuromuscular transmission results in variations (reductions) in the amplitude of the surface potentials contributing to the average. The frequency with which this happens and the magnitude of component drop out in ALS is not known (Carleton and Brown, 1979). The trigger potential represents only a small portion of the muscle fibers making up the motor unit (approximately 1/100) and blocking may be more wide spread in the whole motor unit than appreciated from observation of trigger potentials. The effects of blocking on CMAP amplitude as a decrement to repetitive stimulation can be appreciable (Wang et al., 2001). At discharge rates of 10–20 Hz, blocking at individual neuromuscular junction is observed in post synaptic defects in transmission (myasthenia gravis) (Trontelj and Stålberg, 1990), and similar effects are observed in SMUPs in ALS subjects (Chan et al., 1998). The overall effect of blocking in the STA technique will be smaller SUMP amplitudes, and data in Table 1 indicates that the inclusion of smaller amplitude potentials will have a negligible effect on MUNE values.

Motor unit depth

The depth of SMUPs within a muscle may affect the amplitude of the surface recorded potential due to tissue impedance. The effect is likely to be negligible in thin distal muscles, but could lead to an underestimate of the average SMUP size in thicker proximal muscles. The magnitude of attenuation has been investigated by comparing the depth of the triggering electrode with the amplitude of surface SMUPs. The results are inconclusive, with one study finding no relationship (Bromberg and Abrams, 1995), another study finding a non-significant trend (Brown et al., 1988), and one study finding significantly smaller surface SMUP amplitudes with deeper trigger motor units (Barkhaus and Nandedkar, 1994).

Number of SMUPs averaged

The number of SMUPs collected to obtain the average SMUP value for the MUNE calculation is an important variable. It has been customary with the STA technique to average 10–15 units (Brown et al., 1988), and no significant differences were found between MUNE values calculated from 15 compared to 25 motor units in both normal and ALS subjects (Bromberg, 1993). Similar studies in normal subjects have been performed for the multiple point stimulation technique with no substantial differences reported for sample sizes between 10 and 15 motor units recorded (Doherty and Brown, 1993). This suggests that the pool of motor units available for sampling is relatively homogeneous within a subject. This is supported by data on the distribution of SMUPs with in both normal and ALS subjects (Fig. 3) (Bromberg and Abrams, 1995).

Reproducibility

Test–retest reducibility of MUNE of the STA technique has been assessed in the biceps-brachialis muscle in both normal and ALS subjects (Bromberg, 1993). The range of MUNE values in ALS subjects were generally lower than in normal subjects, with only limited overlap. MUNE values separating normal from abnormal can be set as the lowest value in normal subjects (the lower limit of normal – LLN). Test–retest data are shown in Table 2. No significant differences were found between test and retest MUNE values for either group of subjects. The relative difference was calculated as the absolute difference between test and retest values divided by their mean value and expressed as a percentage. Relative differences were 45.3% for normal subjects and 32.6% for ALS subjects. When the full data points were plotted for normal subjects, an outlying point contributed to the high correlation coefficient of 0.86.

TABLE 2

TEST–RETEST REDUCIBILITY OF STA TECHNIQUE IN NORMAL AND ALS SUBJECTS

	Mean (SD)	Range	*P*-value	Relative difference	Correlation coefficient full (restricted) data
Normal subjects (10)					
Test	553 (380)	235–1580	0.72	45.3%	0.86 (0.07)
Retest	591 (481)	211–1816			
ALS subjects (15)					
Test	149 (87)	53– 354	0.27	32.6%	0.54 (0.65)
Retest	154 (69)	74– 298			

When test–retest data were restricted by removing the outlying point, the correlation coefficient was 0.07. When the full data points were plotted for the ALS subjects, the coefficient was 0.54. Less test–retest variability was observed when MUNE values were low, and when test–retest data were restricted to MUNE values below the lowest value from normal subjects (<235) the correlation coefficient rose to 0.65.

Factors that influence the MUNE value are the CMAP and average SMUP amplitudes. CMAP amplitude relative differences were 20.3% for normal subjects and 21.4% for ALS subjects, with no significant differences for either group. Test–retest SMUP amplitude values were not significantly different for either group. However, tests to determine if the test–retest samples were homogenous indicated inhomogeneity in 7 of 10 normal subjects but in only 2 of 15 ALS subjects. The frequency distribution of SMUP values shows larger values among ALS subjects (Fig. 3). Therefore, the greater homogeneity of SMUP samples among ALS subjects may be explained by the fact that with fewer SMUPs to choose from in ALS subjects it is more likely that the same ones will be chosen. This also explains the high test–retest correlation coefficients in ALS subjects when MUNE values are low (Table 2).

Another source of error in the STA technique is the variability of repeated averages of the same SMUP. This has been studied in a limited number of ALS subjects who had sufficiently stable trigger potentials that the averaging process could be repeated multiple times. The coefficient of variation was less than 10% for SMUPs (Bromberg, 1993).

Comparisons with other measures

MUNE represents the determinant of the number of motor units innervating a muscle. There are other measures that are important in assessing the physiologic state of a muscle, including the CMAP amplitude, fiber density, the motor unit (either in part with quantitative EMG or the whole with macroEMG), quantitative assessment of the interference pattern, and muscle force (Stålberg, 1982). The STA technique is unique in that it can assess many of these measures, and comparisons have been made between them in ALS subjects (Bromberg et al., 1993). Overall, correlations are poor between MUNE and other measures (Table 3). This is felt due to the fact that each measure reflects a different part of the physiologic state of the muscle due to denervation and reinnenration. Further, the effects of denervation and reinnervation in progressive disorders such as ALS are dynamic and change during the course of the disease (Stålberg, 1982). These data led to the conclusion that MUNE provides a unique measure, but a combination of measures will be necessary to fully

TABLE 3

CORRELATIONS BETWEEN MUNE VALUES AND OTHER ELECTROPHYSIOLOGIC MEASURES AND ISOMETRIC ELBOW FLEXION STRENGTH IN BICEPS-BRACHII MUSCLES IN ALS SUBJECTS (FROM BROMBERG ET AL., 1993).

	n	Correlation coefficient	
		r	*P*-value
CMAP amplitude	31	+0.61	0.0003
SMUP amplitude	31	−0.46	0.009
Fiber density	31	−0.40	0.02
Motor unit amplitude	31	−0.39	0.03
Isometric strength	31	+0.37	0.04
Motor unit recruitment	31	−0.36	0.05
Macro EMG amplitude	22	−0.29	0.20
Turns/amplitude ratio	28	−0.02	0.91

characterize changes within a muscle (Bromberg, 1998).

Summary

The STA technique has a number of unique features. These include applicability to perform MUNE in proximal muscles and the ability to collect intramuscular data on the process of collateral reinnervation. The development of decomposition algorithms will permit the acquisition of more data. As such, the STA technique provides the most complete physiological data on motor unit loss and reinnervation.

References

Barkhaus, P. and Nandedkar, S. Recording characteristics of the surface EMG electrodes. *Muscle Nerve*, 1994, 17: 1317–1323.

Bromberg, M. Motor unit estimation: reproducibility of the spike-triggered averaging technique in normal and ALS subjects. *Muscle Nerve*, 1993, 16: 466–471.

Bromberg, M. Electrodiagnostic studies in clinical trials for motor neuron disease. *J. Clin. Neurophysiol.*, 1998, 15: 117–128.

Bromberg M, and Abrams J. Sources of error in the spike-triggered averaging method of motor unit number estimation (MUNE). *Muscle Nerve*, 1995, October: 1139–1146.

Bromberg, M., Forshew, D., Nau, K., Bromberg, J., Simmons, Z. and Fries, T. Motor unit number estimation, isometric strength, and electromyographic measures in amyotrophic lateral sclerosis. *Muscle Nerve*, 1993, 16: 1213–1219.

Bromberg, M., Fries, T., Forshew, D. and Tandan, R. Electrophysiologic endpoint measures in a multi-center ALS drug trial. *J. Neurol. Sci.*, 2001, 184: 51–55.

Brown, W. and Milner-Brown, H. Some electrical properties of motor units and their effects on the methods of estimating motor unit numbers. *J. Neurol., Neurosurg. Psychiatry*, 1976, 39: 249–257.

Brown, W., Strong, M. and Snow, R. Methods for estimating numbers of motor units in biceps-brachialis muscles and losses of motor units with aging. *Muscle Nerve*, 1988, 11: 423–431.

Carleton, S. and Brown, W. Changes in motor unit populations in motor neurone disease. *J. Neurol. Neurosur. Psychiatry*, 1979, 42: 42–51.

Chan, K., Stashuk, D. and Brown, W. A longitudinal study of the pathophysiological changes in single human thenar motor units in amyotrophic lateral sclerosis. *Muscle Nerve*, 1998, 21: 1714–1723.

Doherty, T. and Brown, W. The estimated numbers and relative sizes of thenar units as selected by multiple point stimulation in young and older adults. *Muscle Nerve*, 1993, 16: 355–366.

Galea, V., Fehlings, D., Kirsch, S. and McComas, A. Depletion and sizes of motor units by spinal muscular atrophy. *Muscle Nerve*, 2001, 24: 1168–1172.

Henneman, E., Somjen, G. and Carpenter, D. Functional significance of cell size in spinal motoneurons. *J. Neurophysiol.*, 1965, 28: 560–580.

McComas, A. Invited review: motor unit estimation: methods, results, and present status. *Muscle Nerve*, 1991, 14: 585–597.

McComas, A., Fawcett, P., Campbell, M. and Sica, R. Electrophysiological estimation of the number of motor units within a human muscle. *J. Neurol. Neurosurg. Psychiatry*, 1971, 34: 121–131.

Milner-Brown, H., Stein, R. and Yemm, R. The orderly recruitment of human motor units during voluntary isometric contractions. *J. Physiol.*, 1973, 230: 359–370.

Nandedkar S., and Barkhaus P. Estimation of the number of motor units in human muscle. *Proc. 9th IEEE, Eng. Med. Biol. Soc* Boston, 1987.

Stashuk, D. Decomposition and quantitative analysis of clinical electromyographic signals. *Med. Eng. Phys.*, 1999, 21: 389–404.

Stålberg, E. *Electrophysiological studies of reinnervation in ALS.* Raven Press, New York, 1982.

Stein, R. and Yang, J. Methods for estimating the number of motor units in human muscles. *Ann. Neurol.*, 1990, 28: 487–495.

Strong M., Brown W., Hudson A., and Snow R. Motor unit estimates in the Biceps-brachialis in amyotrophic lateral sclerosis. *Muscle Nerve*, 1988, May: 415–422.

Tandan, R., Bromberg, M., Forshew, D., Fries, T., Badger, G. and Carpenter, J. et al. A controlled trial of amino acid therapy in amyotrophic lateral sclerosis: I. Clinical, functional, and maximum isometric torque data. *Neurology*, 1996, 47: 1220–1226.

Trontelj, J. and Stålberg, E. Single motor end-plates in myasthenia gravis and LEMS at different firing rates. *Muscle Nerve*, 1990, 14: 226–232.

Wang, F., De Pasqua, V., Gérard, P. and Dewaide, P. Prognostic value of decremental responses to repetitive nerve stimulation in ALS patients. *Neurology*, 2001, 57: 897–899.

Motor Unit Number Estimation (Supplements to Clinical Neurophysiology Vol. 55)
Editor: M.B. Bromberg

Chapter 12

MUNE using decomposition-enhanced spike-triggered averaging

Daniel W. Stashuk[a,*], Timothy J. Doherty[b] and William F. Brown[c]

[a]*Department of Systems Design Engineering, University of Waterloo, Waterloo, ON N2L 3G1, Canada*
[b]*Department of Physical Medicine and Rehabilitation, University of Western Ontario, London, ON, Canada*
[c]*Department of Neurology, Tuft's University, Boston, MA, USA*

Introduction

The ability to readily obtain an estimate of the number of motor units (MUs) in a muscle or muscle group can provide important information regarding the severity, course and responsiveness to treatment of many inherited or acquired neuropathies and neuronopathies. The usefulness of this information is directly related to the ease with which it can be obtained and the magnitude of the inherent variability of the estimation technique. Several techniques have been developed for obtaining a motor unit number estimate (MUNE). Some of the more established techniques include, incremental stimulation (IS), multiple point stimulation (MPS), the statistical and spike-triggered averaging (STA) techniques. Each technique has specific advantages and disadvantages with respect to how, when and where it should be used (Doherty et al, 1995; Doherty and Brown, 2002; Shefner, 2001). Unfortunately, not all of the developed techniques are available on any one clinical EMG machine, and it is not currently possible to easily select and apply the most appropriate technique in a specific situation. Instead, a given EMG lab will tend to consistently use just one or two of the available techniques.

All available MUNE techniques are based on the same underlying premise. The electrical response of a muscle to the stimulation of its motor nerve, detected using overlying surface electrodes, is called a compound muscle action potential (CMAP) or M-wave. The CMAP represents the activity of all MUs of a muscle whose axons were excited by the stimulus. If the stimulus is supramaximal, the resultant maximal CMAP represents the concurrent electrical activity of all of a muscle's MUs. The electrical activity of an average sized MU can be represented by a mean surface-detected MU potential (mS-MUP). The mS-MUP can be determined by averaging over a representative sample of S-MUPs. An estimate of the number of MUs in a muscle can be obtained by dividing the value of a size-related parameter of the maximum CMAP by the corresponding value for the mS-MUP. A size-related parameter may be the peak-to-peak voltage (PPAmp), negative peak voltage (NPAmp) or the negative peak area (NPArea). For the estimate to be valid, the maximal CMAP and the sample of S-MUPs used to calculate the mS-MUP must have been detected using the same electrode

**Correspondence to*: Dr. Dan W. Stashuk, Department of Systems Design Engineering, University of Waterloo, Waterloo, ON N2L 3G1, Canada.
Tel.: (519) 888-4567x2982, Fax: (519) 746-4791.
e-mail: stashuk@pami.uwaterloo.ca

doi: 10.1016/S1567-424X(03)00012-6

configuration. In addition, the MUs sampled to calculate the mS-MUP must be representative of the muscle's MU population (Doherty et al., 1995; Doherty and Brown, 2002).

Given this common premise, all current MUNE techniques have a common method for acquiring the CMAP and a common method for calculating the MUNE by dividing size-related parameters of the CMAP (PPAmp, NPAmp or NPArea) by the corresponding mS-MUP parameter value. What separates the various techniques is how they calculate or estimate the mS-MUP and how well the mS-MUP represents the population of S-MUPs that contributed to the maximal CMAP. This chapter describes modifications to the existing STA technique to use the results of the decomposition of a needle-detected EMG signal as a source of spike-triggers for averaging. Preliminary results using the decomposition-enhanced STA (DE-STA) technique are presented and the advantages and disadvantages of the new technique are discussed.

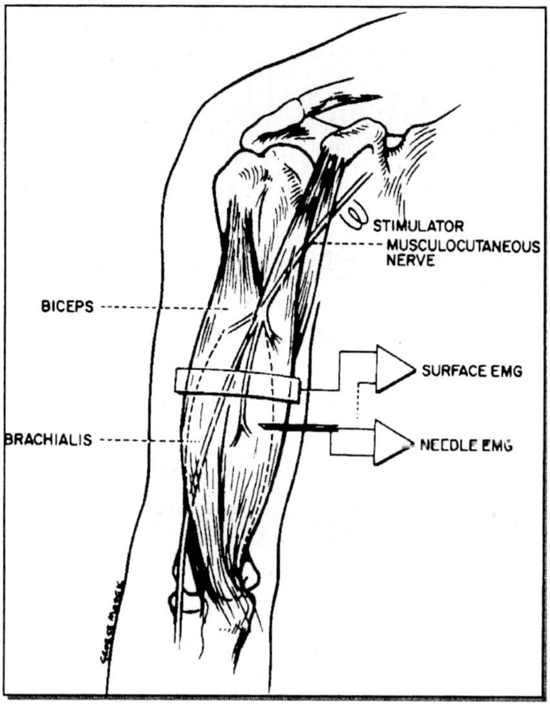

Fig. 1. The conceptual configuration for the surface and intra-muscular detection electrodes for acquiring appropriate EMG signals from the biceps muscles for obtaining a STA-based MUNE is shown schematically (from Brown et al., 1988).

Conventional STA

The goal of STA in MUNE is to acquire a set of S-MUPS that represent the population of S-MUPs that contributed to the maximal CMAP for the estimation of a mS-MUP. During conventional STA, signals are simultaneously detected from the same surface electrodes used for collecting the CMAP and from a selective intramuscular electrode, such as a concentric or monopolar needle (Fig. 1). At the top of Fig. 2, portions of EMG signals simultaneously detected using surface and needle electrodes are shown. Based on volume conduction theory (Malmivuo, 1995), the voltage contributions of a specific MU will be detected virtually simultaneously by the surface and intramuscular electrodes. The selective intramuscular signal is used to determine when a specific MU is active by detecting the occurrence of its MUPs. Isolation of a specific MU is achieved using an adjustable level or window threshold. When using a level threshold, the occurrence of a MUP is detected when its amplitude exceeds an adjustable threshold voltage. When using a window threshold, as shown in the middle of Fig. 2, the width of the window is set by upper and lower voltage levels. A MUP is then detected if its amplitude is above the lower limit but not above the upper limit. The times at which MUPs of a specific MU are detected are used as triggers to select appropriately time-aligned sections of the surface-detected EMG signal (S-EMG). The selected S-EMG sections are then averaged. The averaging is not done along an individual section but rather across the ensemble of selected, trigger-aligned sections. The resulting spike-triggered average, shown at the bottom of Fig. 2, along with an average MUP detected by the intramuscular electrode represents an estimate of the specific MU's S-MUP. Assuming that each MUs is active independently of the other MUs (i.e. there is no synchronization of MU activity), contributions from other MUs to each of the selected sections will, across the ensemble averaging, cancel out and tend to have a net zero contribution to the resulting S-MUP estimate. The intramuscular electrode can be moved to another

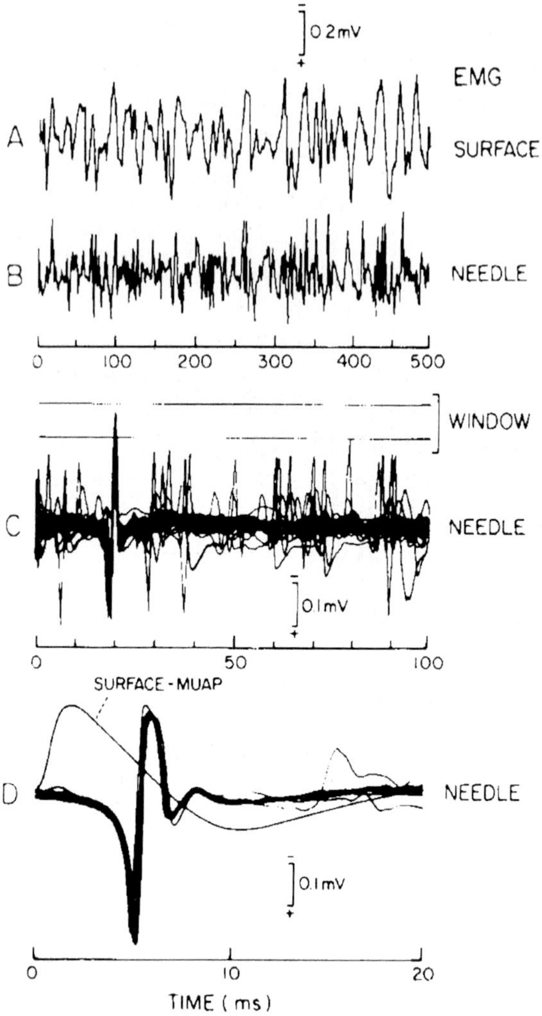

Fig. 2. The relationships between surface and needle detected EMG signals are shown along with superimposed, window-triggered, needle-detected MUPs and the resulting ensemble averaged S-MUP and needle-detected MUP.

position or the level of contraction can be adjusted to select the activity of another MU and its S-MUP estimated. This process is repeated until the requisite number of S-MUPs is acquired (15–20) to calculate a representative mS-MUP.

Decomposition-enhanced STA

The goal of DE-STA with respect to obtaining a MUNE is the same as conventional STA, which is, to acquire a set of S-MUPS that represent the population of S-MUPS that contributed to the maximal CMAP for the estimation of a mS-MUP. During DE-STA, EMG signals are also simultaneously detected using the same surface electrodes used for collecting the CMAP as well as a selective electrode as depicted in Fig. 1. However, the EMG signal from the selective electrode, is decomposed to determine when the specific MUs that made significant contributions to the acquired EMG signal were active. This is accomplished by detecting the occurrence of MUPs in the acquired signal and by classifying each of the detected MUPs as being created by one specific MU. EMG signal decomposition is achieved by a series of signal processing and pattern recognition algorithms. The detected and classified MUPs of a certain MU constitute a MUP train (MUPT) and, as with conventional STA, can be used as triggers to ensemble average suitably selected sections of the corresponding S-EMG signal to estimate a S-MUP for that MU. However, following decomposition, an S-MUP can be estimated for each of the significantly contributing MUs. As with conventional STA, the quality of an estimated S-MUP depends on the amount of interfering activity from other MUs (i.e. the complexity of the S-EMG signals) and on the number of MUPs of its MU that were detected and correctly classified (i.e. the number of correct triggers). EMG signal decomposition allows several (3–10) S-MUPs to be estimated from the EMG signals detected during one contraction. This greatly simplifies and expedites the collection of a suitably sized (10–15) sample of S-MUPs. Typically, depending on the level of contraction and muscle studied, only four to six contractions are required to obtain a suitable MUNE.

Obtaining a MUNE using decomposition-enhanced STA

To obtain a MUNE using EMG signal decomposition techniques the following steps need to be completed:

1. Obtain a maximal CMAP using an active surface electrode positioned over the motor point of the muscle of interest.

2. Using the same surface electrode location and configuration, collect a series of surface and intramuscularly-detected EMG signals during a series of moderate muscle contractions. Before each muscle contraction, re-position the intramuscular electrode to detect the activity of a different set of MUs.
3. Decompose each intramuscularly-detected EMG signal into its MUPTs, the MUPs of which serve as temporal markers for subsequent ensemble averaging of S-MUPs with STA.
4. Once a set of at least 20 S-MUPs have been obtained, align each S-MUP using its negative peak onset and calculate a mS-MUP waveform.
5. Divide the area or PPAmp of the maximal CMAP by the corresponding value of the mS-MUP.

Concepts of EMG signal decomposition

EMG signal decomposition, as depicted in Fig. 3, refers to the separation of a composite signal into its constituent MUPTs. The resolution of a composite EMG signal into its significant, constituent MUPTs requires the ability to detect the discharges (i.e. MUPs) of the MUs significantly contributing to the composite signal and to correctly associate each detected MUP with the MU that created it. EMG signal decomposition therefore involves the two basic steps of detecting MUPs and recognising detected MUPs.

To identify the occurrences of MUPs within a composite signal or to segment the composite signal into portions that contain significant MUPs, common characteristics of MUP shapes, which differentiate them from background signal noise, are used. Criteria to recognise detected MUPs, are that the MUPs produced by the same MU be more similar in shape than MUPs produced by different MUs, that differences in MUP shapes can be measured, and that the distribution of the shapes of the MUPs of each active MU can be characterised. The inherent variability of the MUPs produced by a single MU and the inherent difference between the MUPs of different MUs will depend on aspects of muscle physiology and on the type of electrodes used to detect the EMG signal. The features used to represent MUPs and the similarity measures used to compare MUPs affect the resolution with which differences in MUP shapes can be determined. To characterise and consider the distributions of shapes of MUPs of different

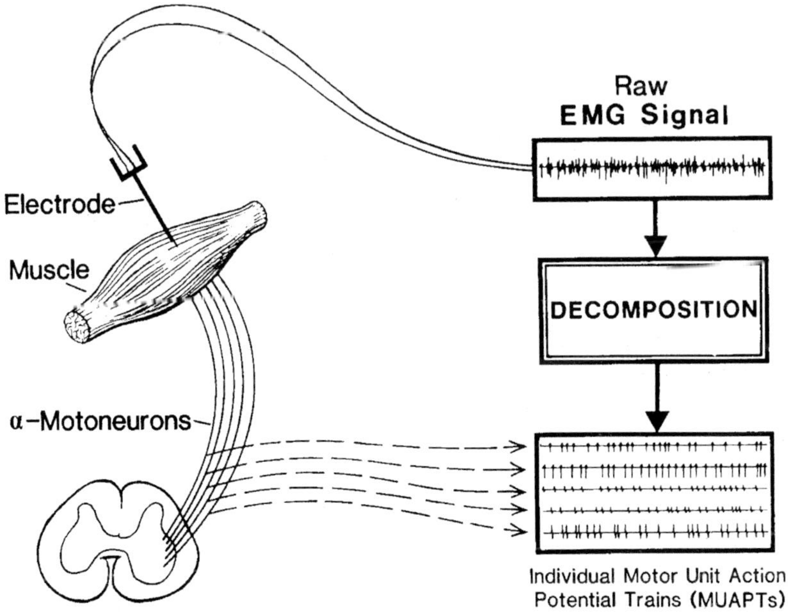

Fig. 3. The concept of EMG signal decomposition are schematically depicted (from DeLuca and Basmajian, 1985).

MUs requires the use of both clustering and supervised classification techniques. Furthermore, MUPs from several MUs can overlap in time or superimpose and therefore their superimposed waveforms may need to be resolved. Finally, because resulting candidate MUPTs represent the activity of MUs, information based on their temporal pattern is also useful.

Successful EMG signal decomposition can therefore involve the following steps: (1) MUP detection or signal segmentation; (2) MUP representation; (3) MUP clustering; (4) supervised MUP classification; (5) resolution of superimposed MUPs; and (6) the discovery of temporal relationships between MUPTs. The specific aspects of each of these steps will not be discussed here. Refer to Stashuk (2001) for a review of EMG signals decomposition techniques and further details. The result of a successful EMG signal decomposition is a group of MUPTs, each of which can be used as a source of triggers for the STA estimation of the S-MUP of a MU that was contributing significant MUPs to the EMG signal decomposed.

Methods

As an initial pilot study a series of MUNEs for the median innervated thenar muscles were obtained using DE-STA from a population of nine normal subjects. Self-adhering, commercially available surface electrodes, cut in strips approximately 1×3 cm were used for detecting S-EMG signals. The active electrode was positioned transversely, in as close proximity to the innervation zone of as many of the median innervated thenar MUs as possible. The reference electrode was located over the metacarpal phalangeal joint of the thumb. A metal plate, positioned over the back of the hand, served as a ground. With the electrodes in this position, S-MUPs voluntarily or electrically evoked are usually simple, bi-phasic, negative–positive potentials and the maximum M-potential has a corresponding initial negative deflection. The thumb was immobilised by tape, to the side of the hand to minimise movement artefact and to facilitate consistent force production during contractions. At the outset of a study, single, supramaximal stimuli were delivered to the median nerve at the wrist and the position of the "active" electrode was adjusted to maximise the NPAmp and minimise the rise time of the maximum M-potential. Following the collection of the maximum M-potential and without moving the surface electrodes, a SEMG signal was detected during a series of three, successive, 1–2 s long, maximal voluntary contractions (MVCs) separated by approximately 2–3 s of rest. This MVC SEMG signal was processed to determine its maximum root mean square (RMS) value over a 1 s interval. The MVC-RMS was then used to gauge the level of subsequent contractions, as the percentage of MVC-RMS of the RMS of the SEMG signal detected during the subsequent contraction. A concentric needle (CN) electrode was then inserted into the thenar eminence and during slight voluntary contraction positioned to detect MUPs with minimal rise times. The subject was then requested to slowly and as isometrically as possible increase the level of contraction until a moderate to full interference pattern was detected. This contraction was maintained for 30 s while the CN and SEMG signals were collected. CN EMG signals were acquired with a band-width of 10 Hz to 10 kHz and a sampling rate of 31.25 kHz. SEMG signals were acquired with a band-width of 5 Hz to 5 kHz and a sampling rate of 3.125 kHz. The collected CN signal was then decomposed using algorithms developed by Stashuk (1999). Each MUPT obtained following the decomposition of the CN EMG signal was then used as a source for triggers for spike triggered averaging the collected SEMG signal and estimating a S-MUP. The needle was then repositioned in the muscle in an effort to acquire a different set of MUs, and another set of CN and surface EMG signals were detected while the subject voluntarily produced a suitable muscle contraction. Three to five contractions were usually required in order to obtain a S-MUP from 20 or more MUs. The level of contraction typically ranged from 3 to 30% MVC-RMS. Each of the S-MUPs were aligned using the negative peak onset and a mS-MUP was calculated across the ensemble of S-MUPs. A MUNE was then calculated by dividing the negative peak voltage or area of the maximum M-potential by the corresponding negative peak voltage or area of the mS-MUP.

Repeatability of the mS-MUP

In an effort to assess the variability in the set of S-MUPs selected to calculate an mS-MUP, needle and surface EMG signals were collected, as described above, during a relatively large series (21–27) of slight and moderate level contractions for each of four subjects. For each of the four subjects, six different subsets of four to seven contractions were chosen from the total set of contractions for a given subject for analysis. The EMG signals acquired during each subset of contractions provided in total approximately 25–32 S-MUPs. The S-MUPs provided by each subset of contractions were then aligned and averaged to create an mS-MUP and MUNE for each subject. Only one CMAP was acquired and the electrodes were not moved between contractions. The level of contractions and the amount of time between contractions were controlled in an effort to minimise fatigue. The coefficient of variation of the MUNEs across the six different sets of contractions for each of the four subjects was then calculated.

Results

Figure 4 shows the results of the decomposition of a CN EMG signal obtained during an 8% MVC-RMS contraction. The decomposition algorithms determined that 5 MUs were significantly contributing to the CN EMG signal. The typical shape of the CN-detected MUP for each MU is displayed in the first column. The second column displays, for each MU, the superposition of its MUPs as detected by the algorithms. The interfering activity of other MUs can be clearly seen in these shimmer plots. The third column displays the estimated S-MUP for each MU and the number of triggers used. The fourth and fifth columns present the firing patterns of the MU as an inter-discharge interval histogram and as individual firing times or instantaneous firing rates, respectively. Figure 5 displays the S-MUPs estimated using the decomposition results shown in Fig. 4, and are the same waveforms displayed in the third column of Fig. 4. Residual baseline noise can be clearly seen in the S-MUPs, even after hundred of averages. This is a consequence of attempting to extract the S-MUP for a single MU from a complex S-EMG signal detected during a contraction created by the activity of a large number of MUs.

Table 1 presents the pilot MUNE data. On average, it took six (range 5–8) contractions (range 3.8–14.7) to obtain a S-MUP from 30 MUs (range 20–34) for an average of five S-MUPs per contraction (range 2.5–6.8). The contraction strengths ranged from 3.8 to 14.7 (mean 8%) RMS MVC. Based on the 11 MUNEs obtained, the average value using NPAmp was 172, with a range of 89–266, a standard deviation of 45.0 and a coefficient of variation of 0.29. The average MUNE value using NPArea was 189, with a range of 108–319, a standard deviation of 64.8 and a coefficient of variation of 0.34.

The results of the repeatability study are shown in Table 2. The total number of contractions for each individual ranged from 21 to 27, with the total number of S-MUPs obtained ranged from 109 to 142. The number of S-MUPs per contraction ranged from 4.6 to 5.7 and the average level of contraction ranged from 7.0 to 15.5% MVC-RMS. Considering the six subsets of contractions chosen to select a suitable number of S-MUPs, from 4.0 to 6.3 contractions were on average selected, yielding on average between 25.7 and 32.7 S-MUPs. The coefficient of variation across the six MUNEs obtained using negative peak voltage ranged from 0.034 to 0.353 and had an average value of 0.143.

Discussion

Decomposition-enhanced STA versus conventional STA

Conventional STA has been used to obtain MUNEs from the biceps brachii and brachialis

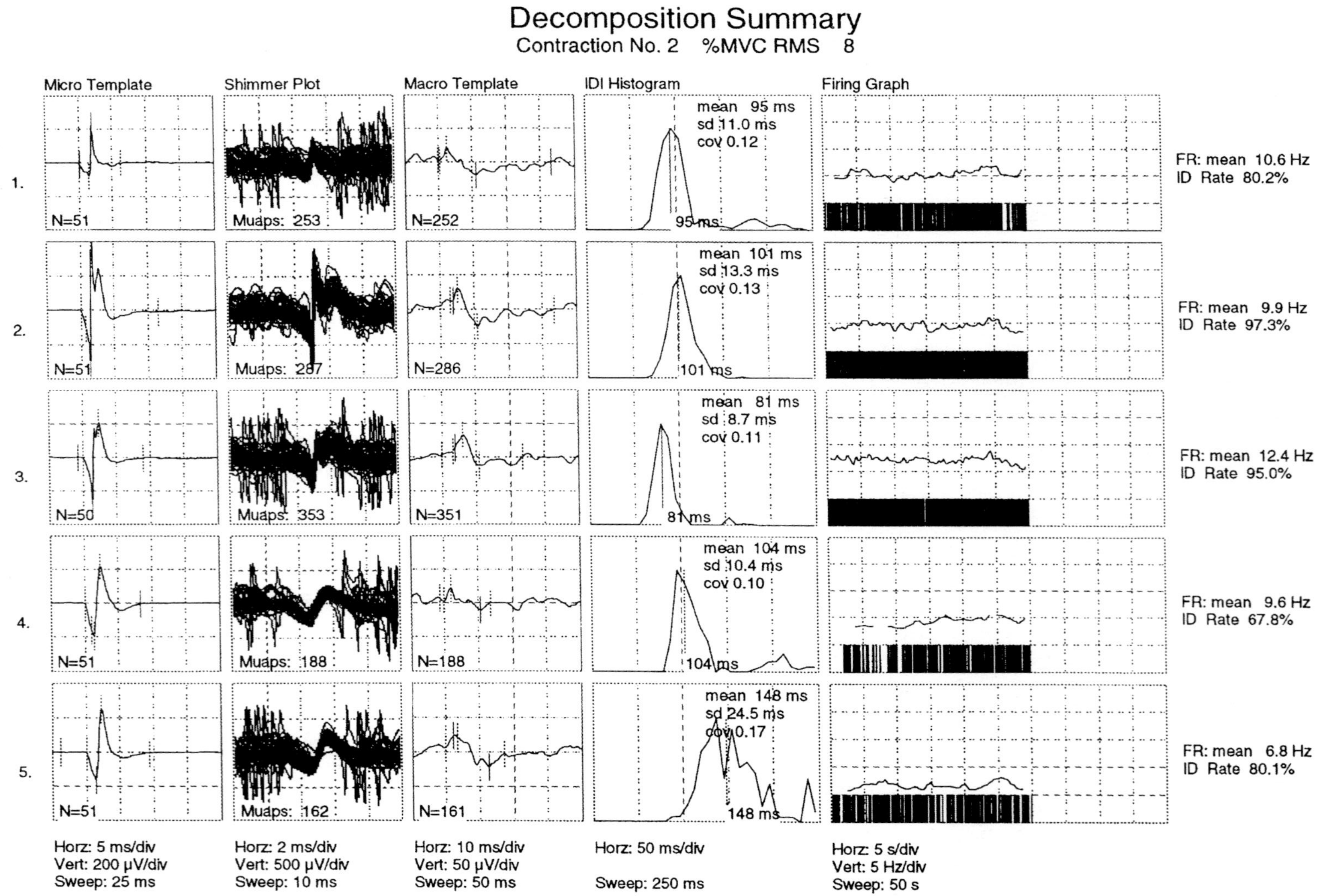

Fig. 4. Typical results of the decomposition of a CN-detected EMG signal are displayed along with the resulting S-MUPs (column 3) obtained from STA of a simultaneously detected surface EMG signal. The signals were detected during a 30 s contraction at an 8% MVC-RMS level of force. See text for further details.

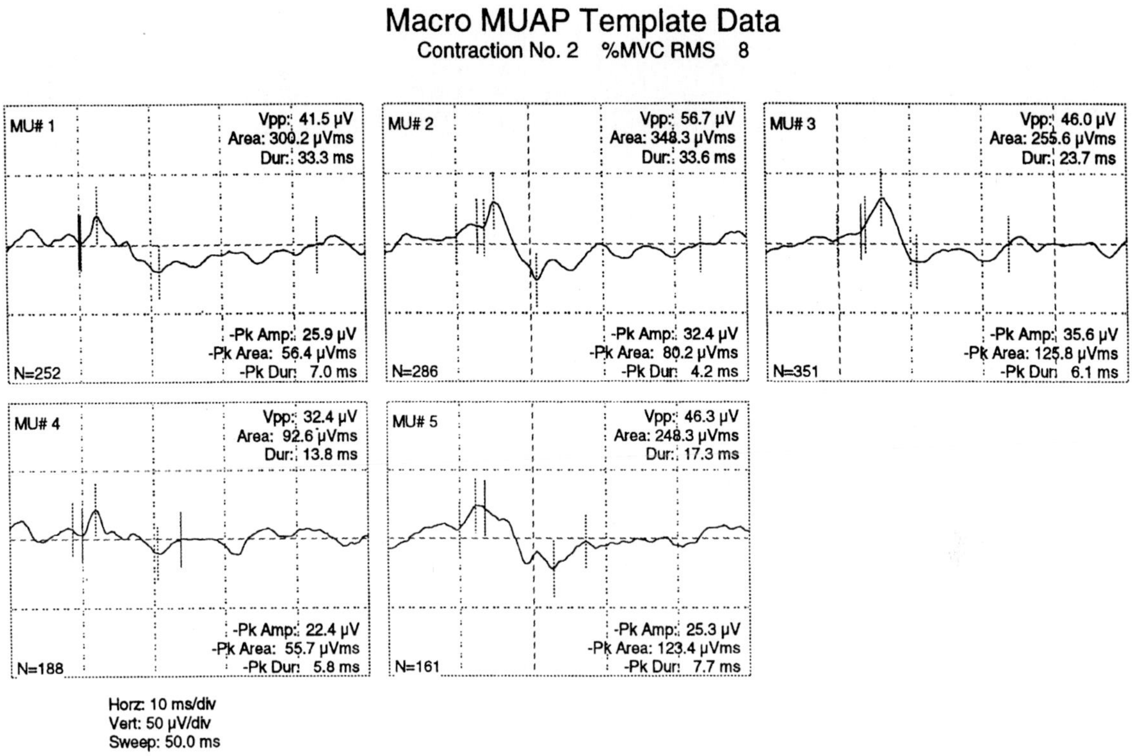

Fig. 5. The five S-MUPs calculated using the decomposition results shown in Fig. 4.

TABLE 1

DE-STA BASED MUNE FOR INNERVATED THENAR MUSCLES OF NORMAL SUBJECTS

Subject	Number of contractions	Number of S-MUPs	S-MUPs per contraction	AVG %MVC-RMS	MUNE V_{pp}	MUNE NPAmp	MUNE NPArea
RL	5	27	5.4	11.4	274	266	319
MO	7	31	4.4	6.5	135	177	148
MF	5	26	5.2	3.8	151	192	161
AHW	7	42	6.0	6.0	132	155	183
TD	5	34	6.8	5.7	176	190	299
YM	6	22	3.7	9.5	140	138	156
DS	8	20	2.5	4.0	142	186	189
AHW1	6	31	5.2	4.6	181	184	191
DWSL1	7	34	4.9	8.5	166	182	186
DWSR1	6	29	4.8	14.7	105	129	136
RTR1	7	34	4.9	9.0		89	108
Averages	6.3	30.7	5.0	7.6	160	172	189
STD	1.0	5.6	1.1	3.4	45.9	45.0	64.8
COV %	16.1	18.2	21.1	44.4	28.7	26.2	34.3

muscles (Brown et al., 1988) as well as from the thenar muscles (Stein and Yang, 1990; Doherty, 1993) and the tibialis anterior muscle (DeKoning et al., 1988). The preliminary results from thenar muscles from nine subjects using DE-STA (MUNE 160 ± 46 using V_{pp}; 189 ± 65 using NPArea) are very similar to those obtained using conventional STA as previously reported by Stein and Yang (1990)

TABLE 2

REPEATABILITY OF THE SET OF S-MUPs CHOSEN TO REPRESENT THE POPULATION OF S-MUPs CONTRIBUTING TO THE CMAP

Subject	Total				Average of six S-MUP sample sets					
	Number of contractions	Number of S-MUPs	S-MUPs per contraction	Average %MVC	Number of contractions	Number of S-MUPs	Average MUNE		MUNE COV %	
							Neg peak voltage	Neg peak area	Neg peak voltage	Neg peak area
AHW	25	142	5.7	7.0	4.0	25.7	178.8	186.3	3.4	6.0
DWSL	27	124	4.6	15.5	5.3	26.0	124.0	150.2	7.8	12.2
DWSR	21	109	5.2	15.2	5.7	29.2	152.5	183.3	10.8	12.9
RTR	24	120	5.0	12.0	6.3	32.7	90.7	101.2	35.3	23.9
							AVG COV %	14.3	13.7	

(MUNE 135 ± 27 using V_{pp}) and Doherty (1993) (160 ± 78 using V_{pp}; 204 ± 100 using NPArea). Conceptually, conventional STA and DE-STA are very similar. They both rely on the fact that a surface and needle electrode detect voltage contributions from the same MUs essentially simultaneously and that the activity of individual MUs is essentially independent. This allows isolated MU contributions detected by the needle electrode to be used to estimate the contributions of that MU to the SEMG signal by ensemble averaging of suitably aligned SEMG signal sections. Nonetheless, each technique has some unique advantages and disadvantages.

Some of the advantages of conventional STA are:

1) There is no alternation and it is well tolerated by both the subject and the operator.
2) It can be applied to proximal and distal muscles and to muscles that are not appropriate for the IS, MPS or F-wave techniques (e.g. biceps brachii and anterolateral compartment muscles of the lower leg).
3) The contraction and averaging can continue until a S-MUP with a suitable signal to noise ratio can be obtained.
4) The interference and possible synchronisation effects caused by other MU activity is small.

Some of the disadvantages of conventional STA are:

1) It requires the use of needle electrodes.
2) The patient must cooperate by maintaining a specific steady contraction and the operator must carefully maintain the needle position during signal collection.
3) One contraction has to be performed for each S-MUP obtained (15–20), which greatly affects the time required to obtain a MUNE.
4) It is not possible to review the consistency or accuracy with which the triggers used actually represent the activity of only one specific MU.
5) In order to confidently track the activity of a single specific MU, the level of contraction must be low (this is less so when using a window threshold) and there is a possible bias toward sampling low-recruitment threshold MUs (the extent of this may change from muscle to muscle).
6) Accurate measurement of S-MUP NPArea may be difficult because of difficulties in establishing the precise onset and baseline of the S-MUP.
7) It is possible that the same MU can be sampled during subsequent contractions.

Some of the advantages of DE-STA include:

1) There is no alternation and it is well tolerated by both the subject and the operator.
2) It can be applied to proximal and distal muscles and to muscles that are not appropriate for the IS, MPS or F-wave techniques (e.g. biceps brachii and anterolateral compartment muscles of the lower leg).
3) Less operator skill and subject cooperation are required compared to conventional STA.
4) Multiple S-MUPs can be obtained from one contraction and therefore fewer contractions are required than for conventional STA.
5) The consistency and accuracy of the MUPs used as triggers for each S-MUP can be reviewed.
6) The level of contraction during EMG signal acquisition can be greater than during conventional STA and therefore larger MUs with higher recruitment thresholds can be studied.
7) It can be confirmed that each S-MUP obtained from a single contraction was created by a unique MU.
8) Other, potentially important, neurophysiological information can be obtained from the results of the EMG signal decomposition.

Some of the disadvantages of DE-STA include:

1) EMG signal decomposition requires specialised algorithms that are currently not widely available.
2) Extracting the activity of one MU from an EMG signal contributed to by many MUs often results in S-MUPs where the activity of other MUs is not sufficiently reduced, possibly due to some degree of synchronisation between MUs, this in turn produces S-MUPs with poor signal to noise ratios (SNRs).

3) Poorly defined or noisy S-MUPs require various degrees of operator interpretation for the determination of S-MUP landmarks (onset, end, positive and negative peak) for the characterisation of S-MUPs in general and specifically, for their alignment for the calculation of the mS-MUP.
4) The need for operator interpretation can lead to greater MUNE variability.
5) To improve the SNR of S-MUP estimates requires the collection of EMG signals during lower levels of contraction or the maintenance of contractions for relatively long periods of time (30–60 s), which may result in some fatigue.
6) It may, relative to conventional STA, be biased to larger S-MUPs and therefore lower MUNEs, or in an absolute sense it may be biased to smaller S-MUPs and therefore larger MUNEs because only relatively low-level contractions are performed during signal detection.
7) The sets of S-MUPS sampled during different levels of contraction may contain different degrees of bias with respect to representing MUs of different recruitment threshold.

Accuracy and reproducibility

The two primary factors that affect the accuracy of a MUNE are the maximal CMAP and the mS-MUP. The factors that affect the maximal CMAP can be well controlled with careful placement of the surface detection and stimulating electrodes. The factors that affect the mS-MUP are more varied and harder to control. The most important factor is how well the sample of S-MUPs used to calculate the mS-MUP represents the population of S-MUPS that contributed to the maximal CMAP. A second, almost equally important factor is how are the sampled S-MUPs processed to estimate the mS-MUP.

Therefore, one of the more important questions with regard to any technique for obtaining a MUNE is whether the S-MUP sample is biased. As first put forward by Henneman and Mendell (1981), it is well established that a size principle exists with regard to the recruitment of MUs such that smaller MUs are recruited at lower levels of force than are larger MUs. Therefore, with regard to STA techniques, it is reasonable to ask if larger S-MUPs are consistently collected during higher-level contractions. This is equivalent to asking if there is a contraction level effect. Henneman's size principle has been demonstrated previously in a number of human studies. However, do larger MUs necessarily create larger MUPs? Dorfman et al. (1988), working with the biceps muscle, have suggested a relationship between average CN-detected MUP size and contraction force (threshold – 30% MVC) using EMG signal decomposition techniques (ADEMG), which indirectly suggests that larger MUs do create larger needle-detected MUPs. Conwit et al. (1997), demonstrated a relationship between force (5–30% MVC) and average S-MUP size in the quadriceps using DE-STA, which indirectly suggests that larger MUs do create larger surface-detected MUPs. However, even though Doherty (1993) has reported a significant relationship between MU twitch force and S-MUP area for thenar MUs of young healthy individuals (correlation coefficient, $r = 0.582$; $P < 0.001$), the relationship is not necessarily tight. In general, this relationship can be confounded by the depth of a MU within a muscle such that small, superficial MUs may have relatively large S-MUPs while large, deep MUs may have relatively small S-MUPs. Therefore, it is most likely that the effect of contraction level on the distribution of S-MUPs sizes, if any, will depend on both the muscle studied and on the S-MUP collection protocol. With regard to STA techniques, this effect can be minimised by trying to position the needle electrode at a different depth for each of the contractions performed.

If it is assumed that smaller MUs create smaller S-MUPs, relative to actual anatomical values, MUNEs obtained using DE-STA may be biased to high values because the MUs sampled will for the most part be smaller, lower threshold units because the EMG signals analysed are only detected during moderate muscle contractions and not during a full range of muscle contractions. This potential physiological bias toward smaller S-MUPs may however be offset by an inherent bias toward larger S-MUPs due to technical factors within the DE-STA protocol. For instance, it is more likely that larger, needle-detected MUPs will be detected and successfully tracked during an EMG signal decomposition, and as reported above, Dorfman et al. (1988) suggested that larger CN-detected MUPs may be created by larger MUs. In addition, it is more likely that larger S-MUPs will have a sufficient number of triggers so that their signal to noise ratio is sufficient to be included in the selected sample of S-MUPs which also possibly favors the sampling of contributions from larger MUs. However, the size or amplitude of a needle-detected MUP is highly dependent on the needle position relative to the contributing muscle fibers of the MU. Further, the size or amplitude of an S-MUP is highly dependent on the depth of the MU within the muscle. These may be greater factors than the theoretical size of the MU itself. This likely explains the often weak relationships reported between MUP size and contraction force. Therefore, the existence and effect of any bias will depend on the muscle studied and on the contraction and needle electrode positioning protocol used to obtain the sample of S-MUPs.

Nevertheless, MUNEs obtained using DE-STA should be more representative than those obtained using conventional STA based on level or window triggering because a wider range of contraction levels can be performed during S-MUP estimation using DE-STA. The preliminary MUNE results from the thenar muscles do not show any significant difference between previous STA-based estimates and those obtained using DE-STA. Perhaps this is because the average level of contraction for the current DE-STA-based estimates was only 7.6% MVC-RMS. Furthermore, the results obtained with STA, DE-STA and MPS are reasonably similar. This suggests that any inherent biases in the methods are either minimal or perhaps overshadowed by other factors such as the relative locations and depths of the MUs relative to the active electrode. Further data needs to be acquired and analysed and specific contraction level effects should be studied.

As shown conceptually in Fig. 2, the extraction of the activity of one MU from the interference pattern detected by a surface electrode, especially during higher levels of contraction, requires STA. The assumption underlying STA is that, on average, the activity of other MUs will cancel out and contribute a net zero voltage to the resulting average. In practice, the amount of cancellation depends on the number of triggers used to calculate the average and the inherent amount of interfering activity. As can be seen in Fig. 5, even after hundreds of triggers the background interference may not be satisfactorily cancelled out (i.e. the baseline before and after the S-MUP is not simply a flat line). This makes estimating the onset and end of the S-MUP difficult. Reviewing and editing marker settings takes time, may be subjective and can require a significant amount of operator interpretation, which can reduce the repeatability of the m-SMUP and therefore the MUNE. It also requires that contractions be maintained for 30–60 s, which may in some circumstances introduce fatigue. Further complicating the estimation of the m-SMUP are artefacts at the beginning of the estimated S-MUPs (initial negative shoulders) that make estimation of the onset difficult (see Fig. 5, MU# 2). The exact cause of these "shoulders" is not known, however, synchronisation of MU firing behaviour is suspected. If synchronisation is a significant factor, extending the length of contractions may not mitigate these affects and in fact may make them worse do to increasing fatigue. Considering these potential difficulties in defining and aligning S-MUPs for calculation of an mS-MUP, objective criteria need to be developed to allow the more automatic determination of when enough triggers have been obtained to sufficiently estimate a S-MUP, suitable marker locations and what to do with small low SNR S-MUPs. With regard to the development of these criteria, relationships between needle and surface detected MUP onsets will be very useful.

Repeatability

Variability in the positioning of the surface electrodes and in the maximal stimulation of the motor nerve can lead to variability in the shape and size of the acquired maximal CMAP. However, the greatest source of variability of a MUNE is in the sampling of the MU population to obtain a set of S-MUPs that are representative of the population of S-MUPs that contributed to the maximum CMAP and in the processing of this sample to estimate a mS-MUP. To study this source of variability, a thenar muscle's MUNE was repeatedly (six times) calculated for each of four different hands using the same maximal CMAP but different sets of S-MUPs obtained from different sets of contractions. On average for each MUNE, five contractions were selected which yielded 28 S-MUPs from which a mS-MUP was calculated. The average MUNE coefficient of variation (COV) across the four different groups of thenar muscle's was 0.143 for NPAmp based estimates and 0.137 for NPArea based estimates (see Table 2). This is a similar amount of variation to that reported by Doherty (1993) for seven repeated thenar muscle's MUNEs obtained using MPS for two different hands (COV 0.167 and 0.12). While these data are preliminary and do not measure the total amount of variation expected, they suggest that, even with the uncertainty of sampling MUs at different levels of contraction and with the difficulty of properly aligning S-MUPs for the calculation of a mS-MUP, the amount of inherent variation expected in MUNEs obtained using DE-STA is no greater then for estimates obtained using other techniques.

Summary

In summary DE-STA is a very useful technique for obtaining MUNEs. It can be performed easily and quickly, it is well tolerated by the subject and operator and is suitably repeatable. Furthermore, it can also provide potentially useful additional information about the size, structure and behaviour of individual MUs. For it to be widely used however, it must be implemented on a wider variety of commercially available systems. In addition, standards for the acceptance or rejection of "noisy" S-MUPs and for the alignment of S-MUPs for the calculation of the mS-MUP need to be developed.

Abbreviations

MU	motor unit
MUP	motor unit potential
MUPT	motor unit potential train
MUNE	motor unit number estimate
MVC	maximal voluntary contraction
MVC-RMS	MVC root mean square
CN	concentric needle
S-EMG	surface detected electromyographic
IS	incremental stimulation
MPS	multiple point stimulation
STA	spike triggered averaging
DE-STA	decomposition-enhanced STA
CMAP	compound muscle action potential
V_{PP}	peak to peak voltage
NPAmp	negative peak amplitude
NPArea	negative peak area

References

Brown, W.F., Strong, M.J. and Snow, R.S. Methods for estimating numbers of motor units in biceps-brachialis and loss of motor units with aging. *Muscle Nerve*, 1988, 11: 423–432.

Conwit, R., Tracy, B., Jamison, C., McHugh, M., Stashuk, D., Brown, W.B. and Metter, E.J. Decomposition-enhanced spike-triggered averaging: contraction level effects. *Muscle Nerve*, 1997, 20: 976–982.

DeKoning, P., Wienke, G.H., van der Most van Spijk, J., van Huffelen, A.C., Gispen, W.H. and Jennekens, F.G.I. Estimation of the number of motor units based on macro-EMG. *J. Neurol. Neurosurg. Psychiatry*, 1988, 51: 403–411.

DeLuca, C.J. and Basmajian, J.V. "*Muscles Alive: Their Functions Revealed by Electromyography*", 5th Ed. William and Wilkins, Baltimore, MD, 1985.

Doherty T.J. Age-related changes in human motor units. PhD thesis, University of Western Ontario, 1993.

Doherty, T.J. and Brown, W.F. Motor Unit Number Estimation: Methods and Applications. "*Clinical Neurophysiology and Neuromuscular Disease*" (W.F. Brown, C.F. Bolton and M.J. Aminoff, Eds.), W.B. Saunders, Philadelphia, 2002, 14: 274–290.

Doherty, T., Simmons, Z., O'Connell, B., Felice, K.J., Conwit, R., Chan, K.M., Komori, T., Brown, T., Stashuk, D.W. and Brown, W.F. Methods for estimating the numbers of motor units in human muscles. *J. Clin. Neurophysiol.*, 1995, 12: 565–584.

Dorfman, L.J., Howard, J.E. and McGill, K.C. Influence of contractile force on properties of motor unit action potentials: ADEMG analysis. *J. Neurol. Sci.*, 1988, 86: 125–136.

Henneman, E. and Mendell, L.M. Functional organization of motoneuron pool and is inputs. "*Handbook of Physiology*" (V.B. Brooks, Ed.), 1981, pp. 423–507. American Physiological Society, Bethesda.

Malmivuo, J. "*Bioelectromagnetism: Principles and Applications of Bioelectric and Biomagnetic Fields.*" Oxford University Press, New York, 1995.

Shefner, J.M. Motor unit number estimation in human neurological diseases and animal models. *Clin. Neurophysiol.*, 2001, 112: 955–964.

Stashuk, D. Decomposition and quantitative analysis of clinical electromyographic signals. *Med. Eng. Phys.*, 1999, 21: 389–404.

Stashuk, D.W. EMG signal decomposition: How can it be accomplished and used? *J. Electromyogr. Kinesiol.*, 2001, 11: 151–173.

Stein, R.B. and Yang, J.F. Methods for estimating the number of motor units in human muscles. *Ann Neurol*, 1990, 28: 487–495.

Motor Unit Number Estimation (Supplements to Clinical Neurophysiology Vol. 55)
Editor: M.B. Bromberg

Chapter 13

Rectified integrated EMG and MUNE

Jack H. Petajan*

Department of Neurology, University of Utah, 50 North Medical Drive, Salt Lake City, UT 84132, USA

Introduction

An ideal method for motor unit number estimation (MUNE) should be applicable to any muscle, be a reasonable estimate of the number of motor units in the muscle, easily applied, and require little time. The method should be sensitive to changes in motor unit number and size so that both myopathic and neurogenic disorders can be assessed. The method should assist in the diagnosis of such disorders. To this date no method achieves these goals. All methods have some inherent errors and limitations. All require too much time to perform, and as a result do not find wide use. Finally, the focus upon motor unit counting may neglect other important electrophysiological characteristics of muscle, such as the relation between force and electrical power generated by the muscle. This simple relationship might be sufficient for determining whether or not a muscle and its innervation are normal. It might be sufficiently sensitive to reduce the numbers of normal needle electrode examinations currently performed.

A linear relation between force and rectified integrated EMG (RIEMG) recorded by means of surface electrodes has been reported by many investigators (Stephens and Taylor, 1973). Fatigue has been investigated with this technique and a decline in power, as well as modal frequency, has been demonstrated (Stephens and Taylor, 1973). Owing to the filtering properties of tissue overlying muscle, distance of the recording electrodes from the potential generator, and lack of standardization of recording conditions, RIEMG has not been applied to the diagnosis of neuromuscular disease. In this chapter, a method for standardization of RIEMG will be proposed and then applied to MUNE. It would be more accurate to call the derived number a "power unit estimate" or PUE, which may be related in some systematic way to the motor unit number. Additional studies comparing this method to other techniques of MUNE will be necessary in order to establish such relationships. Further, it will be suggested that RIEMG may find use along with the neurological examination to more precisely determine the need for needle electrode examination. Finally, the force vs RIEMG relation may provide information helpful in determining whether or not voluntary muscle contraction is maximal or limited by insufficient supraspinal input.

Methods

The biceps brachii muscle was evaluated. One centimeter silver disc recording electrodes were placed over the distal tendon (reference) and center of the muscle belly (active). A ground electrode

**Correspondence to*: Dr. Jack Petajan, Department of Neurology, University of Utah, Salt Lake City, UT 84132, USA.
e-mail: Jack.Petajan@hsc.utah.edu

doi: 10.1016/S1567-424X(03)00013-8

was placed at the wrist. Recordings were made under two conditions: (a) the arm was held against gravity (AG) with the elbow flexed at 45° with the hand gently supinated; and (b) during maximal voluntary contraction (MVC) over a period of 8 s. Co-contraction of antagonistic muscles was excluded during antigravity maintenance of 45° elbow flexion. Surface EMG was recorded with a low pass filter of 10 Hz and a high pass filter of 10 kHz.

RIEMG was displayed as "energy packets", power units, or volt-second integrals of the rectified surface EMG activity. These appeared as uniform vertical lines, with successive lines representing full bins of power. The "energy packet" was 0.16 × sweep × gain yielding volt seconds. At a 500 μV gain, a unit of power was 320 μV displayed at a sweep speed of 10 ms/div. A typical AG recording is shown using the Cadwell Excel RIEMG program (Fig. 1). The gain was lowered if power generated was so high that individual units of power could not be differentiated sufficiently for counting. This sometimes occurred during MVC in normal subjects. During the 8-s recording period, power was seen to increase to a maximum then decline. Power units stored during each second were then scanned and the maximum number selected. For antigravity recording, power units for all 8 s were counted and an average calculated. A stable antigravity recording varied < 10% from 1 s to the next. The triceps muscle sometimes required separate recording because co-contraction could not be ruled out. This was suspected if antigravity recording consistently exceeded normal levels as was often the case in neurogenic atrophy.

It has been established that during maintenance of antigravity posture, single motor units fire at or about the rate of physiologic tremor, or at a recruitment rate of approximately 10 Hz. Using a monopolar 26 g needle electrode, a maximum of 4.5 + 1.7 different motor units are activated within the recording territory of the needle (Petajan, 1990). Motor unit action potentials (MUAP's) were excluded if the rise time of the major spike was greater than 300 μs and the amplitude was less than 100 μV. The amplifier for both RIEMG and MUAP records was set at a gain of 500 μV/div.

Prior to determination of RIEMG during AG and MVC conditions, a monopolar needle electrode was inserted into the mid-belly of the muscle and the maximum number of different MUAP's that could be recorded was determined by moving the electrode to three circumferential recording sites. Focused MUAP's were then counted.

PUE was calculated as the product of the RIEMG MVC/AG ratio and the number of different MUAP's recorded during the AG condition. The result will be henceforth designated as MUNE since we are interested in comparing this technique with others used for MUNE.

An additional recording of RIEMG at three different force levels measured at the wrist was obtained in normal subjects to calculate a slope for the RIEMG force relation. This slope was then compared with the slope obtained from AG vs MVC during measurement of MVC force.

Subjects

Sixty-five male and female subjects with no history of neuromuscular disease in three age categories were studied; Group A: 18–39 years (21 M, 12 F), Group B: 40–60 years (10 M, 10 F), and Group C: greater than 60 years (6 M, 6 F). Patients with amyotrophic lateral sclerosis (ALS) at various stages of disease and followed at 3-month intervals were also studied. Additionally, a small number of patients with a variety of neuromuscular disorders, primarily myopathies, were also studied.

Data analysis

Means and standard deviations were calculated for the number of different motor units recorded during the AG condition. Also, RIEMG MVC/AG ratio, and MUNE for the three groups of normal subjects was calculated. Subjects for the three age groups were compared using the student *t*-test. Patients with neuromuscular disease were compared with the appropriate group of normal subjects. Owing to the varying degrees of involvement, it was not considered reasonable to evaluate patients with ALS and other diseases as groups.

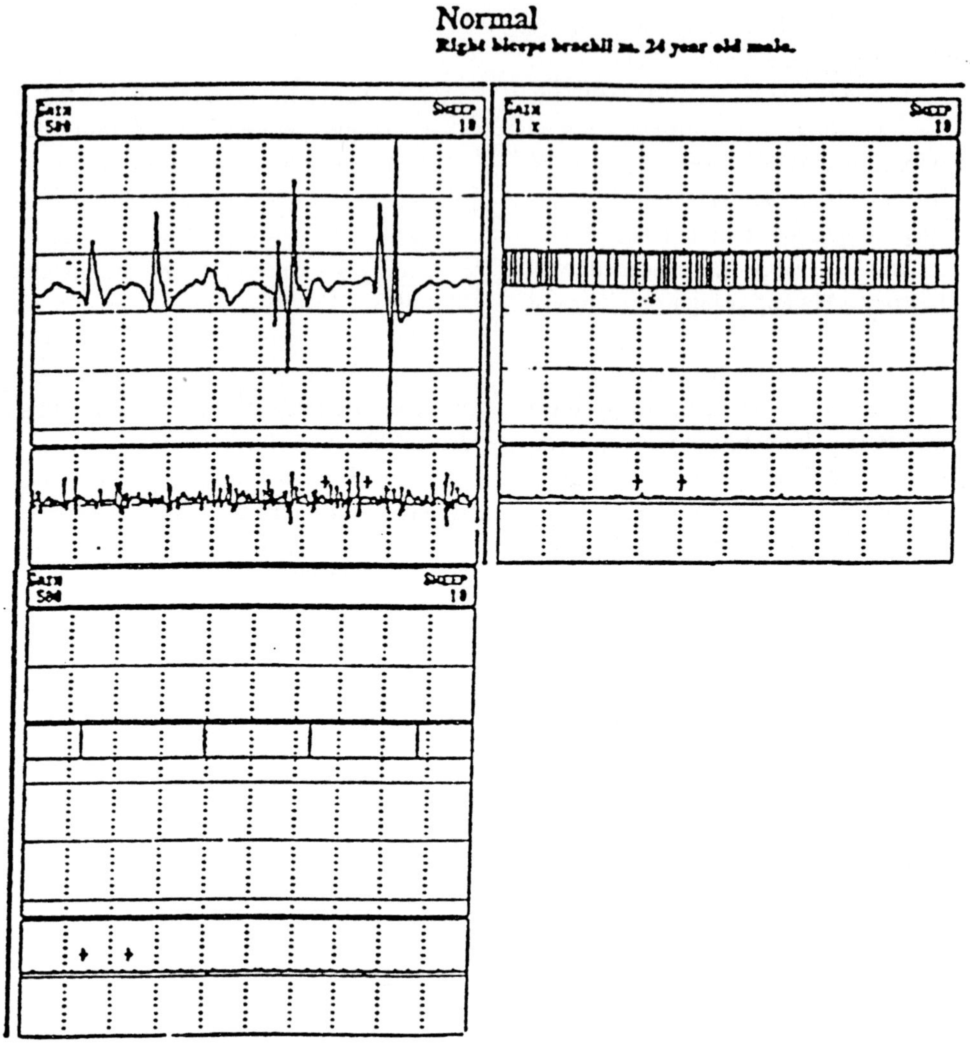

Fig. 1. The number of different MUAPs is shown in the upper left. The segment of the 100 ms epoch that is displayed is bracketed. Ten 100 ms epochs of the eight epochs recorded are shown. Recordings from each of 8 s are scanned and the maximum 100 ms is displayed. An average of the second containing the maximal number of energy packets is determined. RIEMG displayed as 320 μV "energy packets" for the 100 ms epoch are shown for 45° elbow flexion (antigravity posture or AG) and for MVC. The maximal number of energy packets for 100 ms is determined for MVC (RIEMG MVC).

Repeated studies were done on some subjects to assess the reliability of the technique.

Results

Normal subjects

Data for Groups A, B, and C are presented on Table 1. There was no significant difference in the MUAP numbers between groups. The MVC/AG ratio was significantly greater for Group A compared to either Group B or C ($P<0.05$), and Group B was greater than Group C ($P<0.05$), reflecting the decrease in power during MVC generated with advancing age. Similarly, MUNE was significantly greater for Group A in comparison to both Groups B and C. Thus, the greater MUNE values depended to a great extent upon the increased MVC/AG ratio seen in the younger subjects. A typical record of MU numbers and RIEMG at AG and MVC are shown in Fig. 1.

TABLE 1

DATA FROM NORMAL SUBJECTS, DIVIDED BY AGE

Group	MUAP number	RIEMG MVC/AG	MUNE
A	4.6 ± 1.4	31.3 ± 14	140 ± 69
B	4.5 ± 1.8	22.8 ± 10	101 ± 60
C	5.0 ± 1.8	13.4 ± 5	63 ± 28
Total	4.7 ± 1.6	25.4 ± 14	114 ± 67

Group A: 18–39 years; Group B: 40–60 years; Group C: greater than 60 years. MUAP number: number of motor unit action potentials at a given level of muscle activation. RIEMG MVC/AG ratio: rectified integrated EMG activity at maximum voluntary and antigravity levels of muscle activation. MUNE: estimated number of motor units innervating the muscle understudy.

Subjects with denervating pathology

Thirty subjects with ALS and other denervating disorders (15 M, 15 F) with just detectable weakness of elbow flexion were examined. Their age range was 35–64 years, which corresponded approximately in age to Group B normal subjects. Data are shown in Table 2 (McComas, 1991). MUAP numbers are significantly reduced for most subjects, with a mean of 2.1 ± 1.2. The mean MVC/AG ratio was 8.5 ± 5.9, and the mean MUNE value was 19.9 ± 27.4. In this group of patients, two changes account for the decreased MUNE values, a decreased MUAP number and a decreased MVC/AG ratio. Examination of RIEMG values during AG revealed an increase in comparison to controls (2000 ± 1761 vs 1167 ± 442 μV × 100 ms). Further, the value at MVC in ALS subjects was decreased, resulting in significant decrease in the slope of the RIEMG vs force relation. A typical recording is shown in Fig. 2.

A variety of other denervating disorders associated with detectable weakness, such as radiculopathy, acute inflammatory, demyelinating polyneuropathy, etc. had similar findings.

In a smaller group of patients with ALS, MUNE determinations were performed every 2–3 months to follow the course of motor unit loss (Petajan, 1993). The steep decline in MUE is shown in Fig. 3. This rate of decline did not parallel the decline in strength, but seemed to precede it by several months. The loss of motor units as assessed by this technique provided evidence for a more rapid loss of motor units than expected.

TABLE 2

DATA FROM SUBJECTS WITH ALS AND OTHER DENERVATING DISORDERS

MUAP number	Antigravity RIEMG	RIEMG MVC/AG	MUNE
3	5120	2.6	8
4	1056	6.7	27
1	1024	17.6	18
1	1980	11.6	12
2	2380	1.0	2
2	1820	11.8	24
2	1280	7.3	15
2	1184	7.8	16
2	1120	23.4	141
3	704	17.3	52
1	864	17.8	18
2	480	5.6	11
2	1024	10.6	21
2	896	3.6	7
1	2048	3.6	4
2	608	7.4	7
2	1280	5.0	10
1	1792	8.2	8
1	3300	4.1	4
1	1568	10.0	10
2	7040	1.2	2
2	1920	4.8	10
4	2000	18.0	72
1	644	15.4	15
2	1632	7.2	14
1	3328	1.3	1
1	1248	7.4	7
4	2464	7.1	28
2	7680	1.0	2
4	512	7.5	30
Mean 2.1	2000	8.5	20
SD 1.24	1761	5.9	27
$P < 0.01$	< 0.05	< 0.01	< 0.01

MUAP number: number of motor unit action potentials at a given level of muscle activation. RIEMG MVC/AG ratio: rectified integrated EMG activity at maximum voluntary and antigravity levels of muscle activation. MUNE: estimated number of motor units innervating the muscle understudy.

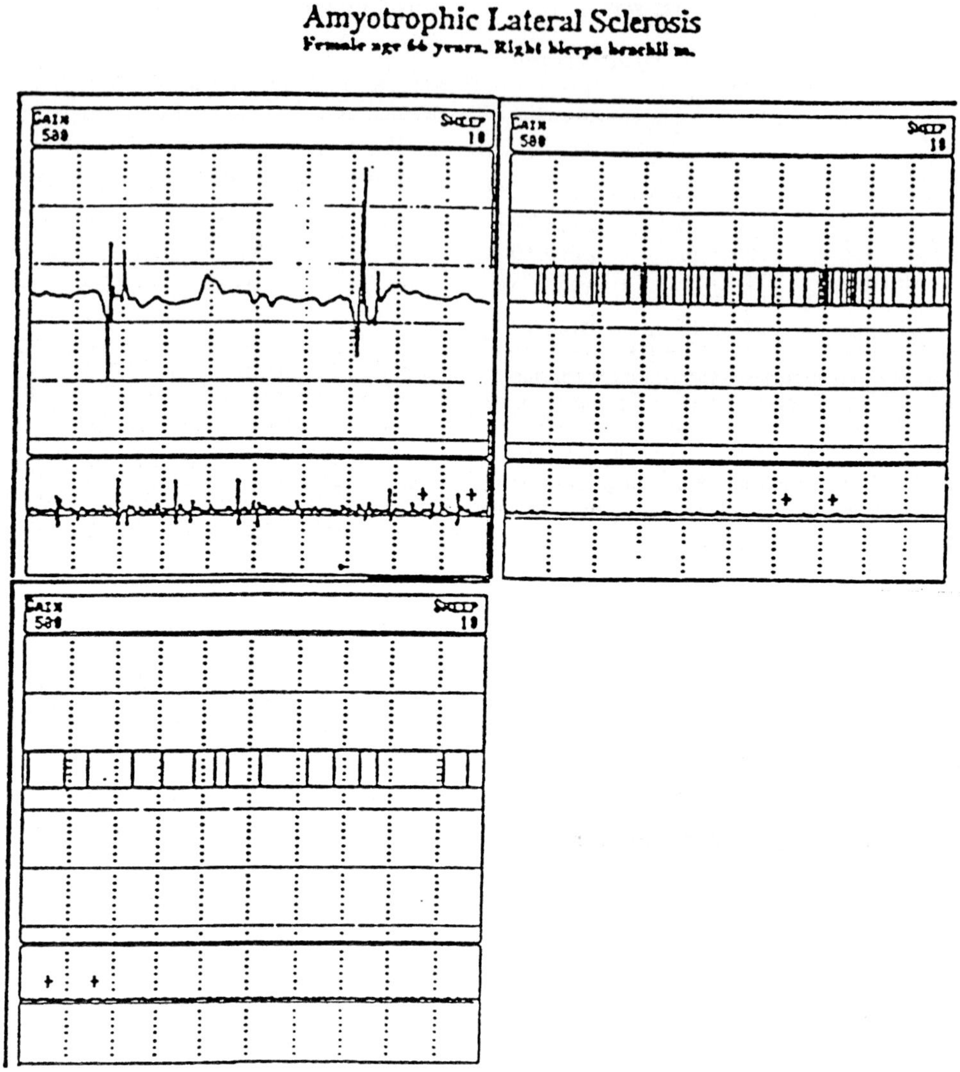

Fig. 2. A recording of biceps brachii m. from an ALS patient with detectable weakness is shown using the format described in Fig. 1.

Subjects with myopathy

Seven patients with different types of myopathies, confirmed by muscle biopsy, were studied. Data are shown on Table 3. All had detectable weakness, increased recruitment seen as an increase in MUAP number during AG recording, and a significant reduction in MUAP amplitude and duration. In association with increased recruitment and the myopathic features of the MUAP's, RIEMG under AG conditions was normal or low and the RIEMG MCV/AG ratio was very low. Three subjects had below normal MUNE values while the remaining subjects had normal values. A recording from a patient with myotonic muscular dystrophy is shown in Fig. 4.

A reduced slope of the RIEMG vs force function was accompanied by a reduced or normal RIEMG at AG, so that the "myopathic line" falls below normal, in contrast to neurogenic atrophy in which RIEMG at AG is usually above normal. Figure 5 shows how the RIEMG vs force function might be altered in neurogenic atrophy and myopathy. Despite a reduced slope of the RIEMG vs

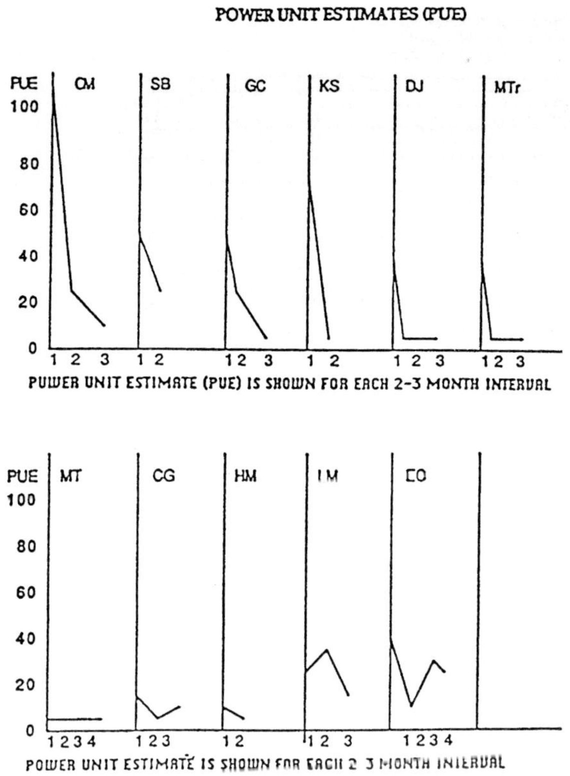

Fig. 3. The rapid decline in PUE and MUE for biceps brachii m. in several ALS patients studied every 2–3 months immediately following diagnosis is shown. There was minimal change in muscle strength over this period.

force function, there is an increase in the number of different MUAP's activated in the AG condition. This increase in recruitment compensates for the reduced RIEMG MCV/AG ratio to increase the MUNE value.

In some cases of myopathy, recruitment is so complete in the AG condition that individual MUAP's cannot be discriminated. When this occurs, it is possible to record RIEMG at lower levels of recruitment and perform the same calculation, since the recruitment firing rate is essentially the same as that in the AG condition. It is only necessary to record simultaneously the number of different MUAP's activated and the RIEMG at that level of recruitment. RIEMG MCV should be obtained under the same conditions of posture

Subjects with myasthenia gravis

Six patients with myasthenia gravis (MG) were studied, five had detectable fatigable weakness with elbow flexion and one had ocular MG. Data are presented in Table 4. All patients demonstrated a reduced RIEMG MCV/AG ratio and a value for the number of different MUAP's slightly above normal. RIEMG in the AG condition was normal.

TABLE 3

DATA FROM SUBJECTS WITH MYOPATHIC DISORDERS, ALL CONFIRMED BY BIOPSY

Age	Sex	Diagnosis	MRC strength	MUAP number	RIEMG AG	RIEMG MVC/AG	MUNE
40	F	L-G	4	6	1972	4.7	28
70	M	Not defined	4	7	816	9.1	64
38	F	Not defined	4	5	2176	4.1	21
27	F	Metabolic	4	9	1428	2.4	112
45	F	Not defined	4	12	650	13.3	160
64	M	PM	4	10	1184	15.6	156
35	F	Myotonic	4	6	800	16.0	96
			Mean	7.9	1289	10.7	91
			Range	5–10	650–2176	4.1–15.6	21–160

Diagnosis: limb-girdle dystrophy (L-G), polymyositis (PM), myotonic dystrophy (Myotonic). MRC strength: Medical Research Council strength 0–5. MUAP number: number of motor unit action potentials at a given level of muscle activation. RIEMG MVC/AG ratio: rectified integrated EMG activity at maximum voluntary and antigravity levels of muscle activation. MUNE: estimated number of motor units innervating the muscle understudy.

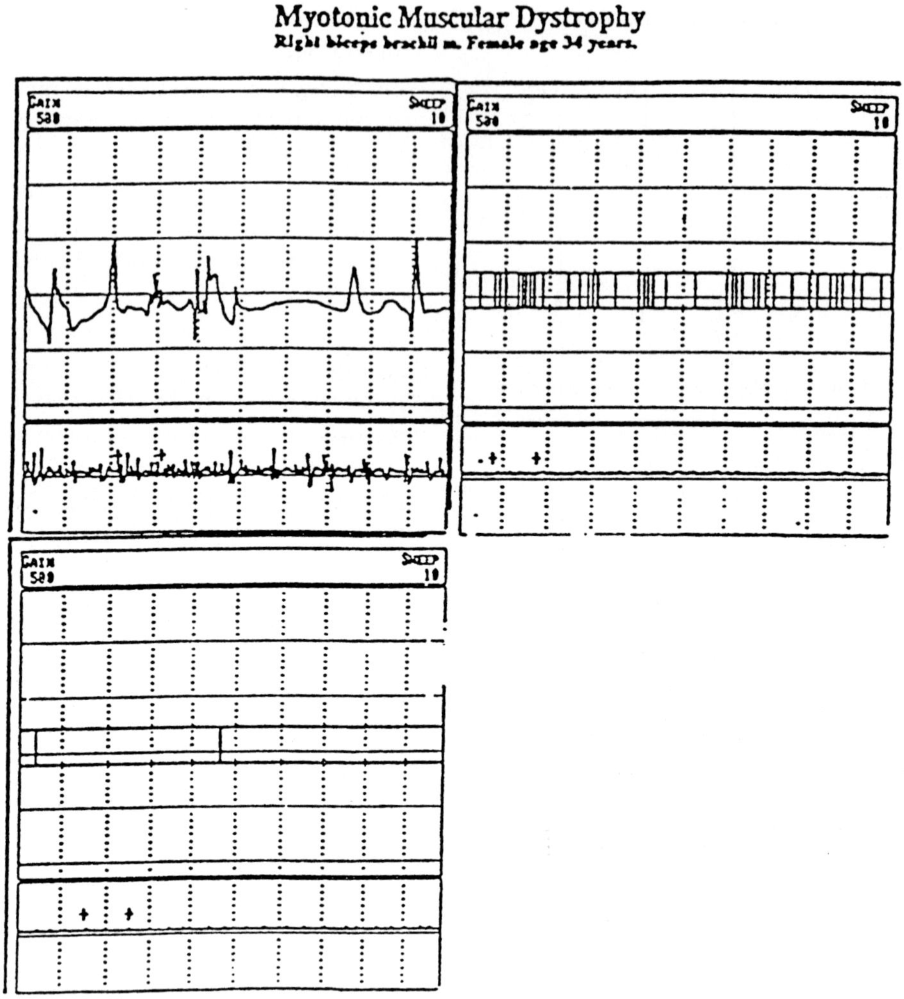

Fig. 4. A recording of biceps brachii m. from a patient with myotonic dystrophy is shown. Note the low RIEMG AG, as well as the reduced value of RIEMG MVC.

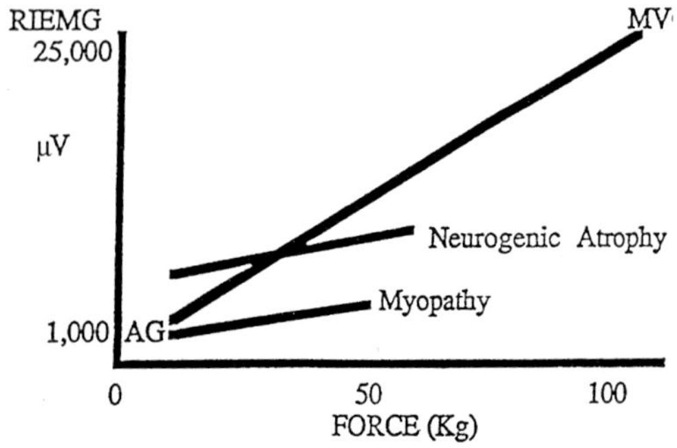

Fig. 5. This hypothetical graph shows how a normal RIEMG (μV/100 ms) vs force function may vary from that of neurogenic atrophy and myopathy. The lower value for each line corresponds to AG (antigravity 45° elbow flexion) and the highest value to MVC.

MUNE in the case of ocular MG was at the lower limit of normal. The single high MUNE value results from a high initial RIEMG during MVC that fatigues rapidly, as shown in Fig. 6. The reduced RIEMG occurring with fatigue would of course result in a lower MUNE. These results emphasize the importance of the fatigue component in MG and its ability to decrease MUNE values.

RIEMG MUNE reliability

There are three components required for PUE and MUNE. The first is an estimate of the

TABLE 4

DATA FROM SUBJECTS WITH MG WITH JUST DETECTABLE WEAKNESS

	MUAP number	RIEMG AG	RIEMG MVC/AG	MUNE
	5	1760	10.2	51
	7	960	27.0	187
	4	1120	7.4	30
	4	1178	9.7	39
	4	1386	7.3	28
	6	800	13.4	80
Mean	5	1200	12.5	69
Range	4–7	800–1760	7.3–27	28–187

MUAP number: number of motor unit action potentials at a given level of muscle activation. RIEMG MVC/AG ratio: rectified integrated EMG activity at maximum voluntary and antigravity levels of muscle activation. MUNE: estimated number of motor units innervating the muscle understudy.

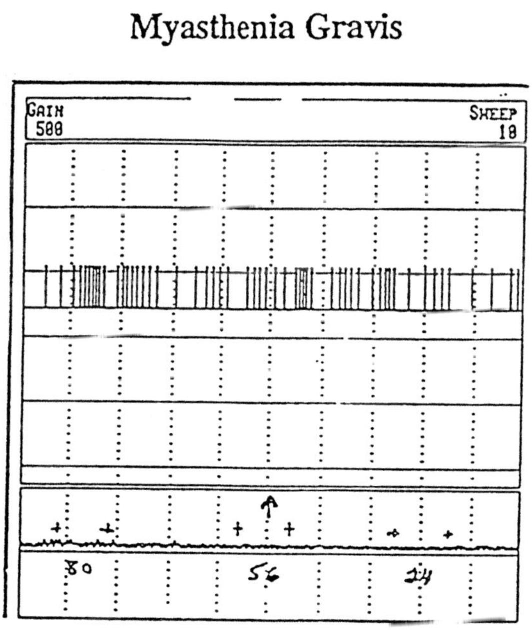

Fig. 6. RIEMG "energy packets" are shown during MVC of biceps brachii m. in a patient with MG. A rapid decline in RIEMG is seen that reflects abnormal fatigue.

number of different MUAP's activated during the AG condition. This value is the most crucial contributor to error. As MUAP number declines into the range of 1–2, a twofold change in MUNE is evident. Fortunately, the decline in RIEMG vs force is so great that even this large a change in the estimate still provides an adequate indication of severe neurogenic atrophy. In a previous study of motor unit recruitment using the AG condition, three examiners assessed the number of different MUAP's firing. Estimates never differed by more than one MUAP (Petajan, 1990). In this study, when recording from different sites, similar observations were made. With regard to the RIEMG ratio MVC/AG, the most significant variation was seen in the MCV value. In seven subjects recorded three or more times, a correlation coefficient of 0.85 was obtained comparing the first with the second and third recording. One can expect the RIEMG at MVC to be as variable as measurement of force during MVC. Recording MVC continuously over a period of 8 s allowed the observer to scan the entire period for the maximum value. MVC is also dependent upon volition. Pyramidal tract disease can affect MVC. Thus, RIEMG MVC is dependent upon the motor neurons that can be activated. Other techniques for obtaining RIEMG MVC may be applied using motor nerve stimulation to record the CMAP.

In general, the greatest contributor to systematic error is the MUAP number, which becomes greater as total number decreases. The greatest contributor to subject error is the variability of RIEMG at MVC. This error can usually be corrected by subject instruction or perhaps by motor nerve

McComas, A.J. An invited review: motor unit estimation: methods, results, and present status. *Muscle Nerve*, 1991, 14,: 585–597.

Petajan, J.H. Antigravity posture for analysis of motor unit recruitment: the "45 degree test". *Muscle Nerve*, 1990, 13: 355–359.

Petajan, J.H. *EMG and motor unit estimation in amyotrophic lateral sclerosis*. Festscrift for Forbes Norris, San Francisco, CA, Sept 11–12, 1993. Smith-Gorden, London.

Stephens, J.A. and Taylor, A. The relationship between integrated electrical activity and force in normal and fatiguing voluntary muscle contraction. "*New Developments in Electromyography and Clinical Neurophysiology*" (J.E. Desmedt, Ed.), Vol. 1, 1973, pp. 623–627. Karger, Basel.

Strong, M.J., Brown, W.F., Hudsin, A.J. and Snow, R. Motor unit estimates in the biceps-brachialis in amyotrophic lateral sclerosis. *Muscle Nerve*, 1988, 11: 415–422.

Motor Unit Number Estimation (Supplements to Clinical Neurophysiology Vol. 55)
Editor: M.B. Bromberg

Chapter 14

Motor unit number index (MUNIX): a pilot study

Sanjeev D. Nandedkar[a,*], Desh S. Nandedkar[b], Paul E. Barkhaus[c] and Erik V. Stålberg[d]

[a]*Oxford Instruments Medical Systems, 12 Skyline Drive, Hawthorne, NY 10532, USA*
[b]*Rensselaer Polytechnic Institute, Troy, NY, USA*
[c]*Medical College of Wisconsin and Milwaukee, VA Medical Center, Milwaukee, WI, USA*
[d]*Department of Clinical Neurophysiology, Uppsala, University Hospital, S-75185 Uppsala, Sweden*

Introduction

Most methods of motor unit number estimation (MUNE) (Nandedkar and Barkhaus, 1987; Brown et al., 1988; Stein and Yang, 1990; Bromberg, 1993; Doherty and Brown, 1993; Stashuk et al., 1994; McComas, 1995; Shahani et al., 1995; Wang and Delwaide, 1995; Slawnych et al., 1996; Lomen-Hoerth and Olney, 2000) identify and record individual surface EMG motor unit action potentials (SMUPs). The mean amplitude (or area) of the SMUPs is divided into the compound muscle action potential (CMAP) amplitude (or area) to estimate the number of motor units (MUs). The SMUPs have small amplitude and hence the recording technique can be tedious and time consuming. In contrast, the statistical method (Daube, 1995) directly estimates the average SMUAP contribution to CMAP from a collection of signals recorded at submaximal stimulation. This makes the recording technique easier. Following the same notion, we have developed a model for MUNE using surface EMG interference pattern (SIP). The result is called motor unit number index (MUNIX). In this communication, we will describe the method of recording and signal analysis. The mathematical model for the computation is briefly summarized in the Appendix. The results of preliminary investigations in the thenar muscle of healthy subjects and patients with amyotrophic lateral sclerosis (ALS) are presented.

Recording technique and computations

MUNIX measurements follow a three step procedure. First, the CMAP is recorded using the standard nerve conduction techniques. We stimulated the median nerve at the wrist and recorded CMAP from the thenar muscle (Fig. 1A). In the second step, the electrodes are maintained at the same position as in step 1. The SIP is recorded when the patient maintains a constant force of contraction. The force is defined by the clinician offering resistance to the tested muscle. We recorded SIP at five force levels: minimal, mild, moderate, submaximal and maximum force (Fig. 1B). Needless to say, this is quite subjective gradation. The subject is allowed a brief rest (10–15 s) before the maximal effort. The process is then repeated to yield 10 SIP signals. Each SIP epoch is 300 ms long. One may also use a single graded contraction to obtain the

**Correspondence to*: Dr. Sanjeev D. Nandedkar. Oxford Instruments Medical Systems, 12 Skyline Drive, Hawthorne, NY 10532, USA.
e-mail: Sanjeev@CASAEngineering.com

doi: 10.1016/S1567-424X(03)00014-X

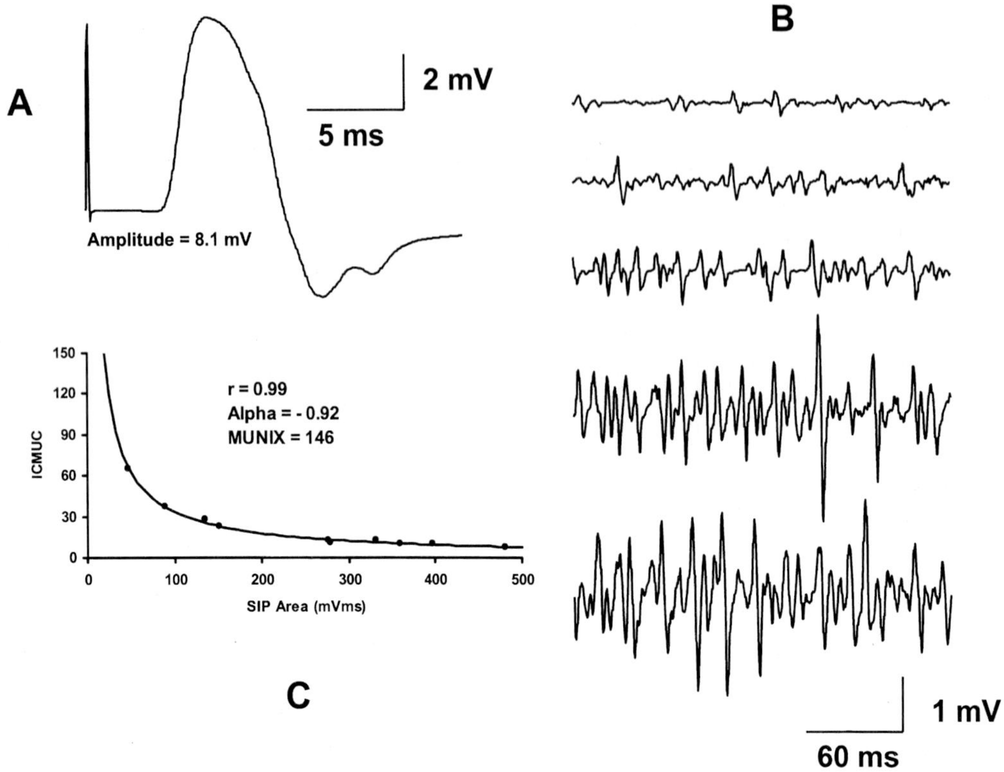

Fig. 1. MUNIX in a normal subject. (A) CMAP shows normal amplitude. (B) The SIP when force of contraction was increased from minimal to maximum in five steps. (C) Analysis of SIP measurements (individual data points) shows an excellent fit with the mathematical model (solid line representing Eq. (2)).

9–10 necessary SIP epochs representing the minimal to maximum effort. In the third step, the signals are analyzed offline. SIPs with excessive noise, interference or other artifacts are excluded from analysis.

The amplitude, area and power of the CMAP are computed from the initial negative peak. The equations for computing the area and power are shown in the Appendix. The area and power of the SIP are measured and normalized for a one-second epoch. The values are used to compute the "ideal case motor unit count (ICMUC)"

$$\mathrm{ICMUC} = \frac{(\mathrm{CMAP\,Power} \times \mathrm{SIP\,Area})}{(\mathrm{CMAP\,Area} \times \mathrm{SIP\,Power})}. \quad (1)$$

Thus, each SIP gives two results: SIP area and ICMUC. Regression analysis is used to define the relationship between SIP area and ICMUC (Fig. 1C) by the following formula:

$$\mathrm{ICMUC} = B(\mathrm{SIP\,Area})^{\alpha}. \quad (2)$$

The parameters B and α obtained from the regression are used to compute MUNIX:

$$\mathrm{MUNIX} = B(20)^{\alpha}. \quad (3)$$

Subjects and testing procedures

All EMG studies were performed at the third author's institution. The protocol was approved by the committee for the human studies. Informed consent was obtained from all subjects. The recordings were performed using a commercially available EMG instrument ("Synergy" by Oxford Instruments, Hawthorne). The signals were saved to the hard disk and then analyzed offline.

Fifteen healthy subjects participated in the study. The MUNIX was measured bilaterally in all subjects. In 10 muscles (six subjects), the MUNIX measurements were repeated to assess the reproducibility of the results. The repeat study was performed roughly 30 min after the first measurement. The electrodes were removed after the first study and re-applied at the time of second investigation. No marks were made on the hand to facilitate identical electrode placements in the study. Furthermore, the data was analyzed after both recording sessions. Thus the investigator did not have knowledge of the measurements (and hence a bias) from the first session before repeating the measurement. For muscles used in the test–retest study, the first measurements were used for the remaining data analysis in this study.

The patient group consisted of 17 patients with definite ALS by Escorial criteria. At the time of examination, the muscle strength was graded using the MRC scale. Scores of 4+, 4− and 3+ were reported as 4.3, 3.7 and 3.3, respectively. In 14 patients MUNIX was measured bilaterally. In 10 muscles (seven patients), the MUNIX measurements were repeated to assess reproducibility. The technique was identical to that described for healthy subjects.

Results

MUNIX measurements in healthy subjects showed a slight decrease with age (Fig. 2). The number of subjects in this study is too small to define the reference values by age. Hence for this pilot study, we have ignored this dependence. In healthy subjects aged less than 60 years, the mean value of MUNIX was 167 and the standard deviation was 57. The lower limit of MUNIX in healthy subjects was chosen to be 70 by which all healthy subjects had a normal MUNIX value. All subjects also had normal CMAP amplitude.

In the patient group, MUNIX values were reduced (Fig. 3). Some muscles had normal CMAP amplitude although MUNIX was reduced. Weaker muscles had a much greater reduction in MUNIX (Fig. 4). Examples of MUNIX are shown in Figs. 5 and 6.

Test–retest measurements showed a strong correlation ($r = 0.9$, $P < 0.01$), as shown in Fig. 7.

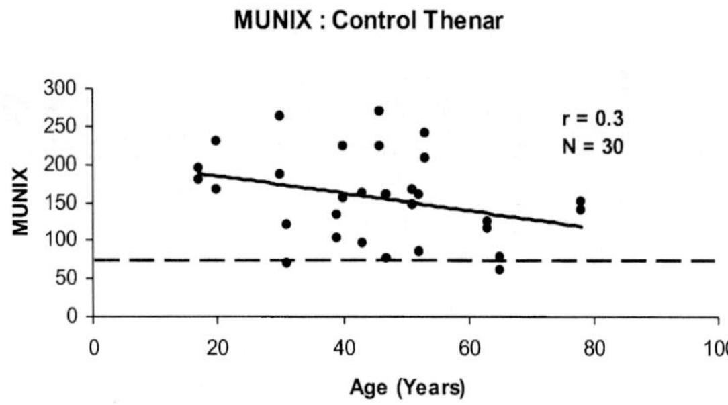

Fig. 2. MUNIX measurements in healthy subjects are plotted against the subject's age. There is a slight trend towards reduced values in elderly patients. The dotted line shows lower normal limit.

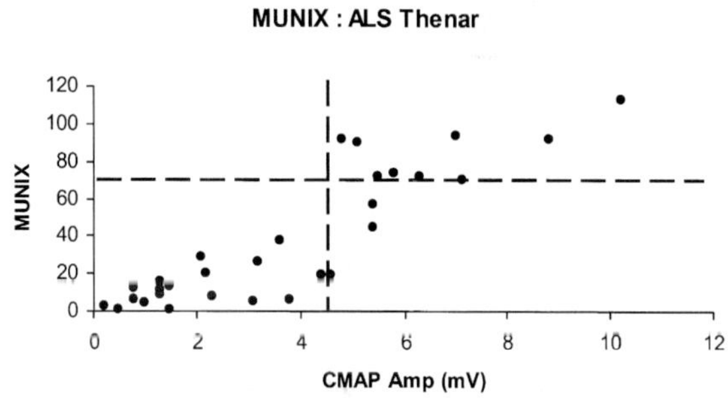

Fig. 3. MUNIX values are plotted against the CMAP amplitude for the ALS patient group. The dotted lines indicate the lower limits of the two measurements.

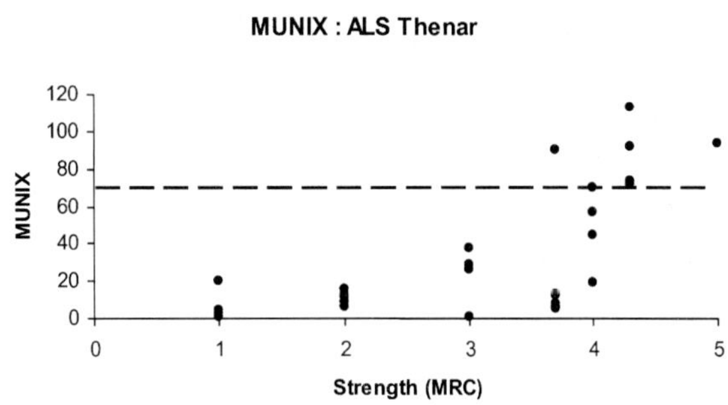

Fig. 4. MUNIX values are plotted against the muscle strength assessed manually. The weaker muscles have lower MUNIX values. The dotted line indicates the lower normal limit of MUNIX.

Discussion

This pilot study demonstrates all the expected relationships between MUNIX and the underlying pathophysiology (McComas, 1995). There was no

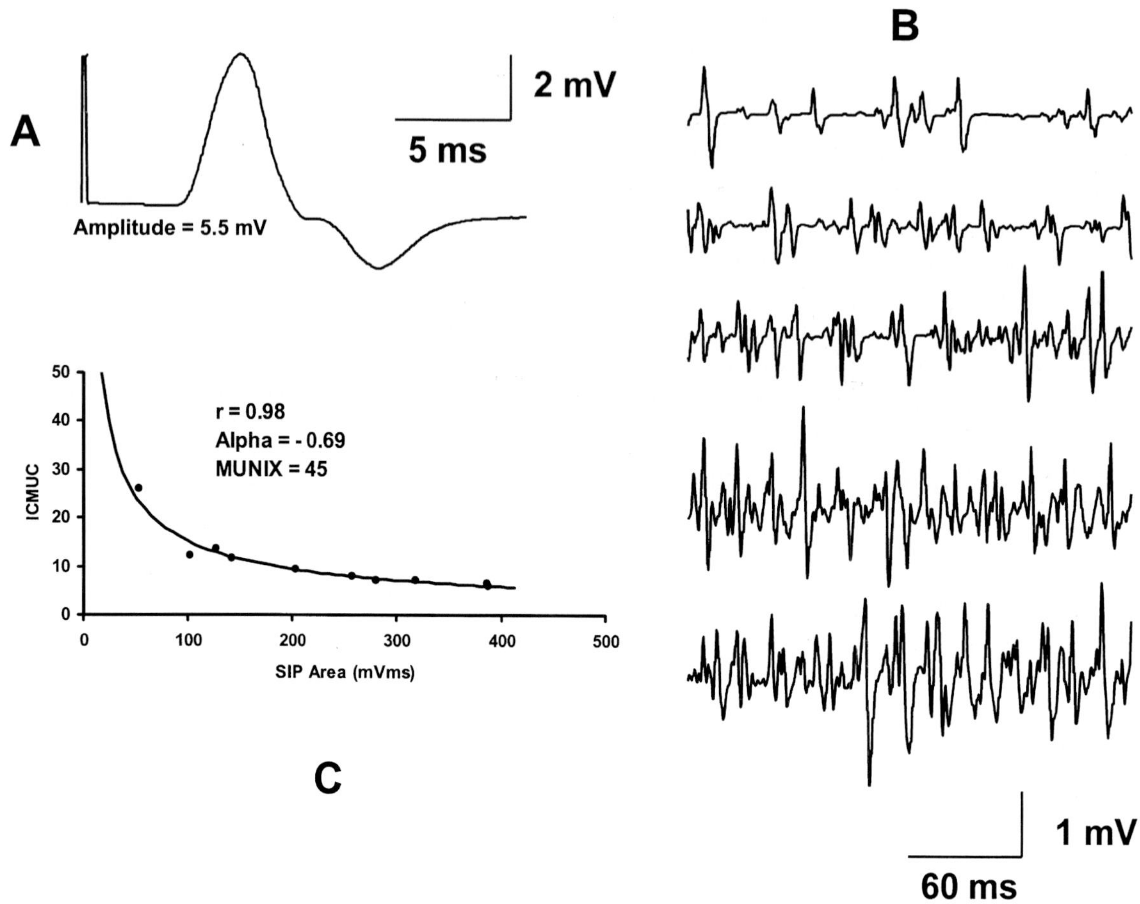

Fig. 5. MUNIX in an ALS patient. (A) CMAP shows normal amplitude. (B) The SIP when force of contraction was increased from minimal to maximum in five steps. Large amplitude spikes (compared to normal, as seen in Fig. 1B) can be recognized by visual assessment at minimal effort. (C) Analysis of SIP measurements. Note the reduced absolute value of alpha and MUNIX

correlation between subject age and MUNIX for healthy subjects aged less than 60 years. There appears to be a slight trend of diminished MUNIX in older patients (Fig. 2). This is consistent with the known loss of MUs in elderly healthy subjects.

MUNIX has good reproducibility based on the test–retest correlation coefficient (Fig. 7). The correlation coefficient ($r = 0.95$) was even higher in the patient group where the number of MUs is reduced. This is also the observation in other methods of MUNE (Armon et al., 1997). MUNIX values (mean = 167, lower normal limit = 70) are similar to those described for the statistical method (mean 153, lower normal limit 70 for 40–50% stimulus level, Daube, 1995).

In the patient group, MUNIX is reduced reflecting the loss of MUs. In some muscles the MUNIX is reduced even though the CMAP amplitude is normal. This indicates the increased MU size is due to reinnervation. In Fig. 5, one can see large amplitude spikes even at minimal effort. However, at maximal effort, the SIP appears "full" by visual assessment, just as in healthy subjects (Fig. 1).

MUNIX and CMAP amplitude decrease with muscle strength (Fig. 4). However, the relationship between the CMAP amplitude and MUNIX is quite variable in the weak muscles. As an example, the recording in Fig. 6 shows a mildly reduced CMAP but with MUNIX of only 5. By visual assessment, one can see discharges and recruitment of

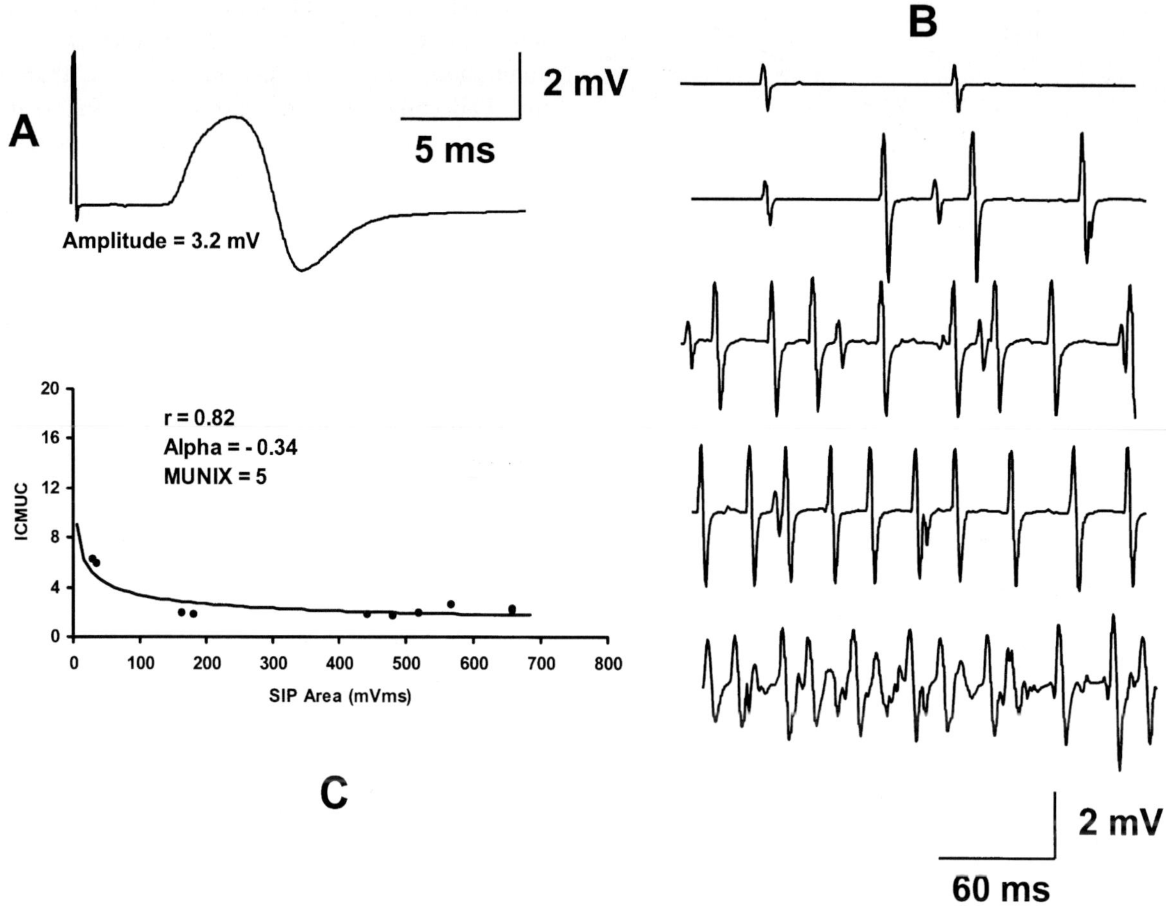

Fig. 6. MUNIX in an ALS patient. (A) CMAP shows reduced amplitude. (B) The SIP when force of contraction was increased from minimal to maximum in five steps. Large amplitude spikes can be recognized by visual assessment at all effort levels. The SIP appears "discrete" by visual assessment. (C) MUNIX and absolute value of alpha are reduced. The minimal change in ICMUC is consistent with the theoretical model.

individual large motor unit potentials. The small MUNIX value is consistent with significant MU loss. In contrast, other muscles had similar MUNIX values but a much lower CMAP amplitude (bottom left corner of Fig. 3). This reflects the different levels of reinnervation in those muscles. In this respect, MUNIX provides additional information of the dynamic changes in the number and size of MUs in diseased state.

The experimental data supports the mathematical model described in the appendix. The correlation coefficient of the regression in Eq. (2) was greater than 0.97 in all healthy subjects. With large number of MUs, there is great superimposition among SMUPs (Figs. 1B and 8C). Hence, ICMUC decreases with force. The absolute numerical value of alpha is high (Fig. 1C). When the number of MUs decreases, there will be less superimposition among the SMUPs (Fig. 6B). The experimental recording conditions become more similar to the "ideal case" portrayed in Fig. 8A. The ICMUC will become less dependent on force. Indeed, in Fig. 6C, we find minimal changes to ICMUC when SIP area increased due to increased force of contraction. The reduced dependence gives a much lower absolute value of alpha and the correlation coefficient of regression also decreased. Intermediate values of alpha and correlation are seen in muscles with modest loss of MUs (Fig. 5).

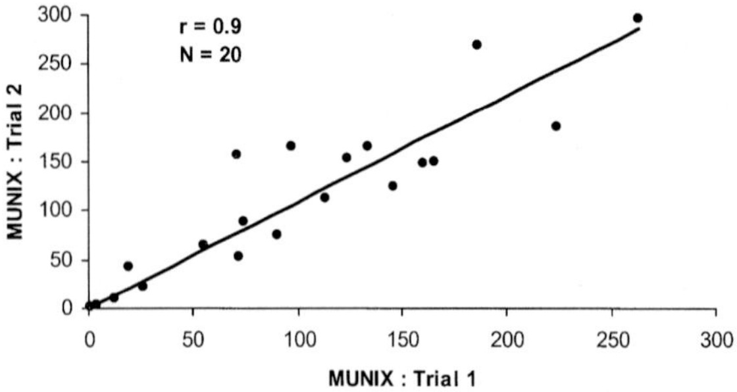

Fig. 7. The test–retest data shows a good correlation coefficient between the MUNIX measurements on two recording sessions.

MUNIX has several practical benefits. It is non-invasive, has minimal discomfort due to stimulation, and can be performed in less than 5 min. This makes it attractive to perform follow up studies in many different muscles of patients with neurogenic diseases. MUNIX also offers some "theoretical" advantages in the MUNE. When the number of MUs is significantly reduced, it would be quite difficult to record SMUPs of different MUs. In the statistical method, it would be difficult to get a suitable stimulation level due to large steps in the "CMAP versus stimulus intensity" plot. The inherent variability of the SMUP and volume conducted potentials also add difficulties to

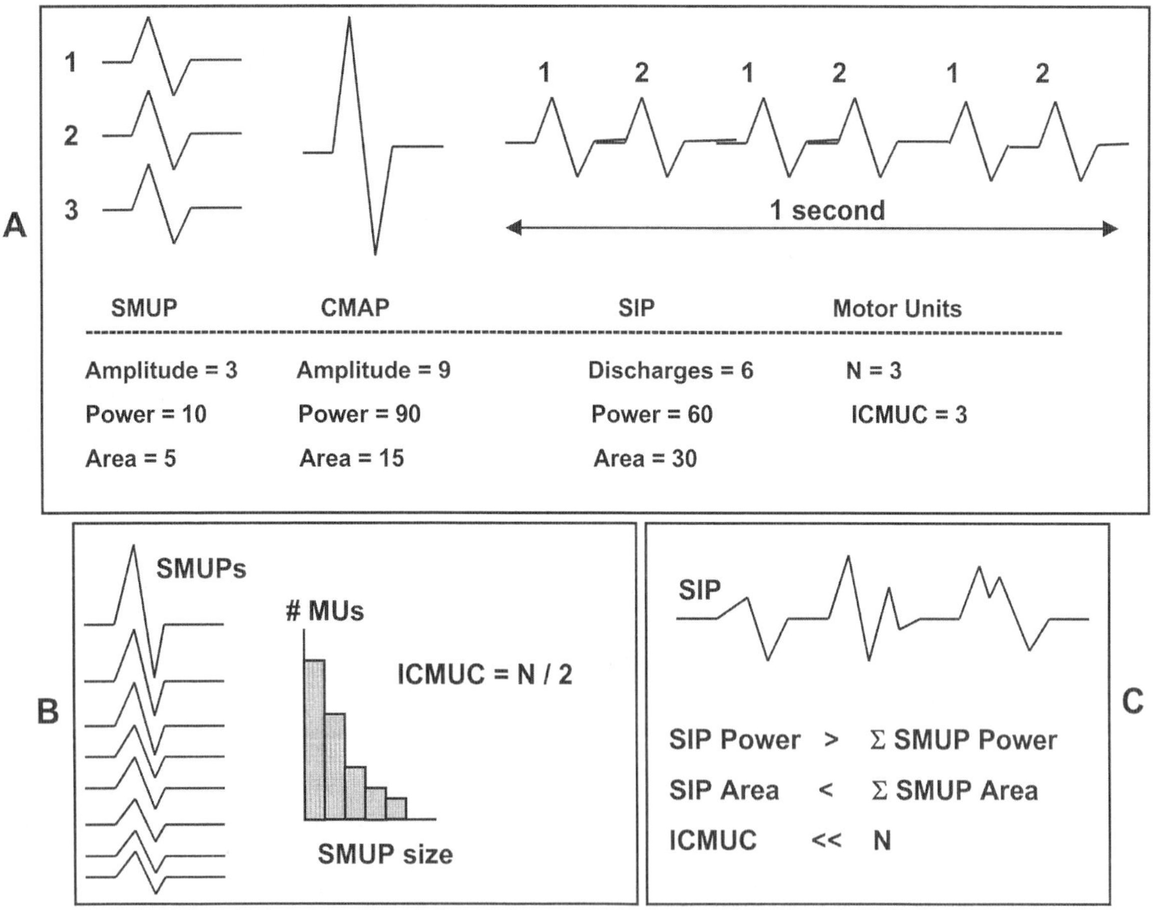

Fig. 8. The theoretical model for MUNIX is explained. (A) "Ideal case" demonstrates that the number of MUs can be estimated by the proposed formula of ICMUC. Arbitrary numerical values are assigned to the SMUP measurements to illustrate the computations based on a muscle with 3 MUs. (B) The variation in SMUP amplitude is modeled by exponential distribution. This adds a scaling factor to the ICMUC formula. (C) Superimposition of SMUPs reduces the ICMUC value significantly compared to the number of motor units.

quantitation. In MUNIX, volume conducted potentials do not appear to have significant effects. The MUNIX is consistently low, as expected, when the CMAP values are significantly reduced (Fig. 3).

Acknowledgements

The first author would like to thank Oxford Instruments for providing support to this project. The third author acknowledges the support in part from Department of Veteran's Affairs. The Center for Academic and Scholastic Achievement (http://www.casaengineering.com) also provided technical support and all illustrations.

References

Armon, C., Brandstater, M.E. and Peterson, G.W. Motor unit number estimates and quantitative muscle strength measurements of distal muscles in patients with amyotrophic lateral sclerosis. *Muscle Nerve*, 1997, 20: 499–501.

Bromberg, M.B. Motor unit estimation: reproducibility of spike triggered averaging technique in normal and ALS subjects. *Muscle Nerve*, 1993, 16: 466–471.

Brown, W.F., Strong, M.J. and Snow, R. Methods for estimating the number of motor units in biceps brachialis muscle and losses of motor units with aging. *Muscle Nerve*, 1988, 11: 423–432.

Daube, J. Estimating the number of motor units in a muscle. *J. Clin. Neurophysiol.*, 1995, 12: 585–594.

Doherty, T.J. and Brown, W.F. The estimated number and relative sizes of thenar motor units as selected by multiple point stimulation in young and older adults. *Muscle Nerve*, 1993, 16: 355–366.

Doherty, T.J. and Brown, W.F. Age related changes in the twitch contractile properties of human thenar motor units. *J. Appl. Physiol.*, 1997, 82: 93–101.

Lomen-Hoerth, C. and Olney, R. Comparison of multi point and statistical motor unit number estimation. *Muscle Nerve*, 2000, 23: 1525–1533.

McComas, A.J. Motor unit estimation: anxieties and achievements. *Muscle Nerve*, 1995, 18: 369–379.

Nandedkar S.D. and Barkhaus P.E. Estimation of number of motor units in human muscle. *Proc. IEEE/9th Annual Conf. of EMBS*, Boston, 1987, 1999–2000.

Shahani, B.T., Fang, J. and Shand, W.R. A new approach to motor unit estimation with surface EMG triggered averaging. *Muscle Nerve*, 1995, 18: 1088–1092.

Slawnych, M., Laszlo, C. and Hershler, C. Motor unit estimates obtained using the new "MUESA" method. *Muscle Nerve*, 1996, 19: 626–636.

Stålberg, E., Chu, J., Bril, V., Nandedkar, S., Stalberg, S. and Ericsson, M. Automatic analysis of the EMG interference pattern. *EEG Clin. Neurophysiol.*, 1983, 56: 672–681.

Stashuk, D.W., Doherty, T.J., Kassam, A. and Brown, W. Motor unit number estimates based on the automated analysis of F responses. *Muscle Nerve*, 1994, 17: 881–890.

Stein, R.B. and Yang, J.F. Methods for estimating the number of motor units in human muscles. *Ann. Neurol.*, 1990, 28: 487–495.

Wang, F. and Delwaide, P.J. Number and relative size of thenar motor unitts estimated by an adapted multiple point stimulation method. *Muscle Nerve*, 1995, 18: 969–979.

Appendix

We begin by considering a theoretical model (Fig. 8A) where the individual surface EMG motor unit potentials (SMUPs) are identical for all MUs. Let $m(t)$ be the SMUP waveform, R_{m} is the SMUP area, and P_{m} is its power. The area and power are computed as:

$$R_{\mathrm{m}} = \int Im(t)/\mathrm{d}t, \tag{4}$$

$$P_{\mathrm{m}} = \int I\, m^2(t)\,\mathrm{d}t. \tag{5}$$

In the CMAP, all SMUPs occur together. If there are N MUs in the muscle, the CMAP waveform is $Nm(t)$. It has area of NR_{m} and power of N^2P_{m}. In the SIP recordings, let us assume that Q MUs are discharging at F Hz. Furthermore, the SMUPs do not superimpose. Thus one-second SIP epoch, contains QF MUP discharges. The SIP area is QFR_{m} and SIP power is QFP_{m}. Substituting these relationship in the formula:

$$\mathrm{ICMUC} = \frac{(\mathrm{CMAP\,Power} \times \mathrm{SIP\,Area})}{(\mathrm{CMAP\,Area} \times \mathrm{SIP\,Power})} = \frac{(N^2P_{\mathrm{m}} \times QFR_{\mathrm{m}})}{(NR_{\mathrm{m}} \times QFP_{\mathrm{m}})} = N. \tag{6}$$

In Fig. 8, the model is demonstrated for following values: $N=3$, $R_{\mathrm{m}}=5$, $P_{\mathrm{m}}=10$, $Q=2$ and $F=3$. The results of computations are also indicated.

The "theoretical" conditions may be satisfied at minimal effort in normal muscle, or in muscles with very few MUs. The SMUPs have different amplitudes reflecting the variation in MU size and the distance between the MU and recording electrode. Electrophysiologic studies (Doherty and Brown, 1997) indicate that a muscle has many small MUs, and fewer large MUs (Fig. 8B). If this is modeled as an exponential distribution, it can be shown that ICMUC is equal to half the number of motor units (ICMUC $= N/2$). Finally, when SMUPs superimpose, the resulting signal has less area and more power than the sum of corresponding measurements of component SMUPs (Fig. 8C). This significantly reduces the ICMUC compared to the number of MUs (ICMUC $\ll N$). This pattern based on theoretical considerations is also seen in experimental recordings.

In normal muscle we have high ICMUC values at minimal effort (Fig. 1). When the force is increased, ICMUC decreases. This reflects the variation in SMUP amplitude (Fig. 8B) and the superimposition of SMUPs (Fig. 8C). Since ICMUC depends on the force of contraction, one must standardize force to compare ICMUC among different subjects. This adds complexity to the method of analysis. Many investigators (Stålberg et al., 1983) have used another electromyographic measurement as an indicator of force. We use the SIP area as a measure of force and plot ICMUC against this variable. In concordance with the theoretical model, ICMUC decreases when SIP area increases (Fig. 1C). Their relationship is characterized by Eq. (2). For comparison among subjects, we evaluate Eq. (2) when SIP area is 20 mV ms, i.e. Eq. (3) for MUNIX. The choice of 20 mV ms is somewhat arbitrary. We chose it because it is roughly the area of the negative peak of CMAP in normal thenar muscles. SIP area reaches 20 mV ms at minimal effort where the ideal conditions of the model are better approximated in the experimental recording. Because the analysis is based on regression, we ignore the scalar factor shown in Fig. 8B in the definition of ICMUC.

Discussion after Section IV

Jasper Daube, Rochester, Minnesota

How much time is required to perform conventional and decomposition spike triggered averaging techniques?

Daniel Stashuk, Waterloo, Ontario

It takes about 30 min for each technique, but more data are generated from the decomposition technique.

Richard Lewis, Detroit, Michigan

With the decomposition technique, with fairly full muscle contraction, there are many more motor units active besides the ones that are being decomposed. Is the high level of electrical activity recorded from the surface electrodes problematic?

Daniel Stashuk, Waterloo, Ontario

The process of spike triggered averaging will eliminate contributions from the other motor units. However, as the interference pattern increases, the signal-to-noise ratio also increases and the estimated surface motor unit action potentials will have more baseline noise. You can diminish this to a certain extent by extending the contraction duration; for example the data I showed were from 30-s contractions which included 200–300 triggers, and one could try to increase this up to 500 triggers. However, theoretically, assuming Gaussian noise and so on, it only drops off as the square root of N. So if you go from 100 to 1000 samples, you are only getting a 10-fold increase.

Mark Bromberg, Salt Lake City, Utah

It is my understanding that the decomposition program will not run when only one or two motor units are being recorded.

Daniel Stashuk, Waterloo, Ontario

The software is currently limited to run with an interference pattern consisting of three or more motor units, but theoretically there is no reason why that has to be.

Timothy Doherty, London, Ontario

I have a question for Jack Petajan. You mentioned that there is a relationship between the root mean square of the integrated EMG and muscle force. With the decomposition technique, we have been looking at the degree of contractile effort at which motor units are recruited. We have been using the root mean square as a surrogate measure of force, and I am interested in your thoughts on how linear this relationship is.

Jack Petajan, Salt Lake City, Utah

It depends upon posture and position, but once these are stable, it is linear. In fact, we have used this relationship as a way of determining whether weakness is factitious or whether there is co-contraction of muscles. These factors can be identified because the maximal force will fall well below the force line that is maintained when the muscle lifts different weights. It is very interesting that antigravity power is the origin of that line. There can be errors at either end of the line. The error at the lower end is that you are underestimating the number of motor units if you put a needle in at low forces. As I indicated, 4 ± 1.4 is not the total number of motor units that are firing when you are holding the limb against gravity. At the upper end, you are overestimating the number of motor units because the firing rate has increased substantially, so these two errors in a sense cancel each other. There was a recent report from the American Academy of Neurology Therapeutics and Technology Assessment Subcommittee (*Neurology*, 2000, 55: 171–177) that reviewed the value of integrated rectified EMG in clinical diagnosis. They were very critical because there can be a difference in impedance between various individuals and there are many different recording techniques making it very difficult to make comparisons. However, if you use a ratio, a lot of these errors cancel out.

Ming Chan, Edmonton, Alberta

Let me return to the question of phase cancellation and positive potentials. Phase cancellation of all components occurs naturally in the CMAP, so I think that phase cancellation should occur in the ensemble average. This will be problematic if one includes only negative peak area.

Daniel Stashuk, Waterloo, Ontario

I do not know what most people are doing, but, as Ming was saying, those potentials have contributed to the CMAP. They should be included as a count of one or whatever.

Jasper Daube, Rochester, Minnesota

In the beginning of my talk, I showed a slide of a lumbrical muscle in which there were probably 50 motor unit potentials that you could isolate coming from that muscle by adjusting the position of the stimulating electrode. Theoretically, I agree they should be included. The suggestion is to do something to eliminate them because they are contributing such a small part and trying to count all 50 or so of them is problematic. How are the people who use the multiple point stimulation technique dealing with them? They will not be included if negative area or amplitude are used.

Ken Arasaki, Tokyo, Japan

They will not be included if you are taking arithmetic averages, like summing up all the negative peak areas of each individual waveform. But the preferred way to do it is to take all the individual SMUPs, align them by their onsets, and then determine an average waveform by taking the negative peak area of that average waveform. In this way, you will get the phase cancellation from these positive waves similar to the phase cancellation that they contributed to in the CMAP.

Jeremy Shefner, Syracuse, New York

That means we need special software to do that if it is not built into the system. The question is not just what do you do with these once you get them, it is what do you sample. It has been my impression that people who do multiple point stimulation do not accept units that have a completely positive waveform.

Mark Bromberg, Salt Lake City, Utah

Well personally, I may reject some, but I also try to include some.

Timothy Doherty, London, Ontario

What we have typically done in practice is to use the software that Bill Brown developed that includes the ability to accept a "null" and an "all" response. In cases where there is a positive baseline potential, which could be generated by a lumbrical or something distant from the active, it is considered the "null". The null is subtracted from the next response, the "all", generated at a higher stimulation intensity that includes a negative onset. In my own experience, potentials that have a small positive onset phase followed by a nice negative phase have been accepted, but potentials that are long lazy positive responses are rejected by calling them the null baseline and subtracting them from the next response. I think the long lazy positive potentials are what Jasper is talking about, and not those with a small positive early component.

Alan McComas, Hamilton, Ontario

My comments are very much in line with those of Ming and Dan. Unless you particularly want to have an estimate which is based on the lumbricals, you just have to get rid of them and, nine times out of 10, you can just by moving the stimulating cathode lateral and closer to the base of the thumb. If you still cannot get rid of them and you are not interested in the lumbricals, then give up. Now, there are other muscles where you cannot avoid some positive contributions. This applies particularly to the plantar muscles, the soleus and sometimes the hypothenar muscles. There, I think you have to go with the philosophy of Ming and Dan that if the positive components are fairly equally represented in the aggregate of your sample and in the shape of your CMAP, then it is quite legitimate to accept them in your calculations.

Jasper Daube, Rochester, Minnesota

It sounds like there is a diversity of opinion that is not going to be solved here. I would suggest that each of us continue to do whatever we think is appropriate, but specific in any publication whether you included or excluded positive potentials.

Mark Bromberg, Salt Lake City, Utah

Are there additional comments on the size of the smallest acceptable potential?

Timothy Doherty, London, Ontario

I think that is a very reasonable, based upon my multiple point stimulation experience that it is very rare to see a unit much smaller than 10 μV. I have data showing the distribution and how much those small units impact on the CMAP. It is their number and not their size that is important with regard to how much impact they had on the CMAP.

Mark Bromberg, Salt Lake City, Utah

I agree that small potentials have a minimal impact after I looked at their effect as spurious triggers in the spike triggered averaging technique.

Ming Chan, Edmonton, Alberta

I am wondering, instead of specifying specific size values for everybody to follow, whether it may not be a more rational to state the smallest unit that cannot be exempted based on baseline noise. That would influence whether someone can reliably and confidently distinguish an action potential from the noise. I think that is the rationale used in single fiber EMG when the spike has to be bigger than a certain amplitude because anything smaller than that cannot be reliably distinguished.

Mark Bromberg, Salt Lake City, Utah

What are our feelings about the number of single motor units that should be sampled to calculate the average potential, at least 10?

Jasper Daube, Rochester, Minnesota

Several presentations have shown that when you reach a certain number of SMUPs, it does not add much to go beyond that. Is there a value of going beyond 20 or 25? Michael, do you have comments?

Michael Slawnych, Calgary, Alberta

It depends on what kind of distribution you are dealing with, so I cannot give you a single number. I think if you take the approach that Tim and others have used of making subestimates from your sample to see how the number affects your MUNE value you can arrive at what a reasonable number is. However, the more, the better.

Mark Bromberg, Salt Lake City, Utah

One quick comment, in patients ALS who are at the end-stages, they may only have two or three or four units. I think we have to make it that clear that there are certain circumstances where it is not possible to record 10 units.

Jasper Daube, Rochester, Minnesota

With the statistical technique, I do not think you would want to suggest that you have to do 10 different stimulus current levels to acquire your data. The phrasing needs to be clear that different rules apply for statistical sampling.

Mark Bromberg, Salt Lake City, Utah

For the question of how to express reproducibility, if we had a roomful of biostatisticians, we would probably get a roomful of different answers. For simple test–retest reproducibility, it can be expressed as the absolute value of the test value minus the retest value divided by the mean of the test and retest values. It can be expressed as a number or it can be multiplied by 100. We need to come up with something for other types of reliability assessment, such as taking the same subject and testing them multiple times. I think the question has to be posed by somebody who is working in the field, because a statistician is not necessarily going to know the kind of environment and the kind of things that we are looking for. So, if you want to approach this question with your statisticians, that would be good.

Timothy Doherty, London, Ontario

I put forward the suggestion, and open for discussion, that the stimulating and recording electrodes be removed and replaced, and the retest be done without knowledge of the first estimate. This will be the situation if a test is repeated weeks, months, years later. There may be situations where for a specific research interest you want to look at the variability from run to run or test to test with the electrodes in the same position, but to answer this question of reproducibility, I think it should be the former.

Mark Bromberg, Salt Lake City, Utah

There are lot of different questions an investigator asks, and I think that is a good point that we need to be very clear what question we are asking. I think these are the main subjects or topics related to a consensus. Hopefully, by the time the proceedings are published, there will be internal agreement as far as guidelines, there will be a number of clinical trials for experience, and we will approach that method in that way.

Section V

MUNE in Normal Subjects

Motor Unit Number Estimation (Supplements to Clinical Neurophysiology Vol. 55)
Editor: M.B. Bromberg

Chapter 15

Establishing normal MUNE values

Victoria H. Lawson*

Department of Neurology, University of Utah, North Medical Drive, Room 3R210, Salt Lake City, UT 84132, USA

Introduction

One of the problems facing investigators using the motor unit number technique (MUNE) is establishing normal reference values from which to make comparisons in disease states. All MUNE techniques have theoretical limitations and assumptions, hence, its name, motor unit number *estimates* rather than motor unit counts. In animal experiments, the distribution of muscle fibers that make up a single motor unit can be visualized using the glycogen depletion method (Kugelberg and Edstrom, 1968), but the number of motor units in the pool innervating the muscle cannot be determined. This makes establishing a gold standard of "normal" motor unit count values challenging. This chapter will review the efforts that have been made to establish these values for MUNE and the difficulties that remain in assigning normal values.

Human anatomic studies

To accept a value as representing "normal", it must have attributes of both *accuracy* and *precision*. Accuracy reflects the degree to which the electrophysiologic measure represents the actual motor unit count, and is subject to observer and instrument bias in addition to biologic variation. Precision reflects the reproducibility of the measure, and is also subject to observer and instrument bias.

To assess accuracy, we may look to human anatomic studies to verify the electrophysiologic measures. Cadaveric studies, however, also require assumptions to obtain an estimate of motor unit counts. Histologic classifications of nerve fibers are based on the difference in diameters between afferent and efferent fibers, and on an estimate of the overlap of afferent diameters in the efferent range. In mixed nerves, an estimate of 40% of large diameter fibers has been considered afferent (Feinstein et al., 1955) based on animal studies (Sherrington, 1894; Eccles and Sherrington, 1930; Rexed and Therman, 1948) and on human de-efferentation studies following old poliomyelitis (Fex and Wohlfart, 1954). Feinstein and colleagues used this proportion in deriving anatomic estimates of the number of efferent fibers in a number of motor nerves. They measured nerve fiber diameters to several different muscles (platysma, brachioradialis, first dorsal interosseous, first lumbrical, anterior tibialis, and the medial head of the gastrocnemius) and found most nerves had a bimodal distribution of diameters (in agreement with previous studies of Eccles and Sherrington, 1930).

**Correspondence to*: V.H. Lawson, Department of Neurology, University of Utah, UT 84132, USA. Tel.: 801-581-6871.
e-mail: victoria.lawson@hsc.utah.edu

doi:10.1016/S1567-424X(03)00015-1

This allowed them to identify a minimum diameter for each muscle above which fibers would be considered large. Based on cross sectional photomicrographs of nerve, counts of the large diameter fibers, less 40% for afferent fibers, gives an estimate of the number of motor units. Using this method, Feinstein and colleagues derived the human anatomic motor unit estimates shown in Table 1.

The 60% proportion of large axons that can be considered motor rather than sensory, however, was challenged by the studies of Boyd and Davey (1968) in muscles of the mammalian hindlimb. These authors found that the proportion of large axons that were alpha motoneurons ranged from 40 to 70%. McComas et al. (1971) counted fibers in the lateral terminal branch of the deep peroneal nerve ($n=2$). They used an estimate of 50% (based on the work of Cooper, 1966) of the fibers greater than 8 μm representing alpha motoneurons, and obtained anatomic counts of 365 and 280 for the EDB (see Table 2). They highlighted the problems of establishing a bimodal distribution of fiber diameters in a nerve and confidently estimating the proportion of large myelinated fibers that represent alpha motoneurons. Lee et al. (1975, see Table 2) converted conduction velocities of alpha motoneurons to fiber diameters of 8.3–11.8 μm, then used 50% of fibers greater than 8.3 μm to derive anatomic counts in the recurrent median nerve of cadavers. This approach circumvents the need for a bimodal distribution but still does not clearly verify that the axons counted represent motor axons.

TABLE 1

ANATOMIC MOTOR UNIT ESTIMATES
(Feinstein et al., 1955)

Muscle	Motor unit estimates
Platysma	1096
Brachioradialis	333[a]
First dorsal interosseous	119
First lumbrical	96[b]
Anterior tibialis	445
Medial head of gastrocnemius	579

[a] Mean of left and right sides in one individual.
[b] Mean of two individuals.

An additional problem that exists for both the electrophysiologic and the anatomic methods is the presence of terminal branching of motor nerve fibers. In an effort to avoid overestimation of the anatomic motor unit count, Feinstein examined more distal sections to evaluate the extent of terminal branching of motor nerve fibers to a different muscle than the one under study. Relatively little branching was found in the nerves to proximal and intermediate muscles (< 1%). However, considerable branching was noted in the distal part of the first dorsal interosseous muscle (37.1% over 3 mm). This suggests that the anatomic estimate made for the first dorsal interosseous and perhaps other distally innervated muscles subject to branching may be an overestimate of the actual motor unit count.

Biologic variability

Another issue is whether individual biologic variability is present in counts obtained histologically, as has been noted in counts obtained electrophysiologically (McComas, 1995). At least two independent reports (Brown et al., 1988; Bromberg, 1993) have described reproducible normal outliers in the Biceps Brachialis muscle by electrophysiologic MUNE. Swallow (1966) found a

TABLE 2

ELECTROPHYSIOLOGIC AND ANATOMIC COUNTS IN HUMANS

Study	Muscle	Electrophysiologic count	Anatomic count
McComas et al. (1971)	Extensor digitorum brevis	199 ± 60[a]	323
Lee et al. (1975)	Thenar muscles	167 ± 16[b]	203

[a] Incremental stimulation MUNE technique.
[b] Spike triggered averaging MUNE technique.

threefold difference in the numbers of nerve fibers in the medial terminal branch of the deep peroneal nerve by anatomic counts. Although the variability between individuals in the MUNE derived electrophysiologically for a specific muscle may in part be due to sampling and technical bias, there exist clear inter-individual biologic differences. These issues have led to attempts to derive a more direct count in animal studies.

Animal studies

Eisen et al. (1974) used the incremental stimulation MUNE technique to obtain estimates in rat soleus and compared these estimates to those derived anatomically from the nerve to the soleus. This was done in normal rats, prior to and after an acute myopathic or neuropathic (after crush or section and re-structure of the sciatic nerve) injury to the solei muscles. Anatomic estimates were obtained by taking one-half of the number of myelinated fibers to the right of the dip in the bimodal distribution of the nerve (that is, greater than 5.5 μm). The authors found good agreement between the estimates obtained using the electrophysiologic and the anatomic method in the normal and neuropathic models (Table 3).

Although the estimates derived electrophysiologically using the incremental stimulation technique and those derived anatomically are very close, the electrophysiologic estimate is larger. This is consistent with expected overestimation by MUNE due to sampling bias with exclusion of large amplitude units (Feasby and Brown, 1974; Brown and Milner-Brown, 1976) and to alternation. Despite these theoretical limitations and the requirement for separate assumptions in deriving an anatomic and physiologic estimate, the numbers are very similar in controlled animal experiments.

TABLE 3

MOTOR UNIT ESTIMATES DERIVED BY ANATOMIC AND ELECTROPHYSIOLOGIC TECHNIQUES IN RAT SOLEUS MUSCLE
(Eisen et al., 1974)

Technique	Normal	Myopathic	Neuropathic
Anatomic	30 ± 4		15 ± 6
Electrophysiologic	32.6 ± 2.5	31.2 ± 5.4	17 ± 8

In an effort to obtain an anatomic estimate that does not depend on the assumptions of Feinstein's studies, Peyronnard and Lamarre (1977) performed the incremental MUNE technique in the extensor digitorium brevis muscle in addition to histologic counts of the peroneal nerve of monkeys after de-afferentation at the level of the L5, L6, L7, and S1 dorsal roots. The absence of large myelinated afferent fibers after de-afferentation was confirmed by histologic examination of a sensory branch of the nerve, and myelinated fiber counts in the motor branch revealed a clearly bimodal distribution. In the de-afferented nerves, the anatomic estimates were above the mean MUNE values but were consistently within the range of the electrophysiologic estimates. The average difference in four of the five animals was 9%, with one animal having a MUNE that was 25% lower than the anatomic estimate, and this was attributed to overestimation of the histologic count due to axonal branching. In the normal nerves, the anatomic estimates were also consistently greater than the mean MUNE value, but only by 12% on average in three of the five animals; the remaining two animals had MUNE values 28 and 39% lower than the anatomic estimates. The larger discrepancy in these animals was thought due to axonal branching (with motor axons from the peroneal nerve running through the extensor digitorum muscle to innervate interosseous muscles). Although the anatomic–physiologic correlation appears relatively close in both groups, it is based on a small number of animals, and was not tested for statistical significance. Further, the presence of alternation in the incremental stimulation technique will overestimate the physiologic count, raising the concern that the difference between the two methods is actually greater than is appreciated from these numbers. This difference may be due to axonal branching although the authors reported serial counts of the large myelinated fibers remaining fairly stable over distances of 30 mm from the entry of the nerve into the muscle.

Arasaki et al. (1997) avoided the assumptions of the anatomic method and the difficulty of axonal branching, and used immunohistochemical staining of cholera toxin in spinal alpha motor neurons after injection of the toxin into the innervated muscle (medial gastrocnemius) in rats. Alpha motor neurons, identified in the lumbar spinal cord by the presence of retrogradely transported cholera toxin, were differentiated from gamma motor neurons by soma size. This allowed a more direct means of obtaining an anatomic count. These counts were compared to MUNE values obtained using mechanical tension and by stimulation of teased single motor axons in the lumbar ventral root. In addition to comparing MUNE values obtained using EMG and using mechanical tension, the authors compared the electrophysiologic MUNE values derived from the arithmetic average of individual single motor unit areas (unprocessed EMG) and those derived from the area of a waveform digitally averaged from the individual units (digitally averaged EMG). The MUNE values obtained by tension (117 ± 21) were not statistically different (using a paired *t*-test, $P > 0.05$) from the digitally averaged MUNE (93 ± 22), but were significantly larger (paired *t*-test, $P < 0.01$) than the MUNE obtained by unprocessed EMG (57 ± 11); the physiologic estimates obtained by tension and digitally averaged EMG were not statistically different (Mann–Whitney test, $P > 0.2$) from the anatomic count (103 ± 16). This study is important in establishing the accuracy of MUNE as it is the first to prove that the anatomic counts clearly represent only motor neurons. Further, the authors were able to show good anatomic–physiologic correlation (statistically insignificant differences) with specific MUNE techniques, and to demonstrate a better correlation with a digitally averaged waveform. This was attributed to the presence of phase cancellation in the arithmetic average of single motor unit action potential amplitudes or areas (used as the divisor to the compound motor action potential).

Human MUNE studies

Although the animal studies have been valuable in examining the relationship between electrophysiologic and anatomic estimates, the limitations of human studies unique to the physiologic method of estimating the number of motor units remain. In Arasaki's work, a teased fiber from the ventral root innervating the muscle was stimulated to evoke a single MAP; six of these MAPs were used to obtain an arithmetic or digital average. Given these fibers were selected by the investigators randomly, no systematic sampling bias was likely introduced. However, in human studies, sampling bias is introduced by the geometric and impedance relationships between the surface location of the stimulating electrode and current fields activating motor nerve axons (incremental stimulation, multiple point stimulation as well as statistical techniques), and by the use of voluntary contraction to recruit motor units (spike triggered averaging technique). Feasby and Brown (1974) showed that stimulation techniques exclude large amplitude units and therefore introduce bias because of a change in activation order with neuropathies; the exclusion of larger units will overestimate the MUNE. Further, contraction methods are also biased toward selecting smaller units as described by the size principle of voluntary recruitment (Henneman et al., 1965a). According to the Henneman size principle smaller units are activated before larger ones in a contraction, again producing an overestimation of the MUNE. Although these limitations are difficult to avoid, it is not clear whether this will introduce bias differentially among normals and among disease processes.

With these limitations in mind, we can return to an assessment of cumulative data in normal individuals. Shefner (2001) and McComas (1995) summarized data on normal thenar muscles in subjects from a number of laboratories using different MUNE techniques. The averages for each technique are presented in Table 4. These electrophysiologic estimates are larger than the anatomic estimates derived by Feinstein for the first dorsal interosseous (119) and the first lumbrical (96) muscles, or by Lee et al. (1975) for the median nerve (203). These discrepancies may be a result of theoretical and practical limitations of MUNE techniques. However, McComas (1995) provides an alternate explanation that is more plausible, at least in the small hand muscles, for MUNE techniques that rely on nerve

TABLE 4

CUMULATIVE DATA ON THENAR MUNE FROM DIFFERENT LABORATORIES (SHEFNER, 2001; MCCOMAS, 1995)

	IST	STA	F-wave	Poisson	MPS
Shefner, 2001					
Mean MUNE	270.4	151	266		251
MUNE/2.5	108.2		106.4		100.4
Number of labs	5	3	3		4
McComas, 1995					
Mean MUNE	342	135		315	288
MUNE/2.5	136.8			126	115.2
Number of labs	1	1		1	1

stimulation. The nerve being stimulated innervates multiple muscles (four, in the case of the hypothenar group; two, with part of a third, in the thenar). If we assume that each muscle is receiving approximately equal innervation, a single intrinsic hand muscle will have, based on this data, between 100 and 137 units, with most estimates falling in the range of 100–120. This is in good agreement with the data obtained in Feinstein's study.

MUNE reproducibility in humans

In the absence of standard normal values, inter- and intra-rater reliability may be evaluated for reproducibility. Given the variability introduced from sampling a population of units, it is valuable to demonstrate that MUNE values on two separate occasions are not significantly different when the true value is unchanged. This reproducibility is essential to the utility of the technique.

Figure 1 shows MUNE values obtained in the thenar muscle group using different techniques by different laboratories. There appears to be reasonably good agreement between the groups within each technique suggesting that inter-rater variability will not have a significant impact on MUNE variability. Intra-rater reliability has been assessed using test–retest studies Doherty and Brown (1993) tested control subjects twice using the multiple point stimulation technique on the thenar muscle group which included changing electrodes between tests. Ten different surface recorded potentials were sampled and the test–retest MUNE was found to be highly correlated ($r = 0.88$). Bromberg (1993) evaluated the spike triggered averaging technique in both control and ALS subjects. As expected, the mean MUNE from the control group was significantly larger ($P = 0.005$) than values from the ALS group, and test–retest values were not significantly different in either group (control, $P = 0.72$; ALS, $P = 0.27$). The correlation coefficient in the control group was higher ($r = 0.86$) until a single outlier was removed, at which time it dropped to $r = 0.07$. This latter value was lower than the coefficient for the ALS group ($r = 0.65$) and it was speculated to be due to re-sampling of the same units in the smaller population of units in ALS subjects. Lomen-Hoerth and Olney (2000) also performed test–retest MUNE on control and ALS subjects using both the multiple point and statistical techniques. The correlation coefficients were 0.90 and 0.98, respectively. Wang and Delwaide (1995) used the adapted multiple point stimulation technique, and obtained a test–retest coefficient of 0.95 in control subjects. Simmons et al. (2001) made the distinction between reproducibility of a group of test–retest data and reproducibility in an individual. To address this, they derived a prediction interval (that is, the range of values expected on retest if the true number of motor units remained the same) for the individuals to evaluate the reproducibility of the statistical technique. A coefficient of variation (which evaluates the relative variation between two sets of data rather than the correlation between two random variables, as in a correlation coefficient) was

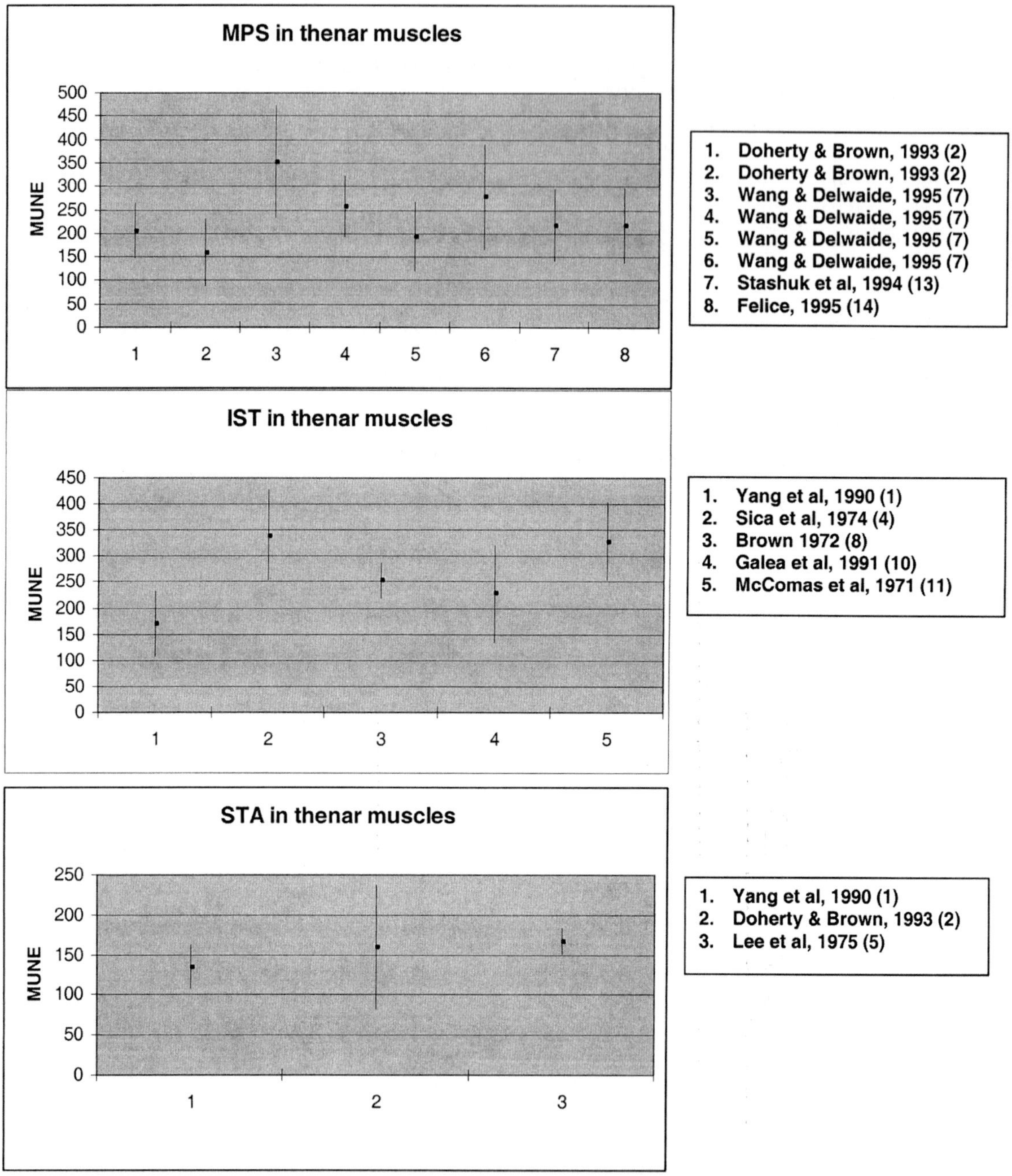

Fig. 1. MUNE values obtained in the thenar muscle group by different laboratories using different techniques.

calculated using the data from 48 individuals (16.48%). By averaging two MUNE values for each determination, weighting averages to calculate an average SMUP size and using a 90% prediction interval (10% false positive rate), the variation was reduced (coefficient of variation 8.77%) and the prediction interval was narrowed to provide the authors with a range that could be used to confirm reproducibility.

Taken together, these data are re-assuring that reasonable reproducibility can be achieved. The data in ALS patients are particularly re-assuring inasmuch as results in this population appear to be even more reproducible than in normal subjects. Thus, despite the assumptions of the various techniques, it can be demonstrated that they can yield a certain degree of precision.

Conclusion

Attempts to establish normal values for MUNE based on anatomic standards have been limited by an inability to clearly establish or recognize the population of nerve fibers that represent motor axons, determine the presence of terminal branching, and the technical difficulties in establishing a bimodal distribution of nerve fibers. Most anatomic data has been obtained in lower extremity or distal muscles. The most definitive anatomic study in humans agrees well with cumulative electrophysiologic data. Unfortunately, anatomic data are not clear enough to establish which MUNE technique is most accurate, and given the assumptions of the anatomic data, does not clearly address the question of biologic variability. This latter concern may be better addressed in animal studies using retrograde labeling as was done in Arasaki's experiments. For these reasons, normal values for MUNE, although influenced by the anatomic data, will likely rely on consistency between laboratories and investigators.

References

Arasaki, K., Tamaki, M., Hosoya, Y. and Kudo, N. Validity of electromyograms and tension as a means of motor unit number estimation. *Muscle Nerve*, 1997, 20(5): 552–560.

Boyd, I.A. and Davey, M.R. *Composition of Peripheral Nerves*. Livingstone, Edinburgh, 1968.

Bromberg, M.B. Motor unit estimation: reproducibility of the spike-triggered averaging technique in normal and ALS subjects. *Muscle Nerve*, 1993, 16(5): 466–471.

Brown, W.F. A method for estimating the number of motor units in thenar muscles and the changes in motor unit count with ageing. *J. Neurol. Neurosurg. Psychiatry*, 1972, 35(6): 845–852.

Brown, W.F. and Milner-Brown, H.S. Some electrical properties of motor units and their effects on the methods of estimating motor unit numbers. *J. Neurol. Neurosurg. Psychiatry*, 1976, 39(3): 249–257.

Brown, W.F., Strong, M.J. and Snow, R. Methods for estimating numbers of motor units in biceps–brachialis muscles and losses of motor units with aging. *Muscle Nerve*, 1988, 11(5): 423–432.

Cooper, S. Muscle spindles and motor units. In *Control and Innervation of Skeletal Muscle* (B.L. Andrew, Ed.), 1966, pp. 9–16. Livingstone, Edinburgh.

Doherty, T.J. and Brown, W.F. The estimated numbers and relative sizes of thenar motor units as selected by multiple point stimulation in young and older adults. *Muscle Nerve*, 1993, 16(4): 355–366.

Eccles, J.C. and Sherrington, C.S. Numbers and contraction values of individual motor units examined in some muscles of the limb. *Proc. R. Soc. Lond.*, 1930, 106: 326–357.

Eisen, A., Karpati, G., Carpenter, S. and Danon, J. The motor unit profile of the rat soleus in experimental myopathy and reinnervation. *Neurology*, 1974, 24(9): 878–884.

Feasby, T.E. and Brown, W.F. Variation of motor unit size in the human extensor digitorum brevis and thenar muscles. *J. Neurol. Neurosurg. Psychiatry*, 1974, 37(8): 916–926.

Feinstein, B., Lindegard, B., Nyman, E. and Wohlfart, G. Morphologic studies of motor units in normal human muscles. *Acta Anat.*, 1955, 23: 127–142.

Felice, K.J. Thenar motor unit number estimates using the multiple point stimulation technique: reproducibility studies in ALS patients and normal subjects. *Muscle Nerve*, 1995, 18(12): 1412–1416.

Galea, V., de Bruin, H., Cavasin, R. and McComas, A.J. The numbers and relative sizes of motor units estimated by computer. *Muscle Nerve*, 1991, 14(11): 1123–1130.

Henneman, E., Somjen, G. and Carpenter, D.O. Excitability and inhibitability of motoneurons of different sizes. *J. Neurophysiol.*, 1965a, 28(3): 599–620.

Henneman, E., Somjen, G. and Carpenter, D.O. Functional significance of cell size in spinal motoneurons. *J. Neurophysiol.*, 1965b, 28: 560–580.

Kugelberg, E.E.L. Differential histochemical effects of muscle contractions on phosphorylase and glycogen in various types of fibres: relation to fatigue. *J. Neurol. Neurosurg. Psychiatry*, 1968, 31(5): 415–423.

Lee, R.G., Ashby, P., White, D.G. and Aguayo, A.J. Analysis of motor conduction velocity in the human median nerve by computer simulation of compound muscle action potentials. *Electroencephalogr. Clin. Neurophysiol.*, 1975, 39(3): 225–237.

Lomen-Hoerth, C. and Olney, R.K. Comparison of multiple point and statistical motor unit number estimation. *Muscle Nerve*, 2000, 23(10): 1525–1533.

McComas, A.J. Motor unit estimation: anxieties and achievements. *Muscle Nerve*, 1995, 18(4): 369–379.

McComas, A.J., Fawcett, P.R., Campbell, M.J. and Sica, R.E. Electrophysiological estimation of the number of motor units within a human muscle. *J. Neurol. Neurosurg. Psychiatry*, 1971, 34(2): 121–131.

Peyronnard, J.M. and Lamarre, Y. Electrophysiological and anatomical estimation of the number of motor units in the monkey extensor digitorum brevis muscle. *J. Neurol. Neurosurg. Psychiatry*, 1977, 40(8): 756–764.

Shefner, J.M. Motor unit number estimation in human neurological diseases and animal models. *Clin. Neurophysiol.*, 2001, 112(6): 955–964.

Sica, R.E., McComas, A.J., Upton, A.R. and Longmire, D. Motor unit estimations in small muscles of the hand. *J. Neurol. Neurosurg. Psychiatry*, 1974, 37(1): 55–67.

Simmons, Z., Epstein, D.K., Borg, B., Mauger, D.T., Kothari, M.J. and Shefner, J.M. Reproducibility of motor unit number estimation in individual subjects. *Muscle Nerve*, 2001, 24(4): 467–473.

Stashuk, D.W., Doherty, T.J., Kassam, A. and Brown, W.F. Motor unit number estimates based on the automated analysis of F-responses. *Muscle Nerve*, 1994, 17(8): 881–890.

Swallow, M. Fibre size and content of the anterior tibial nerve of the foot. *J. Neurol. Neurosurg. Psychiatry*, 1966, 30: 205–213.

Wang, F.C. and Delwaide, P.J. Number and relative size of thenar motor units estimated by an adapted multiple point stimulation method. *Muscle Nerve*, 1995, 18(9): 969–979.

Yang, J.F., Stein, R.B., Jhamandas, J. and Gordon, T. Motor unit numbers and contractile properties after spinal cord injury. *Ann. Neurol.*, 1990, 28(4): 496–502.

Motor Unit Number Estimation (Supplements to Clinical Neurophysiology Vol. 55)
Editor: M.B. Bromberg

Chapter 16

Are motor and sensory responses and MUNE values inherited traits?

Catherine Lomen-Hoerth* and Richard K. Olney

Department of Neurology, University of California, San Francisco, San Francisco, CA 94114, USA

Introduction

Although 90–95% of amyotrophic lateral sclerosis (ALS) cases are sporadic without known etiology and distal symmetric polyneuropathy is commonly idiopathic, hereditary single-gene forms of both diseases are well described (Schenone and Mancardi, 1999; Orrell and Figlewicz, 2001) One hypothesis of the etiology of these diseases is that they are complex genetic diseases in which multiple genes contribute to disease susceptibility. Demonstrating that sensory and motor responses and MUNE are heritable traits would support this hypothesis. A standard method to determine heritability is to compare monozygotic with dizygotic twins. Greater similarity in the trait in monozygotic twins compared with dizygotic twins supports heritability (Piccini et al., 1999; Tanner et al., 2001).

**Correspondence to*: Dr. Catherine Lomen-Hoerth, Department of Neurology, University of California, San Francisco, 505 Parnassus Ave., M348, San Francisco, CA 94114, USA. Tel.: (415) 514-0490, Fax: (415) 514-0491.
e-mail: cathylh@itsa.ucsf.edu

doi:10.1016/S1567-424X(03)00016-3

Methods

Subjects

Twenty-six healthy twin pairs gave informed consent and were enrolled in the study based on their response to a letter sent to all members of the Northern California Twin Registry. We obtained prior approval by our Institutional Review Board. The ages of the twins ranged from 20 to 75. All subjects underwent a neuromuscular history and examination prior to starting testing. One set of twins was excluded due to one twin having diabetes with peripheral nerve involvement, and another set of twins was excluded due to one of the twins having AIDS with peripheral nerve involvement. The remaining 24 twins (7 dizygotic and 17 monozygotic) were analyzed in the study. Two dizygotic twin pairs and one monozygotic twin pair were unable to tolerate the MUNE portion of the study and the studies were terminated prematurely.

Electrophysiological techniques

Bilateral antidromic ulnar and sural sensory nerve conduction studies were performed. Bilateral ulnar and peroneal motor nerve conduction studies were performed with surface stimulation and recording from the hypothenar muscle group and extensor digitorum brevis muscle, respectively. F-wave responses were determined from the peroneal nerve in a standard fashion. The results were averaged for each nerve studied. Motor unit number estimation (MUNE) of the left hypothenar muscle was determined using the weighted statistical method (Shefner et al., 1999). Mean surface recorded motor unit action potential (SMUP) amplitude was measured at several stimulus levels, typically spanning 40% or more of the compound muscle action potential (CMAP) amplitude range. MUNE was calculated by dividing the maximum CMAP amplitude by the weighted mean SMUP amplitude (Lomen-Hoerth and Olney, 2000). Quantitative sensory testing was performed on CASE IV with 4-2-1 algorithm for vibration the cooling detection threshold on bilateral feet and the results were averaged (Dyck et al., 1993).

Statistical analysis

T-tests was used to compare the coefficients of variation between pairs of monozygotic versus dizygotic twins for all electrophysiological tests. A result was considered significant for $P < 0.05$.

Results

Sensory nerve action potentials

Ulnar sensory nerve action potentials (SNAPs) ranged in amplitude from 10 to 76 μV, conduction velocities (CV) ranged from 36 to 54, and distal latencies (DL) ranged from 2.3 to 2.95. Sural SNAP amplitudes ranged from 0 to 43 μV, CV ranged from 36 to 54, and DL ranged from 2.7 to 3.5. The coefficient of variation for dizygotic versus monozygotic was 95 versus 88% ($P < 0.08$) for ulnar SNAP amplitude, 29 versus 4.5% ($P < 0.05$), for ulnar CV, and 7 versus 4% ($P < 0.15$) for DL. The coefficient of variation for dizygotic versus monozygotic was 31 versus 19% ($P < 0.37$) for the sural SNAP amplitude, 8 versus 3.5% ($P < 0.04$) for sural CV, and 68 versus 35% ($P < 0.06$) for DL. Thus, for sensory responses, ulnar and sural sensory nerve CV and ulnar SNAP amplitude were the only variables identified as statistically significantly different between monozygotic and dizygotic twins.

Compound muscle action potentials

Ulnar CMAPs ranged in amplitude from 6 to 14 mV, CV ranged from 44 to 71, and distal motor latencies (DML) ranged from 2.7 to 3.8. Peroneal CMAP amplitudes ranged from 3.5 to 5.9 mV, CV ranged from 41 to 60, and DML ranged from 3.5 to 5.9. The coefficient of variation for dizygotic versus monozygotic was 10 versus 9% ($P < 0.9$) for ulnar CMAP amplitude, 6 versus 3.6% ($P < 0.16$) for ulnar CV, and 3 versus 6% for ulnar DML ($P < 0.13$). The coefficient of variation for dizygotic versus monozygotic was 40 versus 15% ($P < 0.01$) for peroneal CMAP amplitude, 8 versus 3.7% ($P < 0.01$) for peroneal CV, and 11 versus 5.9% ($P < 0.11$) for peroneal DML. Thus for motor responses, peroneal CMAP amplitude and CV were the only statistically significant differences between monozygotic and dizygotic twins. Ulnar CV was likely not statistically significant due to the decreased variability of the response compared with peroneal CV.

F-waves

Peroneal F-waves performed in a subset of twins (4 dizygotic and 13 monozygotic) ranged in minimum latencies from 40 to 52. The peroneal F-waves had a coefficient of variation of 5.3 versus 3.5% ($P < 0.2$) for dizygotic versus monozygotic twins.

Motor unit number estimates

Hypothenar motor unit number estimates ranged from 46 to 65. The coefficient of variation for dizygotic versus monozygotic twins was 6.3 versus 3.3% ($P < 0.06$), just missing statistically significance, however only 5 of the 7 dizygotic twins and 16 of the 17 monozygotic twins underwent MUNE studies, making the numbers smaller than for the nerve conduction studies. Figure 1 plots the differences in MUNE between monozygotic and dizygotic twins. While the dizygotic numbers are small, the 16 monozygotic twins are tightly clustered together with minimal MUNE differences.

Quantitative sensory testing

The detection thresholds for quantitative sensory testing ranged from 6 to 12 JND for cooling and 11–21 JND for vibration. The coefficient of

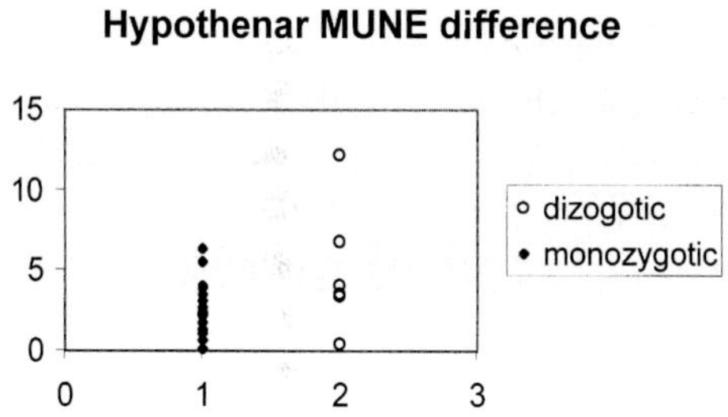

Fig. 1. Plots of the differences in MUNE between dizygotic and monozygotic twins.

variation for dizygotic versus monozygotic twins was 11 versus 9% ($P<0.69$) for vibration and 16 versus 16% ($P<0.99$) for cooling.

Discussion

Because MUNE values and motor and sensory nerve CV have at least twice the variation in dizygotic twins compared to monozygotic twins, the results of this study support the notion that the number of sensory and motor axons in normal subjects is an inherited trait. Amplitude and distal latency differences were not statistically significantly different between the two groups, except for ulnar sensory and peroneal motor amplitudes, but trends were noted that could be statistically significant with a larger sample size. Other confounding factors could be weight and sex between the two groups. When twins were of the same sex, weights tended to be very similar between twins for both mono and dizygotic twins. Two of the dizygotic twins were male–female pairs, and when they were removed from the analysis, the trends remained but the statistical significance decreased, in part due to the small sample size of the dizygotic group. With increased numbers of subjects, we will be able to take into account these variables in our comparison and restrict ourselves to same sex twin comparisons. Interestingly, quantitative sensory testing did not reveal differences between dizygotic and monozygotic twins suggesting that this test may be influenced more by environment than genetics. The differences are greater in the lower limbs than the upper limbs, where greater effects of aging are identified with nerve conduction studies. Perhaps there are genetic differences between the rate at which nerve responses and MUNE values decline with aging. These results support the potential heritability of normal motor and sensory responses and motor unit number estimates, supporting the hypothesis that idiopathic neurodegenerative disease may have a complex genetic basis.

Acknowledgements

This work was supported by a grant from the American Academy of Neurology.

References

Dyck, P.J., O'Brien, P.C., Kosanke, J.L., Gillen, D.A. and Karnes, J.L. A 4,2, and 1 stepping algorithm for quick and accurate estimation of cutaneous sensation threshold. *Neurology*, 1993, 43: 1508–1512.

Lomen-Hoerth, C. and Olney, R.K. Comparison of multiple point and statistical motor unit number estimation. *Muscle Nerve*, 2000, 23(10): 1525–1533.

Orrell, R.W. and Figlewicz, D.A. Clinical implications of the genetics of ALS and other motor neuron diseases. *Neurology*, 2001, 57: 9–17.

Piccini, P., Burn, D.J., Ceravolo, R., Maraganore, D. and Brooks, D.J. The role of inheritance in sporadic Parkinson's disease: evidence from a longitudinal study of dopaminergic function in twins. *Ann. Neurol.*, 1999, 45: 577–582.

Schenone, A. and Mancardi, G.L. Molecular basis of inherited neuropathies. *Curr. Opin. Neurol.*, 1999, 12: 603–616.

Shefner, J.M., Jillapalli, D. and Bradshaw, D.Y. Reducing intersubject variability in motor unit number estimation. *Muscle Nerve*, 1999, 22(10): 1457–1460.

Tanner, C.M., Goldman, S.M., Lyons, K.E., Aston, D.A., Tetrud, J.W., Welsh, M.D., Langston, J.W. and Koller, W.C. Essential tremor in twins: an assessment of genetic vs environmental determinants of etiology. *Neurology*, 2001, 57: 1389–1391.

Motor Unit Number Estimation (Supplements to Clinical Neurophysiology Vol. 55)
Editor: M.B. Bromberg

Chapter 17

MUNE measurement of age-related changes

Timothy J. Doherty[a,]*, Daniel W. Stashuk[b] and William F. Brown[c]

[a]*Department of Physical Medicine and Rehabilitation, University of Western Ontario, London, ON N6A 1Y6, Canada*
[b]*Department of Systems Design Engineering, University of Waterloo, Waterloo, ON N2L 3G1, Canada*
[c]*Department of Neurology, Tuft's University, Boston, MA, USA*

Introduction

It is well established that aging is associated with a substantial decline in neuromuscular performance (Grimby and Saltin, 1983; Roos et al., 1997; Doherty et al., 1993a; Doherty, 2001). Characteristic of this decline is the inevitable reduction in skeletal muscle mass and associated loss of strength that occurs even with "healthy" aging. This decline in skeletal muscle mass, termed *sarcopenia*, is considered a major contributing factor to the loss of functional independence and frailty present in many older individuals (Roubenoff, 2000; Roubenoff and Hughes, 2000; Roubenoff, 2001). Age-associated losses of skeletal muscle mass and strength have received considerable attention in the literature over the past two decades. More recent work has begun to focus on underlying factors contributing to sarcopenia, losses in strength and associated functional impairment. This brief review will focus on the impact of age-related MU loss as indicated by MUNEs.

Aging is associated with a number of changes in the motor system. Starting at approximately 30 years-of-age, in the absence of training, strength declines at a rate of about 10–15% per decade (Vandervoort and McComas, 1986). Since typical activities of daily living require only minimal to moderate muscular contractile efforts, this gradual loss of strength does not become functionally significant until beyond 55–60 years of age for most men and women. Beyond about the sixth decade, the rate of force loss may accelerate, but eventually levels off in the seventh and eighth decades such that men and women in this age group have about 50% of the strength of younger adults (Doherty et al., 1993a). In the absence of disease, further losses in the subsequent decades may be no greater than 10%. This level of strength may approach that necessary to carry out the basic activities of daily living, but leaves little or no safety factor for dealing with concomitant illness or leisure activities requiring higher levels of function (Aniansson et al., 1981; Doherty et al., 1993a; Roos et al., 1997; Roubenoff and Hughes, 2000; Roubenoff, 2001).

Age-related decreases in strength have been well documented in numerous studies (Doherty et al., 1993a). A variety of limb muscles have been

**Correspondence to*: Dr. T.J. Doherty, Department of Physical Medicine and Rehabilitation, University of Western Ontario, St. Joseph's Health Centre, 35 Grosvenor St., London, ON N6A 1Y6, Canada. Tel.: (519) 646-6100x65364, Fax: (519) 646-6174.
e-mail: tim.doherty@sjhc.london.on.ca

doi: 10.1016/S1567-424X(03)00016-3

examined in cross-sectional studies during isometric and dynamic conditions in young, middle-aged, and older men and women. In general, results of these studies suggest that reductions in isometric and dynamic voluntary and electrically evoked contractile strength become substantial by the seventh decade of life, and may accelerate thereafter. Healthy men and women in their seventh and eighth decades demonstrate average reductions of 20–40% in maximal isometric strength in comparison to young controls. On balance, similar reductions have been reported for both men and women for both upper and lower limb muscles. There is some indication that greater losses are present at higher contractile velocities during dynamic contractions and that eccentric force production may be better preserved than concentric (Grimby and Saltin, 1983; Vandervoort et al., 1990; Poulin et al., 1992; Doherty et al., 1993a; Roos et al., 1997).

Age-related losses of strength are directly impacted by, and correlated with, losses of skeletal muscle mass. The total muscle cross-sectional area decreases by about 40% between the ages of 20 and 40 (Doherty et al., 1993a; Porter et al., 1995; Roos et al., 1997). Cross-sectional areas have been determined for various limb muscles using ultrasound, computed tomographic scanning, magnetic resonance imaging, and direct measurement of whole muscle cross sections from cadaveric specimens. For example, Young et al. (1985, 1984) using ultrasonographic imaging, reported 25–35% reductions in the cross-sectional areas of the quadriceps muscles in older men and women as compared to young controls. Computed tomographic scanning has shown similar results for the quadriceps muscle (Klitgaard et al., 1990; Overend et al., 1992), the brachial biceps (Rice et al., 1989; Klitgaard et al., 1990) and triceps (Rice et al., 1989) in men. Additionally, highlighting the inaccuracy of simple anthropometric measures of limb circumference, Rice et al. (1989) found 27, 45, and 81% more non-muscle tissue (fat and connective tissue) for the arm flexors, arm extensors and plantarflexors, respectively.

Vandervoort and McComas (1986) cross-sectionally, examined a rather large cohort of young, middle aged and elderly men and women. Maximal voluntary and electrically evoked maximal twitch forces were determined for both the plantar- and dorsiflexor muscles. Men were stronger than women at all ages and aging was associated with substantial declines in force. These changes were similar for men and women and these declines were similar for both evoked and voluntary contractions. Interestingly, when the values for subjects in the youngest and middle-aged (40–52 years) groups were compared the voluntary torques were similar, with only dorsiflexion in men showing a significant decline. In an attempt to determine the extent to which reduced central drive may contribute to reduced volitional torque production, the twitch interpolation technique was used (Belanger and McComas, 1981). An important finding of this study was that most older men and women were able to maximally activate the lower motor neuron pool for maximal force production. Thus, the reduced volitional forces with aging were attributed to less available muscle mass as opposed to decreased central drive and the inability to adequately recruit the available contractile tissue.

In a second cross-sectional study Frontera et al. (1991) examined the isokinetic torque at 60 and 240°/s for the elbow and knee flexors and extensors in 200 healthy men and women between 45 and 78 years of age. Fat free mass was estimated by hydrostatic weighing and muscle mass was determined in 141 subjects from urinary creatinine excretion. Strength was found to be lower for all muscle groups by 15–27% in the older versus younger age group. However, when strength was adjusted for fat free mass or muscle mass, the age-related differences were eliminated for all muscle groups but the knee extensors at 240°/s. The absolute strength of women ranged from about 40 to 60% of men, but these gender differences were eliminated or minimal when strength was expressed per kg of muscle mass. Therefore, in general from these cross-sectional studies, significant and similar losses occur with aging in men and women. These losses of strength are mainly accounted for by reductions in muscle mass. Taking these findings into account, the next obvious question is what is the cause of the age-related atrophy or sarcopenia?

In attempts to understand the underlying cause of age-related atrophy numerous studies have assessed muscle morphology from tissue obtained using muscle biopsy. The majority of these studies have been undertaken on the vastus lateralis muscle and the overall conclusion is reasonably consistent: average type II fiber size is diminished with age while the size of type I fibers is much less affected (Grimby and Saltin, 1983; Lexell et al., 1988; Lexell and Downham, 1992; Lexell, 1993; Doherty et al., 1993a; Roos et al., 1997). While average reductions in type II area range from 20 to 50%, type I fiber area losses range from 1 to 25%. The variability present in the results of these studies relates to sampling variability, and potential bias with muscle biopsy, and the undoubted inherent biologic variability in the both the older and younger control populations.

The above noted reductions in fiber size, however, are moderate in comparison to the reductions in muscle ass, and therefore reductions in muscle fiber number have been proposed as an explanation for sarcopenia. Lexell et al. (1988) using whole muscle cross-sections from the vastus lateralis obtained post-mortem, reported that by the ninth decade approximately 50% fewer type I and type II fibers were present in comparison to post-mortem tissue obtained from 20 year olds. The fact that similar losses of muscle fibers were present for type I and II fibers stood in contrast to earlier work from muscle biopsy tissue. Further analysis determined that the cross-sectional area of the vastus lateralis, at least, is mainly determined by the total number of fibers and, to a much lesser extent, by the size/and or number of type II fibers (Lexell and Downham, 1992; Lexell et al., 1988).

Thus, it appears that the age-related atrophy, at least for the vastus lateralis muscle is largely dependent on age-related losses of muscle fibers, and less so on atrophy of the remaining fibers. Electrophysiolgic studies, including motor unit number estimation (MUNE) have subsequently shed light on the underlying cause for muscle fiber losses. Earlier studies using the manual incremental stimulation technique indicated significant decline in MU numbers beyond 60 years of age for distal muscles (Table 1). For example, Campbell et al. (1973) reported significant reductions in MUNE values for the EDB in those over 60 years with mean values approaching 50% of control estimates. Brown (1972), Sica et al. (1974) reported similar declines for hand muscles. Our own more recent work has provided similar results for both proximal and distal muscles.

Results

We used the multiple point stimulation (MPS) technique to determine MUNE values for the median innervated thenar muscles in a group of younger (20–40 years) and older (60–80 years) healthy subjects (Doherty and Brown, 1993). As shown in Table 2, the maximum compound muscle action potential (CMAP) sizes were significantly reduced in the older group (about 30%), while the mean single motor unit potential (S-MUP) sizes were significantly larger (about 35%; Fig. 1). MUNE

TABLE 1

AGE-RELATED CHANGES IN MEAN MUNE VALUES

Authors	Muscle groups	Younger age	Older age (> 60 years)
Brown (1972)	Thenar	253 ± 34	< 120
Campbell et al. (1973)	Extensor digitorum brevis	198 ± 58	< 120
Sica et al. (1974)	Thenar	340 ± 87	83 ± 46
	Hypothenar	380 ± 79	177 ± 54
Doherty and Brown (1993)	Thenar	288 ± 95	139 ± 68
Doherty et al. (1993a,b)	Biceps/brachiallis	357 ± 87	189 ± 77

TABLE 2

AGE-RELATED CHANGES IN THENAR MUNE AND TWITCH TENSIONS

Test	Age (20–40 years)	Age (60–80 years)
Maximum CMAP		
Negative peak area (mV ms)	38.2 ± 10.1	25.9 ± 8.4
Average S-MUP		
Negative peak area (μV ms)	145 ± 60	229 ± 132
MUNE	288 ± 95	139 ± 68
Twitch tension		
mN	8.8 ± 7.4	13.4 ± 10.4

Adapted from Doherty and Brown (1993,1997).

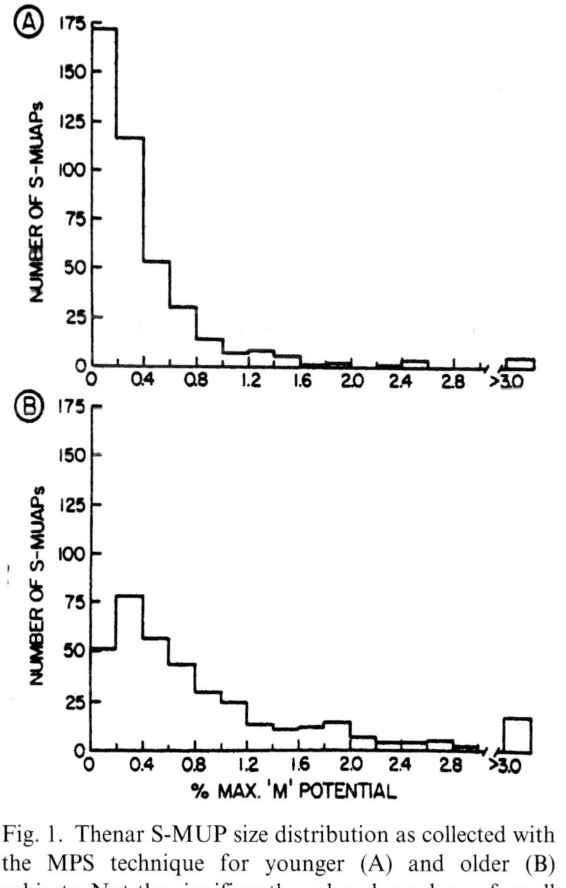

Fig. 1. Thenar S-MUP size distribution as collected with the MPS technique for younger (A) and older (B) subjects. Not the significantly reduced numbers of small S-MUPs in the older subjects.

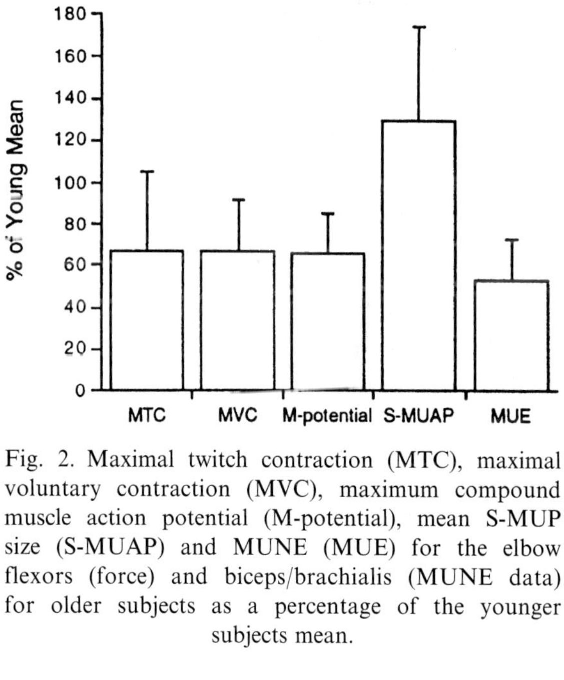

Fig. 2. Maximal twitch contraction (MTC), maximal voluntary contraction (MVC), maximum compound muscle action potential (M-potential), mean S-MUP size (S-MUAP) and MUNE (MUE) for the elbow flexors (force) and biceps/brachialis (MUNE data) for older subjects as a percentage of the younger subjects mean.

values, as a result, were reduced by about 50% on average in the older subjects. Twitch tensions for MUs collected by MPS were similarly increased in the older subjects (Doherty and Brown, 1997).

In the biceps brachii/brachialis of older subjects significant reductions in the maximum CMAP were accompanied by larger average S-MUP sizes, as determined by the STA method (Doherty et al., 1993b). These findings resulted in similar 50% reductions in the MUNE values for this muscle group. In this case, the 30% reductions in the average maximal CMAP were similar to the reduced maximal twitch tensions and maximal voluntary contractile forces noted in the older subjects (Fig. 2).

Discussion

These and other studies have supported the notion that aging is associated with significant losses of motor units or motor neurons and that such losses of MUs, in conjunction with incomplete reinnervation result in the aforementioned losses of muscle fibers and muscle mass. The results of electrophsyiological studies are additionally supported by anatomic studies wherein fewer motor neurons and ventral root fibers were present with ageing (Kawamura et al., 1977; Tomlinson and Irving, 1977). Results of macro EMG studied have provided similar results with significantly larger values reported for older subjects (De Koning et al., 1988; Stålberg et al., 1989). Alternatively, it is noteworthy that very modest age-related changes in the typical needle EMG indices such as amplitude, duration and phases have been reported (Buchtal and Rosenfalck, 1955).

A remaining important question relates to the relationship between the reported losses of MUs based on MUNE – on the order of 50% in most studies – and the rather modest changes noted with ageing in standard needle EMG of control muscles. One explanation for this observation is that the standard needle examination may be insensitive to MU losses of this extent. It has been previously established that the CMAP and muscle strength are relatively well maintained until substantial losses of MUs, perhaps as high as 70%, have occurred (Brown, 1973). There are little data indicating the extent to which the standard needle study will remain subjectively "normal" in the face of such MU losses. Thus, the needle examination may be insensitive to the changes reported in MU populations with normal aging. Further understanding of these relationships will require longitudinal studies combining MUNE, standard, and quantitative EMG techniques.

Summary

Aging is associated with significant declines in muscle strength, which are for the most part secondary to losses of muscle mass. The loss of muscle mass is mainly accounted for by losses of muscle fibers which appear secondary to MU losses. MUNE has significantly contributed to our understanding of the extent to which the MU pool is altered and adapts to aging. In general, proximal and distal muscles appear to have significantly fewer, but larger MUs. On balance, average MUNE values in groups over 60 years of age show reductions of about 50% in comparison to younger controls. Whether this decline is modifiable or an inherent age-related process will require well-planned longitudinal study.

References

Aniansson, A., Grimby, G., Hedberg, H. and Krotkiewski, M. Muscle morphology, enzyme activity, and muscle strength in elderly men and women. *Clin. Physiol.*, 1981, 1: 73–86.

Belanger, A.Y. and McComas, A.J. Extent of motor unit activation during effort. *J. Appl. Physiol.*, 1981, 51: 1131–1135.

Brown, W.F. A method for estimating the number of motor units in thenar muscles and the changes in motor unit count with ageing. *J. Neurol. Neurosurg. Psychiatry*, 1972, 35: 845–852.

Brown, W.F. Functional compensation of human motor units in healthy and disease. *J. Neurol. Sci.*, 1973, 20: 199.

Buchtal, F. and Rosenfalck, P. Action potential parameters in different human muscles. *Acta Physiol. Scand.*, 1955, 30: 125–131.

Campbell, M.J., McComas, A.J. and Petito, F. Physiological changes in ageing muscles. *J. Neurol. Neurosurg. Psychiatry*, 1973, 36: 174–182.

De Koning, P., Wieneke, G.H., van der Most van Spijk, D., van Huffelen, A.C., Gispen, W.H. and Jennekens, F.G. Estimation of the number of motor units based on macro-EMG. *J. Neurol. Neurosurg. Psychiatry*, 1988, 51: 403–411.

Doherty, T.J. The influence of aging and sex on skeletal muscle mass and strength. *Curr. Opin. Clin. Nutr. Metab. Care*, 2001, 4: 503–508.

Doherty, T.J. and Brown, W.F. The estimated numbers and relative sizes of thenar motor units as selected by multiple point stimulation in young and older adults. *Muscle Nerve*, 1993, 16: 355–366.

Doherty, T.J. and Brown, W.F. Age-related changes in the twitch contractile properties of human thenar motor units. *J. Appl. Physiol.*, 1997, 82: 93–101.

Doherty, T.J., Vandervoort, A.A. and Brown, W.F. Effects of ageing on the motor unit: a brief review. *Can. J. Appl. Physiol.*, 1993a, 18: 331–358.

Doherty, T.J., Vandervoort, A.A., Taylor, A.W. and Brown, W. F. Effects of motor unit losses on strength in older men and women. *J. Appl. Physiol.*, 1993b, 74: 868–874.

Frontera, W.R., Hughes, V.A., Lutz, K.J. and Evans, W.J. A cross-sectional study of muscle strength and mass in 45- to 78-yr-old men and women. *J. Appl. Physiol.* , 1991, 71: 644–650.

Grimby, G. and Saltin, B. The ageing muscle. *Clin. Physiol.*, 1983, 3: 209–218.

Kawamura, Y., O'Brien, P., Okazaki, H. and Dyck, P.J. Lumbar motoneurons of man II: the number and diameter distribution of large- and intermediate-diameter cytons in "motoneuron columns" of spinal cord of man. *J. Neuropathol. Exp. Neurol.*, 1977, 36: 861–870.

Klitgaard, H., Mantoni, M., Schiaffino, S., Ausoni, S., Gorza, L., Laurent-Winter, C., Schnohr, P. and Saltin, B. Function, morphology and protein expression of ageing skeletal muscle: a cross-sectional study of elderly men with different training backgrounds. *Acta Physiol. Scand.*, 1990, 140: 41–54.

Lexell, J. Ageing and human muscle: observations from Sweden. *Can. J. Appl. Physiol.*, 1993, 18: 2–18.

Lexell, J. and Downham, D.Y. What determines the muscle cross-sectional area? *J. Neurol. Sci.*, 1992, 111: 113–114.

Lexell, J., Taylor, C.C. and Sjostrom, M. What is the cause of aging atrophy? *J. Neurol. Sci.*, 1988, 84: 275–294.

Overend, T.J., Cunningham, D.A., Paterson, D.H. and Lefcoe, M.S. Thigh composition in young and elderly men determined by computed tomography. *Clin. Physiol.*, 1992, 12: 629–640.

Porter, M.M., Vandervoort, A.A. and Lexell, J. Aging of human muscle: structure, function and adaptability. *Scand. J. Med. Sci. Sports*, 1995, 5: 129–142.

Poulin, M.J., Vandervoort, A.A., Paterson, D.H., Kramer, J.F. and Cunningham, D.A. Eccentric and concentric torques of knee and elbow extension in young and older men. *Can. J. Sport. Sci.*, 1992, 17: 3–7.

Rice, C.L., Cunningham, D.A., Paterson, D.H. and Lefcoe, M.S. Arm and leg composition determined by computed tomography in young and elderly men. *Clin. Physiol.*, 1989, 9: 207–220.

Roos, M.R., Rice, C.L. and Vandervoort, A.A. Age-related changes in motor unit function. *Muscle Nerve*, 1997, 20: 679–690.

Roubenoff, R. Sarcopenia: a major modifiable cause of frailty in the elderly. *J. Nutr. Health Aging*, 2000, 4: 140–142.

Roubenoff, R. Origins and clinical relevance of sarcopenia. *Can. J. Appl. Physiol.*, 2001, 26: 78–89.

Roubenoff, R. and Hughes, V.A. Sarcopenia: current concepts. *J. Gerontol. A. Biol. Sci. Med. Sci.*, 2000, 55: M716–M724.

Sica, R.E.P., McComas, A.J. and Upton, A.R.M. Motor unit estimation in small muscles of the hand. *J. Neurol. Neurosurg. Psychiatry*, 1974, 37: 55–67.

Stålberg, E., Borges, O., Ericsson, M., Essen-Gustavsson, B., Fawcett, P.R., Nordesjo, L.O., Nordgren, B. and Uhlin, R. The quadriceps femoris muscle in 20–70-year-old subjects: relationship between knee extension torque, electrophysiological parameters, and muscle fiber characteristics. *Muscle Nerve*, 1977, 12: 382–389.

Tomlinson, B.E. and Irving, D. The numbers of limb motor neurons in the human lumbosacral cord throughout life. *J. Neurol. Sci.*, 1977, 34: 213–219.

Vandervoort, A.A. and McComas, A.J. Contractile changes in opposing muscles of the human ankle joint with aging. *J. Appl. Physiol.*, 1986, 61: 361–367.

Vandervoort, A.A., Kramer, J.F. and Wharram, E.R. Eccentric knee strength of elderly females. *J. Gerontol.*, 1990, 45: B125–B128.

Young, A., Stokes, M. and Crowe, M. Size and strength of the quadriceps muscles of old and young women. *Eur. J. Clin. Invest.*, 1984, 14: 282–287.

Young, A., Stokes, M. and Crowe, M. The size and strength of the quadriceps muscles of old and young men. *Clin. Physiol.*, 1985, 5: 145–154.

Discussion after Section V

Richard Olney, San Francisco, California

First, I have a comment for Tim about aging studies. Cross-sectional studies, as opposed to longitudinal studies, amplify the effects of aging, so I think most of the changes you referred to were from cross-sectional studies. Second, I would you to comment on the fact that there are limited anatomical studies on cell counts in spinal cords. The studies suggest there is more like a 5–10% loss of anterior horn cells from age 20 to 80, which would be a markedly less than the percent loss from physiological cross-sectional studies. I wonder if you could comment on this.

Timothy Doherty, London, Ontario

Yes, the anatomical work you are probably referring to, Tomlinson and Irving (*J. Neurol. Sci.* 1977, 34: 213–219) and I believe Kawamura (*J. Neuropath. Exp. Neurol.* 1977, 36: 853–860), looked at ventral roots and anterior horn cells. The degree of root and cell loss was less marked, but I think there were difficulties in making these anatomic estimates. They may in fact be facing greater challenges than we are in making electrophysiologic estimates. The point about cross-sectional versus longitudinal data is a good one. To my knowledge, there is no longitudinal study.

Katheryn Swoboda, Salt Lake City, Utah

There must be MUNE data from the investigators who invented these techniques who have done it on themselves repeatedly over years.

Alan McComas, Hamilton, Ontario

Well, good point. If you are interested in data from a study with a sample of one, I have to sadly report that my distal motor unit populations, both in my hand and foot, are only a relatively small fraction of what they were when I was in my 30s.

Jasper Daube, Rochester, Minnesota

I really am hesitant to put myself in the same category of Alan McComas, but I have repeated these studies a number of times on myself and, for whatever it is worth, there is no significant change in my hand muscles. I have not done enough in foot muscles.

Tim, a question for you. When we look at a new technique such as MUNE, it is valuable to compare data with data from other techniques. The change in motor unit size (amplitude) in the biceps muscle with aging in standard EMG is nowhere near as great as 50%. Further, it is my experience with estimating motor unit recruitment in normal subjects of different ages that it is not reduced by 50%. My initial thought is that the lesser amount is correct and there are probably some other errors creeping into your data. Do have any comparisons with changes in EMG on the same subjects in whom you are doing motor unit number estimates?

Timothy Doherty, London, Ontario

I have not systematically studied this issue. However, in my own biceps data I did look at motor unit duration, amplitude, and phases, and changes were not as dramatic as the changes reported from MUNE. I wonder whether the difference just reflects the fact in normal aging motor unit loss is less dramatic compared to rapidly progressive disorders. This would lead to a lesser degree of collateral reinnervation and a lesser increase in motor unit potential duration and size.

Victoria Galia, Hamilton, Ontario

I published the results of a cross-sectional study of normal subjects to age 80 using the automated incremental MUNE technique (*J. Clin. Neurophysiol.* 1996, 13: 253–260). I found MUNE values in the thenar muscle group to be similarly low. However, values did not decline in the biceps muscle.

Mark Bromberg, Salt Lake City, Utah

I want to make a point that there are very few correlations between neurophysiologic and quantitative estimates. The only data shown for recruitment verses MUNE values is based on subjective 1+, 2+, 3+ estimates of recruitment.

Jeffrey Metter, Baltimore, Maryland

I have a question related to the effects of changes in muscle mass on electrophysiologic properties. There can be as much as much as a 30–40% loss of mass between ages 20 and 80 year-old. I would suspect that this is would have an impact on some of the electrical measures. Any thoughts?

Timothy Doherty, London, Ontario

There are two points. If you are looking at it strictly from an MUNE standpoint, we are looking at ratios, and the CMAP potential would be reduced. We found a correlation between the CMAP, total cross-sectional area and force. From the standpoint of other motor unit measures, such as intramuscular potentials or macro potentials, there are a number of issues. There is not a tight relationship between intramuscular needle-detected potentials and other measures of motor unit force, for example, twitches. The needle-detected potential is affected by many other factors. Thus there is a relationship, but it is not tight. The other issue is that if you recall Lexell's data, the cross-sectional area of individual fibers is not affected as much as the overall loss of fibers. So individual action potentials are potentially going to be affected less than the motor unit number estimate.

Section VI

MUNE in Disease States

Motor Unit Number Estimation (Supplements to Clinical Neurophysiology Vol. 55)
Editor: M.B. Bromberg

Chapter 18

MUNE in ALS: natural history and implications

John Turnbull, Joan Martin, Jane Butler, Victoria Galea and Alan McComas*

Department of Medicine (Division of Neurology) and School of Rehabilitation Science (Dr. Galea), McMaster University, Hamilton, ON L8N 3Z5, Canada

Introduction

MUNE (motor unit number estimation) provides the only means of determining the number of motor units, and hence the number of functioning motoneurons, during life. For this reason it has the potential to provide valuable information concerning the natural history of denervating disorders, including amyotrophic lateral sclerosis (ALS). In this review we first present the motor unit populations that are present at the initial diagnostic EMG examination, together with the relative sizes of the units, assessed in terms of their motor unit potential (MUP) amplitudes. Next, we show the rate at which the motor unit populations decline, first for individual muscles and then for the pooled populations. Lastly, we discuss the possible significance of these last results in terms of the pathogenesis of the disease. Some of these data were presented in an earlier publication (Dantes and McComas, 1991).

**Correspondence to*: Dr. Alan J. McComas, Division of Neurology (4U1), McMaster University Medical Centre, 1200 Main Street West, Hamilton, ON L8N 3Z5, Canada. Tel.: (905) 525-9140x22519, Fax: (905) 521-2656.
e-mail: mccomas@fhs.mcmaster.ca

doi:10.1016/S1567-424X(03)00018-7

Methods

Patients

The initial data were obtained from 123 patients attending the diagnostic EMG Clinic at McMaster University Health Sciences Centre from 1972 onwards, and these formed the basis for our first neurophysiological survey (Dantes and McComas, 1991). To these we have added results from a further 43 patients attending the ALS Clinic at McMaster Health Sciences Centre. This clinic, established in 1996, serves as a referral center for virtually all new cases of ALS in the Hamilton-Wentworth and surrounding regions, and draws on a population base of more than 1 million. Altogether 97 men and 69 women were studied, and the mean ages for the onset of symptoms were 58.3 SD $\pm$ 12.2 and 56.8 $\pm$ 15.0 years, respectively (see also Discussion section). The median interval between the onset of symptoms and the first EMG examination was approximately 12 months. There was considerable variation, however, and five of the patients had had symptoms for at least 10 years prior to examination, so that the mean interval was appreciable (22.0–29.0 months). A further three patients, also with typical clinical and EMG features of ALS, survived for 10 years while under our care. The nature of the presenting symptoms has been described for the patients in the initial report (Dantes and McComas, 1991).

Of the 166 patients in the enlarged study, there were four with a history of ALS in a parent. As would be expected of an elderly population, there was a high incidence of associated conditions. These included parkinsonism (three cases), cardiac and cerebrovascular disease (five), cervical spondylosis and radiculopathy (seven), lumbar disc degeneration and lumbosacral radiculopathy (11), old polio (one), diabetes (six), cancer (four), carpal tunnel syndrome (10), and fibromyalgia (two). Although a history of trauma was not sought, in one case symptoms of ALS followed soon after a motor vehicle accident, and in another after complications during epidural anesthesia (see Discussion section).

MUNE

All of the values reported here were obtained with the incremental method, and nearly all of these examinations were performed manually (McComas et al., 1971a), either by the same electromyographer or by one of three EMG technologists with considerable experience in MUNE. The muscles investigated were those of the thenar and hypothenar groups in the hand, and the extensor digitorum brevis (EDB) and plantar muscle group in the foot; the soleus and biceps brachii were studied less frequently. The data now presented come from a total of 607 distal muscles. The recording electrodes were strips of silver foil or, more recently, self-adhesive EKG electrodes that had been cut in half. For each muscle or group of muscles, the active electrode was placed over the end-plate zone(s), or as close to it as possible. All of the patients also underwent a conventional EMG examination, which included needle studies.

Results

Motor unit estimates

Figure 1 shows the estimated numbers of motor units, at the time of the initial EMG, in the thenar, hypothenar and EDB muscles, together with the lower limits of the corresponding ranges for healthy subjects below the age of 60 years. In view of the motor unit attrition which occurs above this age, due to the normal aging process (Campbell et al., 1973), the results for the older patients have been shown separately. The most striking feature of Fig. 1 is the severe denervation that has usually taken place by the time of the first electrophysiological assessment. In comparing the muscle groups, there were significantly more values still within the normal range for the hypothenar muscles than for the thenar ones (30 vs 5) and the normalized means differed significantly (39.2 ± 32.4 and $19.9 \pm 19.7\%$, respectively; $P < 0.001$) when the MUNE values in the same 62 hands were considered. Similarly, the plantar muscles (not shown) retained a greater proportion of motor units than the EDB (respective means, 57.6 ± 49.1 and $27.8 \pm 35.6\%$, $P < 0.001$, in 51 feet).

MUP amplitudes

The mean amplitudes of the MUPs generated by the surviving motor units were calculated for all the muscles examined, and the results for EDB are shown as a function of the corresponding MUNE values in Fig. 2. It can be seen that the largest potentials were found in the muscles with the greatest denervation, but that not all of these muscles exhibited such potentials.

Rate of motor unit loss

In 38 muscles MUNE studies were performed on two or more occasions and the majority of the values are given in Fig. 3. In 20 of these muscles there were 100 or more units present at the first examination, and in 12 the initial estimates were within the respective control ranges. These muscles were of special interest in that they provided information concerning the rapidity of the disease process in ALS from the beginning of involvement of the motoneuron pool. Accordingly the results for these muscles were segregated, with the second and subsequent MUNE values being expressed as percentages of the initial ones. Since the testing was

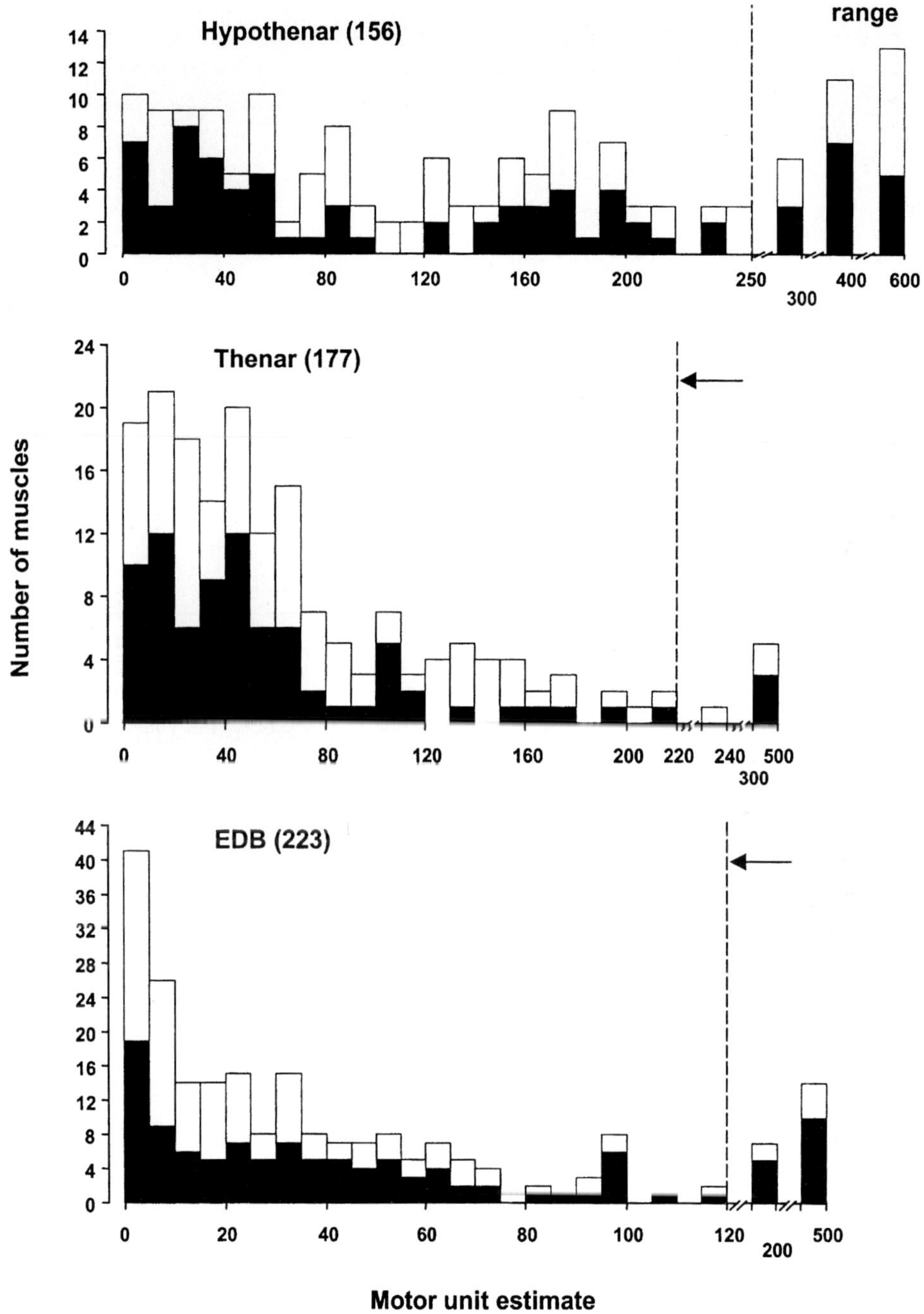

Fig. 1. Motor unit numbers in 556 distal muscles of the hand and foot in ALS patients, at the time of their first EMG examination (51 plantar values not included). Results for patients above and below the age of 60 years are shown by open and filled columns, respectively.

performed at irregular intervals, it was usually necessary to intrapolate in order to obtain values for each 3-month period. The averaged results for these 20 muscles are shown in the initial part of the composite curve in Fig. 4, together with the number of muscles used in each average. The later part of the curve (after 18 months) continues to show averaged values, but this time from a different population,

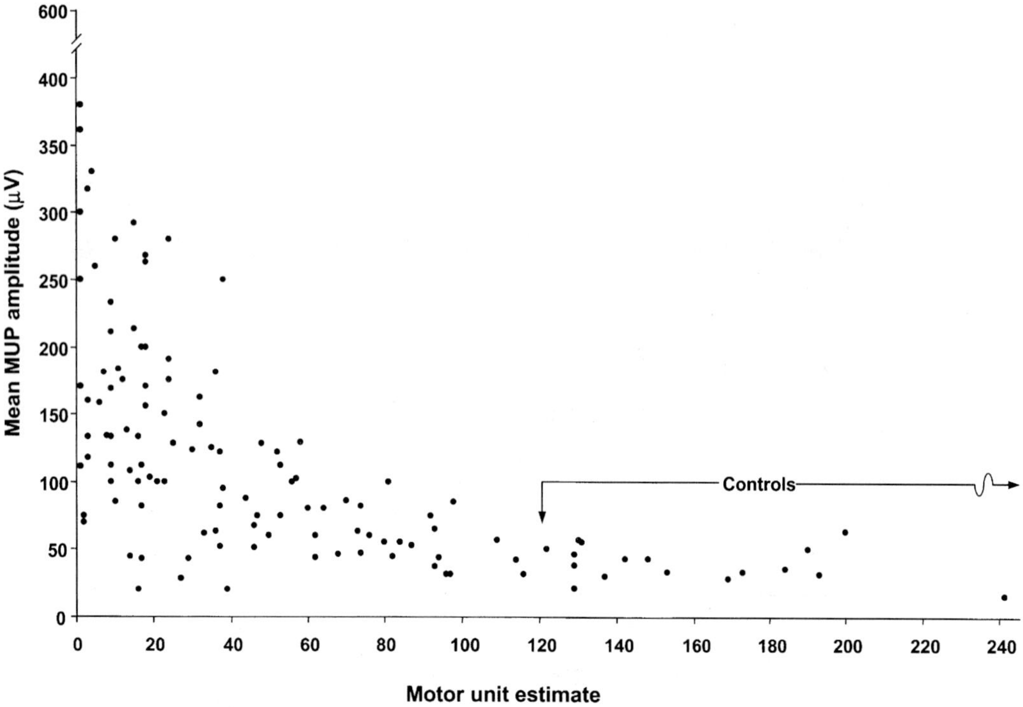

Fig. 2. Mean motor unit potential amplitudes at different stages of denervation in 122 EDB muscles of ALS patients under the age of 70 years.

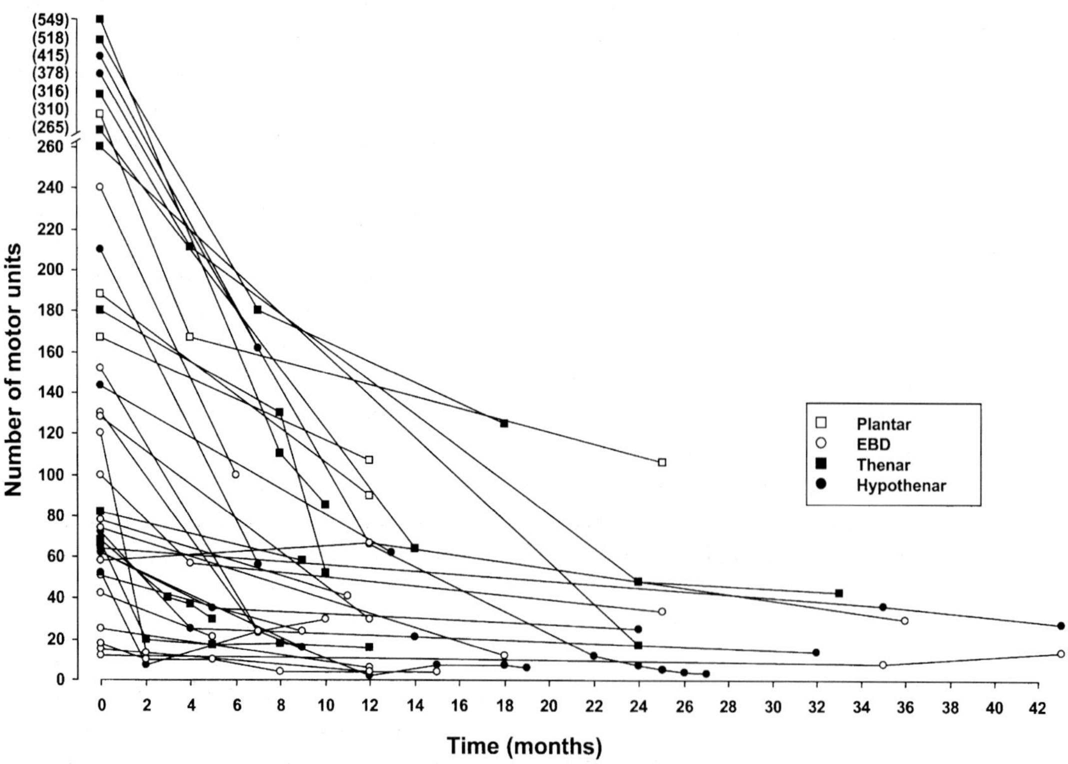

Fig. 3. Rate of loss of motor units in ALS patients, shown for individual muscles of the extremities.

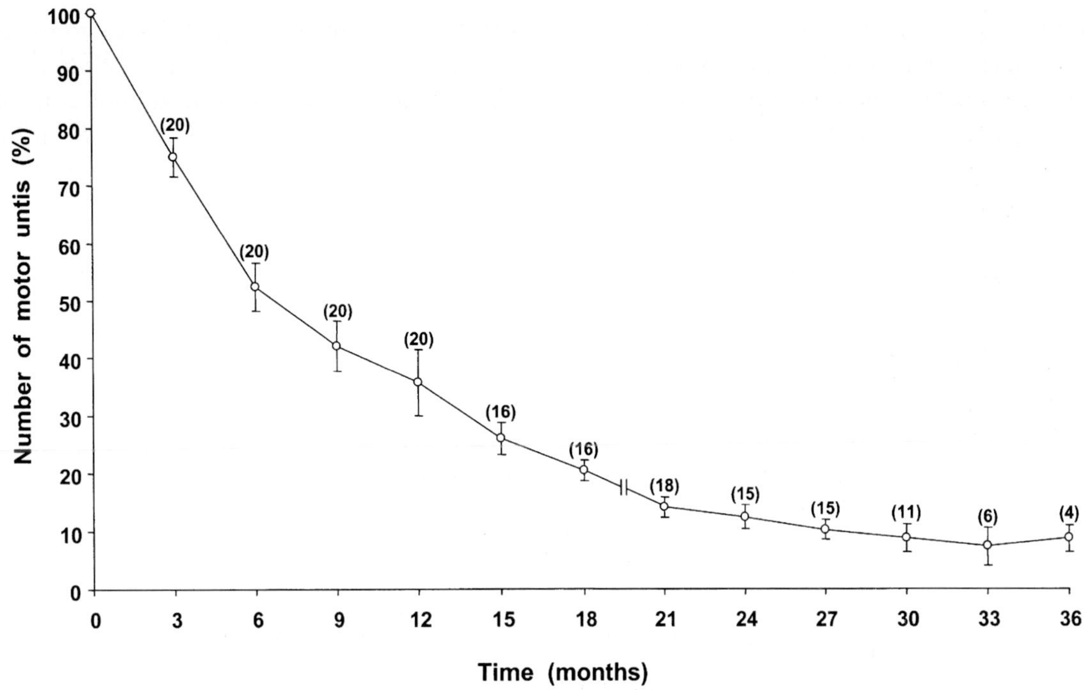

Fig. 4. Mean rate of motor unit loss (with standard errors) after normalization of data in Fig. 3. Numbers of muscles used for means are given in parentheses. See text.

comprising 18 muscles, in which there was already substantial denervation at the time of the first examination. These values are given as percentages of the mean MUNE (245) for the 20 muscles with least denervation.

Discussion

Patient population

The present study confirms previous ones in showing a preponderance of males in the patient population, and the mean ages of onset of ALS symptoms in men and women, 58.3 and 56.8 years, respectively, are consistent with other reported values (Bonduelle, 1975; Caroscio et al., 1987). Our population was also typical in that only a small proportion of cases, less than 3%, was familial.

Choice of MUNE technique

While the manual incremental technique has inherent limitations, as described elsewhere (McComas et al., 1971a), it has the great advantage of convenience and the control values, at least for the hypothenar muscles, are those nearest to anatomical estimates for the same muscles (Santo Neto et al., 1998). Moreover, when denervation is severe, as it was in most of the muscles examined in this study, the reliability of the method is increased, since the units in the sample form a large part of the total population. Indeed, in some muscles it was possible to see the incremental responses of the entire populations of units.

Natural history of ALS

Even though the cause of death in ALS is directly related to the severity of muscle denervation, mortality curves give a poor indication of the rate of motor unit and motoneuron loss across a population of patients. The correlation is particularly low for the earliest stages of the disease, since appreciable denervation will already have occurred in the most affected patients before any deaths start to appear in the curve. On the other hand, the presence of a distinct tail in the mortality curve, due to a minority of patients with slower forms of the disease, indicates that some motor units are less susceptible to the ALS process than others.

In comparison with mortality data, it would be expected that serial determinations of muscle function would be better related to losses of motoneurons and motor units. Studies of this type are those of Tourtellotte et al. (1965), Appel et al. (1987), and of Munsat and colleagues (Andres et al., 1986). In addition to timed motor activities, including speech, the latter workers measured pulmonary function and isometric muscle strength in nine muscle groups on both sides of the body. They found that there was a linear deterioration of muscle function with time, and from this they concluded that the rate of motoneuron loss was also linear (Munsat et al., 1988). This conclusion is questionable, however, since it does not take into account the ability of collateral reinnervation to maintain force and muscle mass in the presence of substantial motor unit loss. For example, in an earlier study of partially denervated muscles, including some of ALS patients, we found that the maximal twitch tensions of the extensor hallucis brevis muscle did not fall below the normal range until the MUNE values (in EDB) were reduced by at least 80% (McComas et al., 1971b). While it is possible that such muscles might fatigue more rapidly than normal during prolonged voluntary contractions, it is clear that measurements of muscle force and mass may seriously underestimate the extent of denervation. In keeping with this caveat are the findings of Felice (1997), who performed MUNE determinations on the thenar muscles of ALS patients and found that these values were more sensitive of disease progression than other tests, including grip strength.

The present study, like its predecessor, has enabled the loss of motor units, and functioning motoneurons, to be determined directly. The study is far from perfect, since it has made use of intrapolation to obtain MUNE values at selected time intervals, and it has linked two curves, for motoneuron pools starting with minimal and moderate denervation, respectively. Nevertheless, a visual comparison of the MUNE results for individual muscles, in Fig. 3, with the composite curve for the pooled data, in Fig. 4, leaves no doubt as to the validity of the latter. The composite curve shows that, once a motoneuron pool is involved by the degenerative process in ALS, there is usually a rapid disappearance of functioning motor units, such that, on average, half are lost within 6 months and half of the remainder within another 6 months. A similarly rapid loss of units in the first 6 months of study has recently been reported by Wang and Delwaide (1998). The composite curve continues to decline exponentially, leaving a small residuum of units, approximately 10%, which appear resistant to the disease process. This part of the curve must be interpreted cautiously, however, and a distinction made between what happens in an individual population of motoneurons, and in a series of motoneuron pools. Thus, it does not follow that, in every motoneuron pool, there is a small number of ALS-resistant cells, for some muscles do become completely denervated, as shown most convincingly by the absence of an evoked response on motor nerve stimulation. At the other extreme, there is a minority of patients in whom the disease runs a slow course, and it is the inclusion of these data which strongly affects the tail of the composite curve. To resolve this uncertainty a prospective study of individual motoneuron populations in ALS is clearly needed, in which serial MUNE studies are performed at regular intervals throughout the remainder of the patient's life, so that intrapolation and averaging can be avoided.

It is known that neurons in Onuf's nucleus do not degenerate in ALS and the present study provides other evidence that, at a stage of the disease when motoneuron degeneration is widespread, some cells are more resistant to the ALS process than others. For example, in the hand, the hypothenar muscles usually have higher MUNE values than the thenar ones, and the same is true in the foot, for the plantar muscles in comparison with EDB. The difference between the hypothenar and thenar muscles has also been noted by Kuwabara et al. (1999) using MUNE and by Eisen (1993). There is no obvious explanation for these differences in neuronal vulnerability, and the problem is made more intriguing by the fact that similar differences are a feature of such diverse conditions as the normal aging process, poliomyelitis, thyrotoxicosis, toxic neuropathies, and myotonic dystrophy (McComas, 1977). Unfortunately, this puzzle is one that will be difficult to solve, especially since it may not be suited to animal experiments.

Finally, the MUNE results presented here have resolved one of the uncertainties in ALS, the duration of the illness before symptoms first appear. Thus, if 80% of motoneurons must be lost before there is muscle atrophy and weakness (McComas et al., 1971b), then Fig. 3 indicates that no more than 12 months would be required for these symptoms to occur in the majority of patients. In contrast, fasciculations and cramps might well be noted sooner, since these would be expected to appear as soon as the motoneurons started to degenerate.

Pathophysiology

The amplitudes of the MUPs, determined as part of the MUNE studies, are significant for an understanding of the pathogenesis of ALS, for they indicate the relative sizes of the surviving motor units. While the units appear of normal size or even diminished in some muscles with advanced denervation, as pointed out by Dengler et al. (1989; see also Emeryk-Szajenska et al., 1997), there are other muscles in which very large units are found and in which the mean sizes are increased, as shown in Fig. 2 for the EDB muscle. Similar results, but with a more obviously hyperbolic relationship between the numbers and mean MUP amplitudes, have previously been reported for the hypothenar muscles (Dantes and McComas, 1991). Since collateral reinnervation would require increased protein synthesis, both for the new axonal sprouts and for the additional axoplasmic transport, the participating motoneurons must surely be healthy until involved by the ALS process. Taken in conjunction with the data on the rate of motor unit loss (see above), the time between ALS involvement of a cell and the death of the cell cannot be more than a few months and may even be a matter of a few days or weeks. It is here that the serial physiological studies of individual motor units, as already begun by Chan et al. (1998), promise to be especially informative.

Although we have not analyzed the matter statistically, our MUNE studies in ALS are entirely consistent with the clinical impression that weakness and wasting, having started in part of a limb, spreads to involve neighboring regions (Caroscio et al., 1987). Thus, MUNE values may initially be normal in the hand but reduced in the foot, and vice versa, before the losses of units become generalized. We interpret this to mean that the disease process, having begun somewhere in the spinal cord or brainstem, also spreads locally.

Pathogenesis

The similarity between the onset of ALS symptoms and the temporal pattern of motor unit loss with age is quite striking, as Fig. 5 indicates. In this figure we have taken the normalized numbers of motor units in muscles of the hand and foot at different ages, reported earlier (McComas et al., 1973), and have calculated how many additional units are lost in each decade. At the bottom of the figure are the ages of onset of ALS symptoms, also

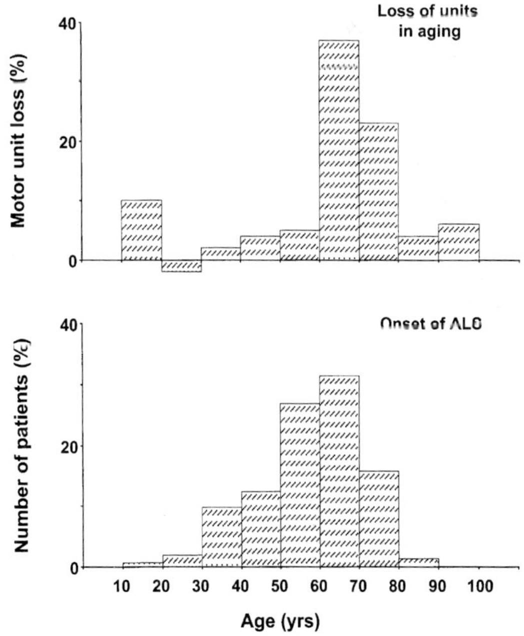

Fig. 5. *Top:* Percentage of motor units lost, through normal aging, in each decade. (Data from McComas et al., 1973.) *Bottom:* Ages of onset of ALS symptoms in 166 patients.

shown in decades. The similarity between the two sets of data led us to propose that ALS was an extreme form of the normal aging process, though we left open the nature of the cellular mechanism involved (McComas et al., 1973). We now recognize that there are at least three qualitative differences between aging and ALS that makes this hypothesis untenable. First, upper motoneuron signs are absent in healthy elderly subjects even though the numbers of units may be severely depleted. Second, it is now clear that, while no limb muscles are immune to ALS, some muscles, such as the biceps brachii, may not show any significant motor unit loss in aging (Galea, 1996). Finally, there are the instances of ALS in young patients that are difficult to reconcile with an aging hypothesis. Rather than discard aging as an etiological factor in ALS entirely, we now postulate that it has an indirect role (see below).

In proceeding further, it is prudent to accept that there may be several etiological factors in ALS, in addition to genetic and immunological ones (Rowland, 1982), and multiple mechanisms of cell death (Bromberg, 1999). It would be surprising, for example, if the basis of the typical rapidly progressive form of ALS was the same as that for those patients in whom the disease runs a very prolonged course. One distinction which may be possible, however, is between a process in which there is a cumulative change of some kind in the motoneurons, and one in which random events affect susceptible neurons. In the former, Clarke et al. (2000) have pointed out that there is an increasing risk of neuronal death with time, while in the latter the risk remains constant ("one-hit" model). If cell death in ALS was due to the accumulation of toxic radicals, as originally envisaged for familial cases with SOD deficiency, then the increasing risk should result in a sigmoid decline in the number of motoneurons. However, as we have shown, in most sporadic cases of ALS the reduction in motor unit number is exponential and must begin soon after the first appearance of the ALS process in the central nervous system. Therefore, if the arguments of Clarke et al. (2000) are applicable to the MUNE results, then a single event must be involved, acting on motoneurons which have become vulnerable, most probably on account of their age. The motoneurons of the distal muscles of the limbs may be especially vulnerable, for not only do these muscles show more aging changes than proximal ones, but ALS is most likely to present with distal symptoms, such as weakness of grip or footdrop, when the limbs are affected (Jokelainen, 1977).

What might the etiological event be? While there are other possibilities, we are increasingly attracted to the concept of activation and infection of a motoneuron pool by a neurotropic virus. The viral hypothesis is admittedly an old one (see Johnson and Brooks, 1984), but it would be consistent with the rapidity and topographical pattern of spread of the ALS process throughout the brainstem and spinal cord (see above and Hudson et al., 1986). Further, there are obvious similarities between ALS and herpes zoster, a known viral disease in which the virus resides in the dorsal root ganglia and can be activated in various ways. In both diseases, there is destruction of neurons and an increased risk with advancing age. Again, trauma is accepted as one of the precipitating factors in herpes zoster and, while there is controversy over their significance (Kurland et al., 1992), it is difficult to ignore striking reports of ALS following injury (Gawel et al., 1983; Riggs, 1985), or the following case:

Among our own patients there was a 35-year-old woman, who had been perfectly fit until she injured her right knee skiing. During an arthroscopic examination under epidural anesthesia one month later she developed acute weakness of both legs and a burning discomfort over her buttocks and thighs. On discontinuing the anesthetic the burning sensation resolved but the strength in the right leg never recovered fully. Instead, after some months the weakness began to increase in that leg and then, over the next 5 years, to affect the other leg, and eventually both arms. During this period the presence of increasing denervation in the affected limbs was established by serial MUNEs (McComas, 1995). With the appearance of upper motoneuron signs, and with typical EMG findings, the diagnosis of ALS was made, and death resulted 7 years after the onset of her leg weakness.

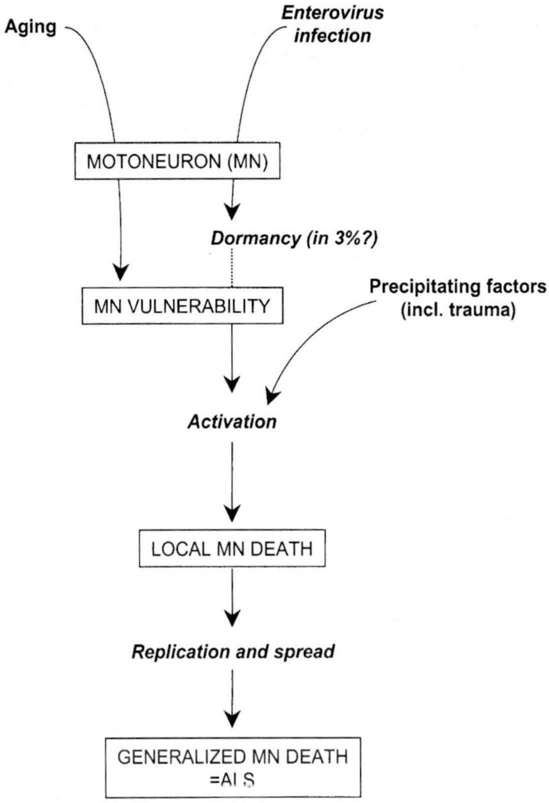

Fig. 6. Hypothetical scheme to show how aging might make motoneurons vulnerable to activation of a neurotropic virus, with or without the intervention of some precipitating factor (e.g. trauma).

In reviewing cases such as this, the issue is surely not so much whether trauma is a frequent, statistically significant, cause of ALS, but whether it is a cause at all for, if it were, it would still shed new light on the pathogenesis of the disease.

Although initial attempts to detect traces of virus in the spinal cords of ALS patients were unsuccessful (as they were in the affected dorsal root ganglia of patients with herpes zoster), Berger et al. (2000), using highly sensitive techniques, have recently reported the presence of enteroviral RNA sequences in 88% of spinal cords of ALS patients and in only 3% of controls. Obviously, many important questions remain (Karpati and Dalakas, 2000) but in the meantime a tentative scheme for the etiology and pathogenesis of ALS would be that depicted in Fig. 6.

Conclusions

Incremental MUNE has been applied to 607 distal limb muscles in 166 patients with ALS and in the majority of muscles significant denervation was already present at the time of the first investigation. However, while the MUNE values were always lowest in the clinically affected limb(s), there were local differences as well. In the hand, denervation was more pronounced in the thenar muscles than in the hypothenar ones, and in the foot EDB was more affected than the plantar muscles. As the MUNE values dropped, the mean amplitudes of the potentials of the surviving motor units increased in most, but not all, muscles. Serial MUNE studies showed that the mean rate of loss of units was exponential and was initially high, with half of the units disappearing in the first 6 months after a motoneuron pool had become involved. These results indicate that, in most patients, the disease must have started within a year of the appearance of weakness and wasting. The exponential loss of units is consistent with a one-hit model of neuronal degeneration, in which a susceptible motoneuron is affected by a single event, rather than by a cumulative change of some kind. A plausible explanation for this event is that it is infective, and follows the activation of a neurotropic virus.

Acknowledgements

We are indebted to Rebecca Newberry for technical assistance. Dr. Marita Dantes' earlier analysis of some of the data is very much appreciated.

References

Andres, P.L., Hedlund, W., Finison, L., Conlon, T., Felmus, M. and Munsat, T.L. Quantitative motor assessment in amyotrophic lateral sclerosis. *Neurology*, 1986, 36: 937–941.

Appel, V., Stewart, S.S., Smith, G. and Appel, S.H. A rating scale for amyotrophic lateral sclerosis: description and preliminary experience. *Ann. Neurol.*, 1987, 22: 328–333.

Berger, M.M., Kopp, N., Vital, C., Redl, B., Aymard, M. and Lina, B. Detection and cellular localization of enterovirus RNA sequences in spinal cord of patients with ALS. *Neurology*, 2000, 54: 20–25.

Bonduelle, M. Amyotrophic lateral sclerosis. In: *Handbook of Clinical Neurology* (P.J. Vinken and G.W. Bruyn, Eds.), Vol. 22, 1975, pp. 218–338. Elsevier, Amsterdam.

Bromberg, M. Pathogenesis of amyotrophic lateral sclerosis: a critical review. *Curr. Opin. Neurol.*, 1999, 12: 581–588.

Campbell, M.J., McComas, A.J. and Petito, F. Physiological changes in ageing muscles. *J. Neurol. Neurosurg. Psychiatry*, 1973, 36: 174–182.

Caroscio, J.T., Mulvihill, M.N., Sterling, R. and Abrams, B. Amyotrophic lateral sclerosis. Its natural history. *Neurol. Clin.*, 1987, 5: 1–8.

Chan, K.M., Stashuk, D.W. and Brown, W.F. A longitudinal study of the pathophysiological changes in single human thenar motor units in amyotrophic lateral sclerosis. *Muscle Nerve*, 1998, 21: 1714–1723.

Clarke, G., Collins, R.A., Leavitt, B.R., Andrews, D.F., Hayden, M.R., Lumsden, C.J. and McInnes, R.R. A one-hit model of cell death in inherited neuronal degenerations. *Nature*, 2000, 406: 195–199.

Dantes, M. and McComas, A. The extent and time course of motoneuron involvement in amyotrophic lateral sclerosis. *Muscle Nerve*, 1991, 14: 416–421.

Dengler, R., Konstanzer, A., Hesse, S., Schubert, M. and Wolf, W. Collateral nerve sprouting and twitch forces of single motor units in conditions with partial denervation in man. *Neurosci. Lett.*, 1989, 97: 118–122.

Eisen, A. Comments on the lower motor neuron hypothesis. *Muscle Nerve*, 1993, 16: 820–822.

Emeryk-Szajenska, B., Kopeć, J. and Karwanska, A. The reorganization of motor units in motor neuron disease. *Muscle Nerve*, 1997, 20: 306–315.

Felice, K.J. A longitudinal study comparing thenar motor unit number estimates to other quantitative tests in patients with amyotrophic lateral sclerosis. *Muscle Nerve*, 1997, 20: 179–185.

Galea, V. Changes in motor unit estimates with aging. *J. Clin. Neurophysiol.*, 1996, 13: 253–260.

Gawel, M., Zaiwalla, Z. and Rose, F.C. Antecedent events in motor neuron disease. *J. Neurol. Neurosurg. Psychiatry*, 1983, 46: 1041–1043.

Hudson, A.J., Vinters, H.V., Povey, R.C., Hatch, L.A., Percy, D.H., Noseworthy, J.H. and Kaufmann, J.C.E. An unusual form of motor neuron disease following a cat bite. *Can. J. Neurol. Sci.*, 1986, 13: 111–116.

Johnson, R.T. and Brooks, B.R. Possible viral etiology of amyotrophic lateral sclerosis. In: *Neuromuscular Diseases* (G. Serratrice, D. Cros, C. Desnuelle, J.-L. Gastaut, J.-F. Pellissier, J. Pouget and A. Schiano, Eds.), 1984, pp. 353–359. Raven Press, New York.

Jokelainen, M. Amyotrophic lateral sclerosis in Finland. 2. Clinical characteristics. *Acta Neurol. Scand.*, 1977, 56: 194–204.

Karpati, G. and Dalakas, M.C. Viral hide-and-seek in sporadic ALS. A new challenge. *Neurology*, 2000, 54: 6–7.

Kurland, L.T., Radhakrishnan, K., Smith, G.E., Armon, C. and Nemetz, P.N. Mechanical trauma as a risk factor in classic amyotrophic lateral sclerosis: lack of epidemiologic evidence. *J. Neurol. Sci.*, 1992, 113: 133–143.

Kuwabara, S., Mizobuchi, K., Ogawara, K. and Hattori, T. Dissociated small hand muscle involvement in amyotrophic lateral sclerosis detected by motor unit number estimates. *Muscle Nerve*, 1999, 22: 870–873.

McComas, A.J. In "*Neuromuscular Function and Disorders*", 1977, 364 pp. Butterworths, London.

McComas, A.J. Motor unit estimation: anxieties and achievements. *Muscle Nerve*, 1995, 18: 369–379.

McComas, A.J., Fawcett, P.R.W., Campbell, M.J. and Sica, R.E.P. Electrophysiological estimation of the number of motor units within a human muscle. *J. Neurol. Neurosurg. Psychiatry*, 1971a, 34: 121–131.

McComas, A.J., Sica, R.E.P., Campbell, M.J. and Upton, A.R.M. Functional compensation in partially denervated muscles. *J. Neurol. Neurosurg. Psychiatry*, 1971b, 34: 453–460.

McComas, A.J., Upton, A.R.M. and Sica, R.E.P. Motoneurone disease and ageing. *Lancet*, 1973, 2: 1477–1480.

Munsat, T.L., Andres, P.L., Finison, L., Conlon, T. and Thibodeau, L. The natural history of motoneuron loss in amyotrophic lateral sclerosis. *Neurology*, 1988, 38: 409–413.

Riggs, J.E. Trauma and amyotrophic lateral sclerosis. *Arch. Neurol.*, 1985, 42: 205.

Rowland, L.P. Diverse forms of motoneuron disease. In: *Human Motor Neuron Disease* (L.P. Rowland, Ed.), 1982, pp. 1–13. Raven Press, New York.

Santo Neto, H., DeCarvalho, V.C. and Marques, M.J. Estimation of the number and size of human flexor digiti minimi muscle motor units using histological methods. *Muscle Nerve*, 1998, 21: 112–114.

Tourtellotte, W.W., Haeren, A.F., Simpson, J.F., Kuzma, J.W. and Sikorski, J. Quantitative clinical neurological testing. I. A study of a battery of tests designed to evaluate in part the neurological function of patients with multiple sclerosis and its use in a therapeutic trial. *Ann. N.Y. Acad. Sci.*, 1965, 122: 480–505.

Wang, F.C. and Delwaide, P.J. Number and relative size of thenar motor units in ALS patients: application of the adapted multiple point stimulation method. *Electroencephalogr. Clin. Neurophysiol.*, 1998, 109: 36–43.

Motor Unit Number Estimation (Supplements to Clinical Neurophysiology Vol. 55)
Editor: M.B. Bromberg

Chapter 19

Using MUNE to make linear estimates of rate of progression in ALS[1]

Carmel Armon*

Department of Neurology, Loma Linda University School of Medicine, Loma Linda, CA 92354, USA

Introduction

The rate at which amyotrophic lateral sclerosis (ALS) progresses varies greatly among patients, making it difficult to individualize prognostic information for patients and ascertain beneficial effects of new treatments developed to slow disease progression. This leads to the requirement of large sample sizes in clinical trials. Prognostic factors which have emerged from population-based observational studies are patient age at onset of ALS (worse if older) and site of disease onset (worse if bulbar onset) (Armon, 1994). The role of additional putative factors, such as patient mood and morale, is harder to quantify and document. Nevertheless, clinical observations suggest that most patients maintain an individual rate of progression. Isometric myometry data (Brooks et al., 1991; Munsat et al., 1991; Bryan et al., 1995), showing that most patients enter a linear phase of progression of their disease, support these clinical observations. However, when patients are seen at one point in time, such as at entry into a clinical trial, it is not possible to determine if they are in the linear phase of disease progression.

We first introduced the concept of linear estimates of rate of disease progression (LEP) (Armon and Moses, 1998). LEP can be derived from a measurement of strength or function at a single point in time, an estimate of its value at the time of disease onset, and disease duration at the time the patient is evaluated (Fig. 1). These linear estimates may be considered equivalent to the first term of the Taylor expansion of the true functions representing rate of disease progression, even when the functions themselves are unknown, recalling that the first term of the Taylor expansion of any function is linear. The use of calculated linear estimates avoids the necessity of determining that patients are actually progressing linearly, or their true rate of progression. We proceeded to establish the utility of LEP in predicting patient survival. As a first step, we determined utility of LEP in predicting survival from disease onset, because in our opinion this was the most plausible hypothesis. To mimic the situation when a patient was first seen or

[1]Presented in part at the 45th annual meeting of the American Association for Electrodiagnostic Medicine, Orlando, Florida, October, 1998, and at the First International Symposium and Workshop on Motor Unit Number Estimation, July 2001, Snowbird, UT, USA. Previously published, in part, in *Muscle and Nerve* 1999; 22: 1571–1575 and 2000; 23: 874–882, from which some of the text, tables and figures are reproduced.

**Correspondence to*: Carmel Armon, Department of Neurology, Loma Linda University School of Medicine, 11175 Campus Drive, Coleman Pavilion, Room 11108, Loma Linda, CA 92354, USA.
Tel.: (909) 558-4907, Fax: (909) 558-0207.
E-mail: res0tna7@verizon.net

doi: 10.1016/S1567-424X(03)00019-9

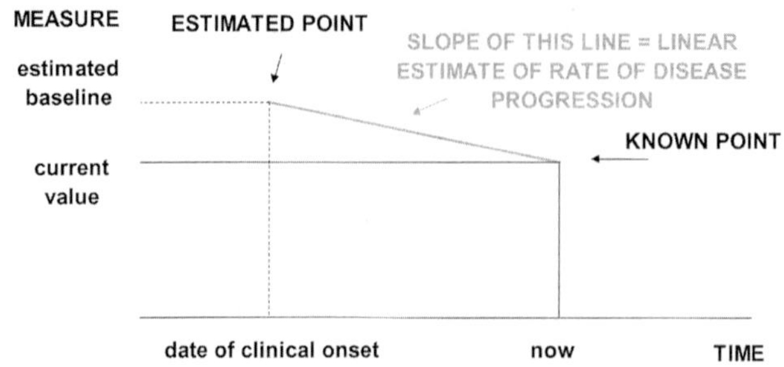

Fig. 1. Diagram to illustrate the concept of a linear estimate of rate of disease progression.

enrolled in a clinical trial, we examined whether the LEP calculated from one point in time could predict survival from that time. We found LEP to predict survival from the date of measurement if they were based on forced vital capacity expressed as percent of predicted value (FVC%) or foot dorsiflexion strength, but not grip strength. We checked the general applicability of our initial observations by applying these methods and results to data from two additional patient groups, one that had been studied earlier and one later than our initial patient group (Armon et al., 2000). We demonstrated that LEP (based on FVC% or foot dorsiflexion strength) predicted survival from the date of measurement only in the later group. This group had been enrolled in a clinical trial based on criteria similar to those of our initial patient group (which are comparable to contemporary clinical trial enrollment criteria), and had more complete disease duration and survival data.

We had reported that motor unit number estimates (MUNE) were highly correlated with isometric myometry assessment of strength in regionally-concordant weak distal muscles of 21 patients (Armon et al., 1997). We were able to validate this observation in 13 additional patients for upper extremity MUNE, but not for lower extremity MUNE (in nine of the 13 patients in whom lower extremity MUNE were obtainable) (Armon and Brandstater, 1997). The number of patients in this second series was small.

MUNE probably represent the primary consequence of ALS (loss of lower motor neurons) more closely than isometric myometry or measures of function such as forced vital capacity (FVC) (which reflect also the effects of reinnervation of muscles by surviving motor neurons and compensatory strategies that patients may apply). Consequently, we set out to examine whether the LEP derived from MUNE might also predict survival (Armon and Brandstater, 1999). Secondary objectives were to determine the significance of biologic variables, once MUNE-based LEP were accounted for, and to compare MUNE-based LEP to those based on isometric myometry or FVC%. In this chapter we also examine, in a preliminary fashion, the potential impact of applying LEP-based considerations to the design and analysis of clinical trials in patients with ALS.

Methods (Armon and Brandstater, 1999)

ALS patients were participants at the Loma Linda, California center in one of two multi-center Phase III clinical trials in ALS (Miller et al., 1996; Bradley, 1999) who had MUNE studies performed (Armon and Brandstater, 1997; Armon et al., 1997). Although inclusion criteria for the two trials differed, no patient was ultimately thought to have a diagnosis other than ALS. The agents tested did not show efficacy and treatment assignment was not taken into consideration in the present analysis.

FVC and demographic and disease-specific data were obtained as part of both study protocols. Isometric myometry was performed as part of one study's protocol in all the patients (Miller et al., 1996), and was obtained for select muscle groups (grip, foot dorsiflexion) in a subset of the patients in the other study (Bradley, 1999). MUNE studies of thenar, hypothenar and extensor digitorum brevis (EDB) muscles were performed according to the unmodified manual method of McComas (McComas et al., 1971; McComas, 1991). Eight to 11 incremental responses were recorded in each muscle if there were at least that number of units present. If there were fewer units, all were counted. The worst affected limb was selected, unless it was affected to the point of complete, or near-complete, paralysis. Values for grip and foot dorsiflexion strength were normalized using the method of Andres et al. (1988). FVC was expressed as percent of predicted (FVC%). MUNE were standardized by dividing the raw estimate by the lower limit of normal for each muscle taken as 100 for thenar and hypothenar and 85 for the EDB muscles (Daube, 1995). Patients were followed beyond the duration of the studies until they died or received tracheostomy, or until contact with them was lost. LEP based on grip strength and foot dorsiflexion strength and FVC% were derived as reported previously (Armon et al., 2000). MUNE-based LEP were calculated as:

$$\text{MUNE-based LEP} = \frac{\text{(standardized MUNE-2)}}{\text{duration of disease from onset}}. \quad (1)$$

Disease onset was defined as the time the patient noted weakness at any site.

Statistical analysis was performed using the Statistical Package for the Social Sciences (SPSS, 1996). The principal hypothesis tested was that MUNE-based LEP would be predictive of tracheostomy-free survival from disease onset. The primary dependent variable was time from disease onset to death or tracheostomy. Probability of tracheostomy-free survival was calculated using the Kaplan–Meier method. Thenar, hypothenar, and EDB MUNE and the linear estimates for their rates of decline, gender, age at onset, site of onset (bulbar vs. spinal), height and weight were tested as independent variables, or risk factors, within a Cox proportional hazards model, using stepwise regression techniques, which enable bivariate and multivariate analyses. Within secondary analysis, MUNE-based LEP were compared to regionally-concordant strength or FVC%-based LEP. In addition we conducted exploratory analysis to examine if MUNE-based LEP could be used to predict patient survival from the date they were derived.

Results

Thirty-four ALS patients were included, of whom 26 were men, and 28 had spinal and six had bulbar onset. Age at the time of MUNE ranged from 30.8 to 79.1 years (mean 59.5, SD 12.2). Disease duration at the time MUNE were obtained was 0.5–5.5 years (mean 2.1, SD 1.0). By the time the analysis was performed, 21 patients (62%) had died or received tracheostomy. Time from disease onset to death, tracheostomy or censoring was 1.4–6.6 years (mean 3.4, SD 1.5). Median survival was 3.6 years. A histogram of the distribution of hypothenar-based LEP is shown in Fig. 2. The mean hypothenar-based LEP was −0.95/year, SD 0.70/year. Range and percentile data for hypothenar, thenar, and EDB-based LEP are summarized in Table 1.

Testing each independent variable individually for statistical significance as a risk factor in a Cox proportional hazards model showed that each of the MUNE-based LEP was highly significant. Site of onset (bulbar vs. spinal) was also statistically significant (Table 2). Using stepwise regression,

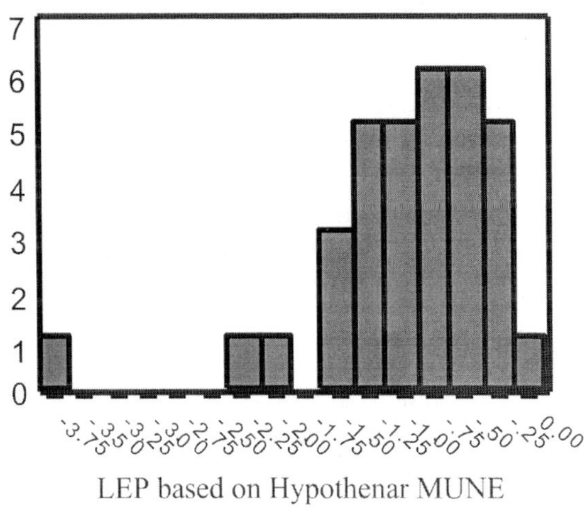

Fig. 2. Histogram of distribution of LEP based on hypothenar MUNE in 34 patients with ALS. The units of LEP (horizontal axis) are derived from standardized MUNE divided by time, in years. See Methods section for definition.

TABLE 1

SUMMARY DATA FOR MUNE-BASED LINEAR ESTIMATES OF RATES OF DISEASE PROGRESSION (LEP) IN 34 PATIENTS WITH ALS

MUNE site	Minimum	Maximum	Percentiles		
			25.0000	50.0000	75.0000
EDB LEP	−2.66	−0.24	−1.3135	−0.8797	−0.6047
Hypothenar LEP	−3.72	−0.11	−1.2527	−0.8088	−0.5229
Thenar LEP	−3.82	−0.14	−1.3131	−0.9982	−0.5970

EDB, extensor digitorum brevis. The units for LEP are derived from standardized MUNE, divided by time, in years. See Methods section for definition.

TABLE 2

INDIVIDUAL EVALUATION OF ALL INDEPENDENT VARIABLES AS RISK FACTORS FOR PATIENT DEATH (OR TRACHEOSTOMY), FROM DATE OF ALS ONSET

Variable	Wald χ^2 score	*P* value
Estimated rate of hypothenar MUNE decline	27.8117	<0.00005
Estimated rate of thenar MUNE decline	23.1137	<0.00005
Estimated rate of EDB MUNE decline	18.1204	<0.00005
Hypothenar MUNE	1.1261	0.2886
Thenar MUNE	0.9105	0.3400
EDB MUNE	0.3968	0.5287
Age at onset	0.0367	0.8480
Gender	1.6172	0.2035
Site of onset (bulbar vs. spinal)	4.0570	0.0440
Weight	1.3400	0.2470
Height	0.4269	0.5135

EDB = extensor digitorum brevis; MUNE = motor unit number estimate.

a highly significant two-variable model emerged ($\chi^2 = 31.6$, $P < 0.00005$). The two variables in the model, each of which was independently significant, controlling for the other, were rate of hypothenar MUNE decline ($P < 0.00005$), and bulbar (vs. spinal) onset ($P = 0.0217$). The nine variables not in the model were not significant as add-ons (residual $\chi^2 = 7.726$, d.f. = 9, $P = 0.5620$).

Estimated rate of decline in hypothenar MUNE was found to be the most significant variable in predicting survival, both by itself and in the multivariate analysis. This may be illustrated by comparing tracheostomy-free survival for the patient group progressing faster than the median, stratifying by LEP based on hypothenar MUNE, to survival of the group progressing slower than the median (Fig. 3). The median tracheostomy-free survival of the 17 faster-progressing patients was 2.6 years, less than half of the 5.5 years' survival of the 17 slower-progressing patients, or a difference of almost 3 years. Exploratory analysis, looking at tracheostomy-free survival from the date of the MUNE study, shows that the median survival for the slowly-progressing group was 2.5 years, double that of the faster progressing group (1.2 years, Fig. 4). Comparison of MUNE-based LEP to regionally-concordant strength or function-based LEP shows that the χ^2 values are larger, and the *P*-values smaller, for MUNE-based LEP, compared to regionally-concordant strength or function-based LEP (Table 3). This supports the conclusion that MUNE reflect better than strength or function

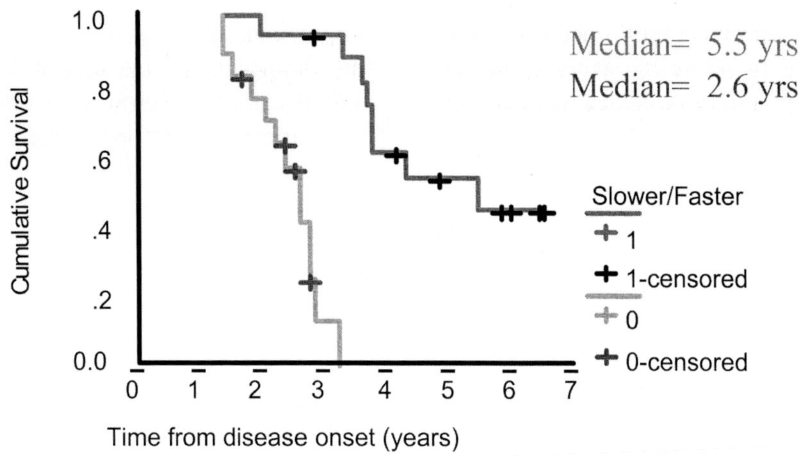

Fig. 3. Cumulative survival from disease onset, stratifying patients using hypothenar MUNE-based LEP. *Upper curve:* survival of the 17 patients with estimated rates of progression slower than the median; *lower curve:* survival of the 17 patients with estimated rates of progression faster than the median.

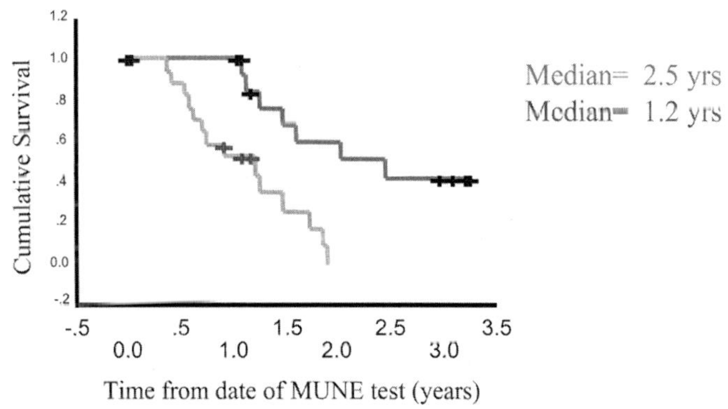

Fig. 4. Cumulative survival from date of measurement, stratifying patients using hypothenar MUNE-based LEP. *Upper curve:* survival of the 17 patients with estimated rates of progression slower than the median; *lower curve:* survival of the 17 patients with estimated rates of progression faster than the median.

TABLE 3

COMPARISON OF MUNE-BASED LEP TO REGIONALLY-CONCORDANT STRENGTH OR FUNCTION-BASED LEP AS RISK FACTORS FOR PATIENT DEATH (OR TRACHEOSTOMY), FROM DATE OF ALS ONSET

Variable	Wald χ^2 score	*P* value
Estimated rate of EDB MUNE decline	16.7660	< 0.0005
Estimated rate of foot dorsiflexion strength decline	9.9100	0.0016
Estimated rate of hypothenar MUNE decline	26.7877	< 0.00005
Estimated rate of thenar MUNE decline	22.4957	< 0.00005
Estimated rate of grip strength decline	18.3687	< 0.00005
Estimated rate of FVC% decline	10.9330	0.0009

EDB = extensor digitorum brevis; MUNE = motor unit number estimate.

the biologic process of loss of motor neurons resulting from ALS and therefore the expectation that MUNE-based LEP should be better predictors of survival.

Discussion

Linear estimates of rate of disease progression based on thenar, hypothenar and EDB MUNE were highly predictive of survival from time of disease onset in this select population of patients with ALS enrolling into two clinical trials. MUNE-based LEP were statistically more significant, and hence are likely better predictors of survival, than LEP based on regionally-concordant measures of strength or function. The approach used in Figs. 3 and 4 to represent hypothenar MUNE-based LEP as predictors of survival shows separation in the two survival curves greater than that obtained using any other variable reported to date. Our LEP studies confirm the clinical observation that patients with a faster course die (or need tracheostomy) sooner. It is intriguing that regardless of whether LEP are based on myometry, FVC, or MUNE, all predict survival. This suggests that they capture the rate of disease progression in patients with ALS. Nevertheless, the MUNE-based LEP performed best, perhaps because they are closest to reflecting the rate of the core process of anterior horn cell loss in patients with ALS. Replication of these findings is needed. Some of the methodologic limitations of these results are discussed elsewhere (Armon and Brandstater, 1999); they do not detract from the findings: hypothenar MUNE-based LEP perform better than all previously-available predictors of survival in ALS, including LEP based on isometric myometry or FVC (Armon et al., 2000).

This suggests that drug trial designs which take into consideration MUNE-based LEP may be able to demonstrate therapeutic effect with fewer patients even than those potentially attainable by taking into consideration LEP based on isometric myometry or FVC (Armon et al., 2000). LEP may be used to permit stratified randomization to treatment or placebo arms based on rate of disease progression, resulting in arms better balanced on this important variable, and the analysis technique may be chosen to permit controlling for LEP. The latter approach has been largely endorsed by the recommendations of the statistics working group in a recent conference of investigators with interest in clinical trials in patients with ALS (Second Airlie House Workshop, 1998). These recommendations support the use of techniques appropriate for survival analysis which permit controlling for relevant covariates specified a priori in order to test for treatment effect, but do not mention specifically rate of disease progression or LEP as covariates which should be controlled for in all studies.

Evaluating the potential impact of incorporating such LEP-based considerations to achieve efficiencies in clinical trial study design can be done using a heuristic, or "Monte Carlo" approach. This requires access to large datasets of actual patients in whom disease duration, myometry, FVC, MUNE, and survival data are available, so that LEP can be calculated and their role evaluated. It is possible, within such datasets, to test in an iterative fashion the impact of hypothetical treatment effects, and to evaluate how taking LEP data into consideration results in reduction of sample size to detect a given treatment effect, all expressed in probabilistic terms. In the absence of access to such independent datasets I have performed rudimentary calculations using artificially-produced datasets, derived by duplication of my existing datasets. Due to the severe methodologic limitations that attend testing hypotheses in such datasets, all results are tentative, and should be viewed at best as preliminary or exploratory. They suggest that a 25% reduction in sample size requirements may be realized if two treatment arms are balanced according to LEP and if LEP are taken as a covariate and controlled for in Cox proportional model-based survival analysis. Evaluation of this number in independent datasets is needed.

In conclusion, it is intriguing that an estimate that may be off by up to 30%, as suggested by comparing MUNE values derived using different techniques and algorithms (McComas, 1991; Daube, 1995; Bromberg, 1998), may be used to generate such an outstanding predictor of survival – hypothenar MUNE-based LEP. In the land of the blind, the one-eyed person is king. Sharing of access to existing datasets, greater collaboration between investigators than has been achieved to date, and identification of a broad basis of common ground will be needed if the field of MUNE is to advance. Although MUNE is currently viewed as a time-consuming electrophysiologic technique, restricted to aficionados and fraught with methodological limitations, the technique has the potential to play a pivotal role in patient diagnosis, patient prognosis, and improving the efficiencies of clinical trials of disease-modifying treatments for patients with ALS.

References

Andres, P.L., Finison, L.J., Conlon, T., Thibodeau, L.M. and Munsat, T.L. Use of composite scores (megascores) to measure deficit in amyotrophic lateral sclerosis. *Neurology*, 1988, 38: 405–408.

Armon, C. Motor neuron disease. "*Handbook of Neuroepidemiology*" (P.B. Gorelick and M. Alter, Eds.), 1994, pp. 407–456. Marcel Dekker, New York.

Armon, C. and Brandstater, M.E. Motor unit number estimates and quantitative muscle strength: a validation study. *Muscle Nerve*, 1997, 20: 1072–1073.

Armon, C. and Brandstater, M.E. Motor unit number estimate-based rates of disease progression of ALS predict patient survival. *Muscle Nerve*, 1999, 22: 1571–1575.

Armon, C. and Moses, D. Linear estimates of rates of disease progression as predictors of survival in patients with ALS entering clinical trials. *J. Neurol. Sci.*, 1998, 160(Suppl. 1): S37–S41.

Armon, C., Brandstater, M.E. and Peterson, G.W. Motor unit number estimates and quantitative muscle strength measurements of distal muscles in patients with amyotrophic lateral sclerosis. *Muscle Nerve*, 1997, 20: 499–501.

Armon, C., Graves, M.C., Moses, D.E., Forte, D.K., Sepulveda, L., Darby, S.M. and Smith, R.A. Linear estimates of disease progression predict survival in patients with amyotrophic lateral sclerosis. *Muscle Nerve*, 2000, 23: 874–882.

Bradley W.G. for the BDNF Phase III Study Group. A controlled trial of recombinant methionyl human BDNF in ALS: The BDNF Study Group (Phase III). *Neurology*, 1999 Apr 22, 52(7): 1427–1433.

Bromberg, M.B. Electrodiagnostic studies in clinical trials for motor neuron disease. *J. Clin. Neurophysiol.*, 1998, 15(2): 117–128.

Brooks, B.R., Sufit, R.L., DePaul, R., Tan, Y.D., Sanjak, M. and Robbins, J.A. Design of clinical therapeutic trials in amyotrophic lateral sclerosis. "*Advances in Neurology*" (L.P. Rowland, Ed.), Vol. 56, 1991, pp. 521–546. Raven Press, New York.

Bryan, W.W., Barohn, R., Murphy, J.R., Armon, C., Miller, R. G., Goodpasture, J., Parry, G.J., Petajan, J., Ross, M.A. and Stromatt, S. and the ALS/SSNJV Study Group. Placebo versus natural history in an ALS clinical trial. *Neurology*, 1995, 45(Suppl. 4): A280–A281.

Consensus Guidelines for the Design and Implementation of Clinical Trials in ALS Appendix 5, Statistical Considerations. Second Airlie House Workshop, 1998. http://www.wfnals.org.

Daube, J.R. Estimating the number of motor units in a muscle. *J. Clin. Neurophysiol.*, 1995, 12: 585–594.

McComas, A.J. Invited review: motor unit estimation: methods, results, and present status. *Muscle Nerve*, 1991, 14: 585–597.

McComas, A.J., Fawcett, P.R.W., Campbell, M.J. and Sica, R. E.P. Electrophysiological estimation of the number of motor units within a human muscle. *J. Neurol. Neurosurg. Psychiatry*, 1971, 34: 121–131.

Miller, R.G., Petajan, J., Bryan, W.W., Armon, C., Barohn, R. J., Goodpature, J.C., Hoagland, R.J., Parry, G.J., Ross, M. A. and Stromatt, S. and the rhCNTF ALS Study Group. A placebo-controlled trial of recombinant human Ciliary Neurotrophic Factor (rhCNTF) in amyotrophic lateral sclerosis. *Ann. Neurol.*, 1996, 39: 256–260.

Munsat, T.L., Hollander, D., Andres, P. and Finison, L. Clinical trials in ALS: measurement and natural history. "*Advances in Neurology*" (L.P. Rowland, Ed.), Vol. 56, 1991, pp. 515–519. Raven Press, New York.

*SPSS Base 7.5 for Windows. User's Guide. SPSS Inc., Staff. C. 1996. Pap. text ed. 41.00 (0-13-657214 6) P-H.

Motor Unit Number Estimation (Supplements to Clinical Neurophysiology Vol. 55)
Editor: M.B. Bromberg

Chapter 20

MUNE in spinal muscular atrophy

Kathryn J. Swoboda* and Mark B. Bromberg

Department of Neurology, University of Utah School of Medicine 3R210, 50 North Medical Drive, Salt Lake City, UT 84132, USA

Introduction

Spinal muscular atrophy (SMA) is characterized by the loss of lower motor neurons, resulting in diffuse weakness and muscular atrophy. Patients present most frequently in infancy and early childhood, and are divided into types based on severity of weakness (Munsat and Davies, 1997). The degree of lower motor neuron loss in the different types is predominantly inferential and cannot be determined from clinical assessments (Russman et al., 1983; Zerres and Rudnik-Schöneborn, 1995; Iannaccone et al., 2000). Clinical observations suggest a period of rapid loss followed by prolonged periods of stability in some individuals (Russman et al., 1983; Zerres and Rudnik-Schöneborn, 1995; Crawford, 1996; Iannaccone et al., 2000), but subsequent rates of lower motor neuron loss are unknown. Life expectancy varies between and within types, and the relationship between degree of lower motor neuron loss and survival is unknown (Zerres and Rudnik-Schöneborn, 1995). We previously reported our preliminary observations in a small group of patients (Bromberg and Swoboda, 2002). Our purpose here is to review our ongoing experience with MUNE in SMA, including cross-sectional and longitudinal data in 31 patients with a wide range of age and SMA phenotype.

Motor unit number estimation (MUNE) is an electrophysiologic method to estimate the number of lower motor neurons innervating a group of muscles supplied by a nerve (McComas, 1991). MUNE values are calculated from the ratio of the maximal compound muscle action potential (CMAP) to the average single motor unit potential (SMUP). MUNE principles and assumptions have been reviewed (Brown and Milner-Brown, 1976; Slawnych et al., 1990; McComas, 1991). We chose the multiple point stimulation technique due to its ease of application in infants and young children.

Methods

A description of our methods have been outlined previously (Bromberg and Swoboda, 2002). The results we report are only those obtained with surface multipoint stimulation, although initially we had evaluated whether nerve near stimulation might be better in chubby infants. Responses were considered all-or-none if they were present and stable at one current level without fractionation (minimum of eight independent observations) and absent at a lower level. MUNE calculations were based on negative peak area.

**Correspondence to*: Dr. Kathryn Swoboda, Department of Neurology, University of Utah School of Medicine 3R210, 50 North Medical Drive, Salt Lake City, UT 84132, USA. Tel.: 801-588-3385, Fax: 801-588-3392.
e-mail: swoboda@genetics.utah.edu

doi: 10.1016/S1567-424X(03)00020-5

Conscious sedation with midazolam was used in some infants and children. No complications occurred from sedation or MUNE testing. Subjects tolerated the procedure with minimal or no visible discomfort. All subjects or their parents expressed willingness to return for repeat testing.

Results

All SMA subjects had homozygous deletions in the telomeric copy of the survival motor neuron gene on chromosome 5 (Lefebvre et al., 1995), except subject 23, who has one deletion and a presumed point mutation. This group includes one patient with congenital arthrogryposis, nine SMA I patients, 12 SMA II patients, eight SMA III patients, and a 9-month old of as yet uncertain status.

MUNE values were readily obtained except in one neonate with arthrogryposis (subject 8) in whom no CMAP or muscle twitch was elicited. Every attempt was made in each subject to obtain at least 10 units. However, this was not possible in many SMA I subjects. Between 5 and 13 were collected in each subject. The same SMUP, defined as having an identical waveform, could frequently be activated from multiple sites along the nerve.

Low MUNE values were found in all symptomatic subjects (Table 1). A 9-month-old infant (subject 2) diagnosed prenatally and studied prior to symptom onset had a normal MUNE value. Follow-up testing at 28 months of age revealed a greater than 60% reduction in MUNE value. Her symptomatic brother (subject 1) with SMA studied at 3.5 years of age had markedly reduced values. Reevaluation at just over 4 years of age revealed a substantial drop in MUNE values. Subject 10, a clinically normal 2-week-old neonate diagnosed prenatally (two siblings with SMA type I died by 6 months of age) had a normal CMAP amplitude but a MUNE value less than 50% of expected, suggesting lower motor neuron loss with compensatory collateral reinnervation in utero. She died by 5 months of age. Subject 11, a 45-year-old SMA II patient, had a very low MUNE value, supporting prolonged survival of motor neurons in some cases. Reevaluation a year later revealed a stable MUNE value. Overall, lowest MUNE values were found in SMA I patients, but there was considerable overlap of values among SMA II and III patients (Fig. 1).

Test–retest reliability is generally good, and clearly higher at lower MUNE values (Table 1, Fig. 2). CMAP amplitude values ranged widely, and although they correlated in a general sense with MUNE values, they did not correlate with SMA type or subject age. The CMAP and MUNE value in the 6.5-year-old control subject and in a neonate and 11-month-old with other neuromuscular disorders were very much higher than in symptomatic SMA subjects. SMUP values in SMA subjects vary widely, depending on their age at testing and SMA sub-type.

Discussion

Our continuing experience with MUNE confirms our earlier impressions that MUNE appears to be a reliable, non-invasive tool which can be used to assess SMA patients over time. It is particularly helpful in the assessment of infants and young children, and provides additional information that cannot be obtained from clinical observation or tests of function (Crawford, 1996; Iannaccone et al., 2000; Bromberg and Swoboda, 2002).

MUNE has been infrequently applied in SMA patients, and rarely in the setting of evaluation of patients very early in infancy (Hausmanowa-Petrusewicz and Krawanska, 1986; Bromberg and Swoboda, 2002). Our data demonstrate that MUNE can provide very important information in this setting regarding the time course of motor neuron loss in SMA. The multiple point stimulation technique addresses the issue of alternation, uses low stimulation intensities to collect SMUPs, and can be performed on any EMG machine (Doherty and Brown, 1993). The test requires approximately 20–30 min to perform, is well-tolerated, and can be readily used in patients less than 2 years of age.

We believe our results are technically sound. How accurately our numbers reflect the number of surviving lower motor neurons is unknown at this time, since we are using an end organ target of these neurons, the muscle, to make inferences regarding

TABLE 1

MUNE, CMAP, SMUP AND FUNCTIONAL STATUS

Case	SMA type	Age at testing	MUNE value NP_{area}	CMAP $NP_{area}^{mVms}/NP_{amp}^{mv}$	Average SMUP $NP_{area}^{mVms}/NP_{amp}^{mV}$	Functional status
8[a]	0	1 day	Not possible	NR – absent		Joint contractures; ventilator from birth
						Died 2 weeks
10[a]	I	16 days	87	16.9/5.9	0.18/0.05	*Normal: pre-symptomatic*
						Died 5 months
15[a]	I	23 days	268	11.5/4.1	0.04/0.02	*Normal: pre-symptomatic*
		9 weeks	12	1.8/0.6	0.15/0.06	G-tube placed; bipap trial
		Retest	8	2.8/1.0	0.36/0.06	Died 4½ months
20[a]	I	7 weeks	4	0.46/0.16	0.06/0.03	No antigravity mvmt
		Retest	3	0.55/0.15	0.12/0.04	
		10 weeks	2	0.27/0.10	0.16/0.07	CPAP dependent
		Retest	1	0.36/0.14	0.22/0.10	RF; died 10 weeks
3[a]	I	3.5 months	9	1.6/0.23	0.07/0.03	No antigravity mvmt
		4.3 months	4	1.1/0.20	0.07/0.04	Ventilator dependent
		Retest	6	0.8/0.20	0.13/0.05	Died 4.5 months
7	I	4 months	10	2.4/0.9	0.24/0.12	Upper extremity antigravity
		Retest	8	2.4/0.9	0.29/0.13	
		12 months	10	0.4/0.19	0.04/0.02	
		21 months	10	0.3/0.16	0.03/0.03	
		Retest	8	0.3/0.19	0.03/0.02	Very weak; recurrent respiratory arrest; bipap (night)
9[a]	I	6 months	5	1.2/0.54	0.23/0.11	Upper extremity antigravity only; died 8.5 months
		8 months	3	0.9/0.48	0.26/0.13	
26	I	7.5 months	9	0.7/0.2	0.08/0.03	Some antigravity arms
		Retest	9	0.8/0.18	0.09/0.04	G-tube; bipap
16	I	16 months	5	0.59/0.32	0.12/0.06	Some antigravity arms
4	I	21 years	12	2.6/0.70	0.22/0.08	Wheelchair bound
		Retest	9	2.9/0.73	0.31/0.10	
		22 years	7	2.8/0.60	0.42/0.12	Tracheostomy/ventilator
		23 years	9	5.1/1.35	0.59/0.14	Some progressive weakness
23	I/II?	9.5 months	21	5.0/1.8	0.24/0.10	Antigravity arms and legs, not yet sitting
28	II	20 months	8	0.5/0.34	0.07/0.04	No longer sits (maximum 10 s), poor head control; G-tube
		Retest	7	0.5/0.29	0.07/0.04	

2	II	9 months	401	16.1/6.7	0.04/0.03	*Normal: pre-symptomatic*
		28 months	142	15.2/5.1	0.11/0.05	Walks with walker
29	II	12 months	17	3.0/0.9	0.18/0.07	No longer sits
		Retest	16	3.1/1.1	0.20/0.07	
27	II	17 months	52	4.8/2.2	0.09/0.06	Antigravity shoulder; sits but falls easily
		Retest	45	4.7/2.5	0.11/0.08	
21	II	18 months	7	1.2/0.5	0.17/0.08	Sits when placed; tenuous
		Retest	8	1.0/0.4	0.13/0.06	? G-tube
18	II	19 months	45	6.8/3.0	0.15/0.07	Crawls; sits
		23 months	13	3.3/1.6	0.23/0.10	Crawls; sits
1	II	3.5 years	48	5.0/1.7	0.10/0.06	Sits if placed
		5.1 years	45	3.5/1.3	0.08/0.04	Sits if placed
33	II	8 years	19	3.3/0.60	0.11/0.07	Wheelchair bound
14	II	15 years	20	3.3/1.4	0.17/0.08	Sat briefly at 5–6 months; Wheelchair bound
5	II	19 years	9	15.8/5.3	1.77/0.6	Wheelchair bound
		20 years	20	12.2/4.6	/0.6	Wheelchair bound
		21 years	15	10.5/4.1	0.63/0.2	Wheelchair bound
11	II	45 years	6	6.5/2.1	1.2/0.04	Wheelchair bound
		46 years	5	6.7/2.2	1.4/0.04	Wheelchair bound
17	III	2.5 years	71	12.8/4.7	0.18/0.05	Walks independently
		3 years	87	10.0/3.5	0.12/0.03	Walks independently
		Retest	95	11.3/3.5	0.12/0.04	
22	III	6.5 years	26	6.8/2.7	0.26/0.10	Wheelchair bound
13	III	17 years	76	9.0/3.6	0.12/0.07	Wheelchair by 9 years; Scoliosis
19	III	28 years	116	38.4/10.4	0.33/0.12	Walks independently
		28.4 years	126	39.4/10.7	0.31/0.11	
12	III	4.5 years	50 R	20.4/7.5	0.41/0.13	Walks independently
		5 years	66 L	18.7/6.3	0.28/0.10	Heel cord contractures
6	III	10 years	103	22.2/6.8	0.22/0.12	Walks with assistance
		11 years	104	19.8/6.4	0.19/0.10	Wheelchair bound
		12 years	113	18.5/4.7	0.16/0.06	Wheelchair bound
31	III	23 years	100	11.3/4.6	0.11/0.05	Assisted ambulation
30	III	50 years	125	32.9/10.4	0.25/0.10	Onset teens; skied into 20s Walks independently
Ctrl1	N/A	6.5 years	311	39.0/13.3	0.13/0.04	Normal strength
Ctrl2	N/A	11.5 months	365	11.1/5.3	0.03/0.02	Infant with myopathy
Ctrl3	N/A	6 weeks	251	10.9/5.7	0.04/0.03	Cervical spine trauma

Subjects 1 and 2, and subjects 4, 5, and 6 are siblings; 30 is the parent of 31.
[a] Deceased.

motor neuron numbers. Since we are assessing a distal muscle in the hand, broad generalization of our results is difficult. Reduced numbers of voluntarily activated SMUPs supports severe lower motor neuron loss. Our normal subject data remain limited and in infants and young children will remain primarily limited to patients referred for a variety of suspected neuromuscular conditions. However, our values are similar to adult MUNE values and consistent with anatomic estimates from infants.

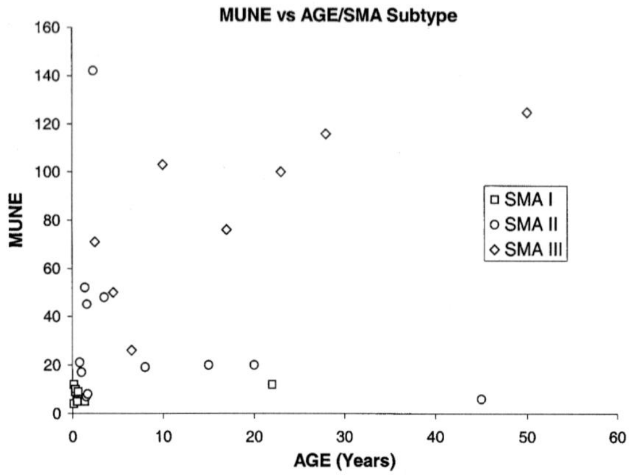

Fig. 1. Plot of MUNE values against patient age and SMA subtype.

Our goal in refining MUNE testing in SMA infants and children is to assess the natural history of lower motor neuron loss. These data suggest that MUNE values fall rather quickly to low levels early in the progression of weakness, especially in type I and II patients. The few cases in which we have been able to test patients pre-symptomatically (subjects 2, 10 and 15) suggest that onset of symptoms follows a sometimes substantial period of motor unit loss. Recruitment of additional subjects, and continued longitudinal MUNE testing and correlation with functional status and other factors known to modify phenotype are in progress. Informative endpoint measures for clinical SMA trials are problematic, and MUNE may be promising, especially for pre-symptomatic patients, infants and young children.

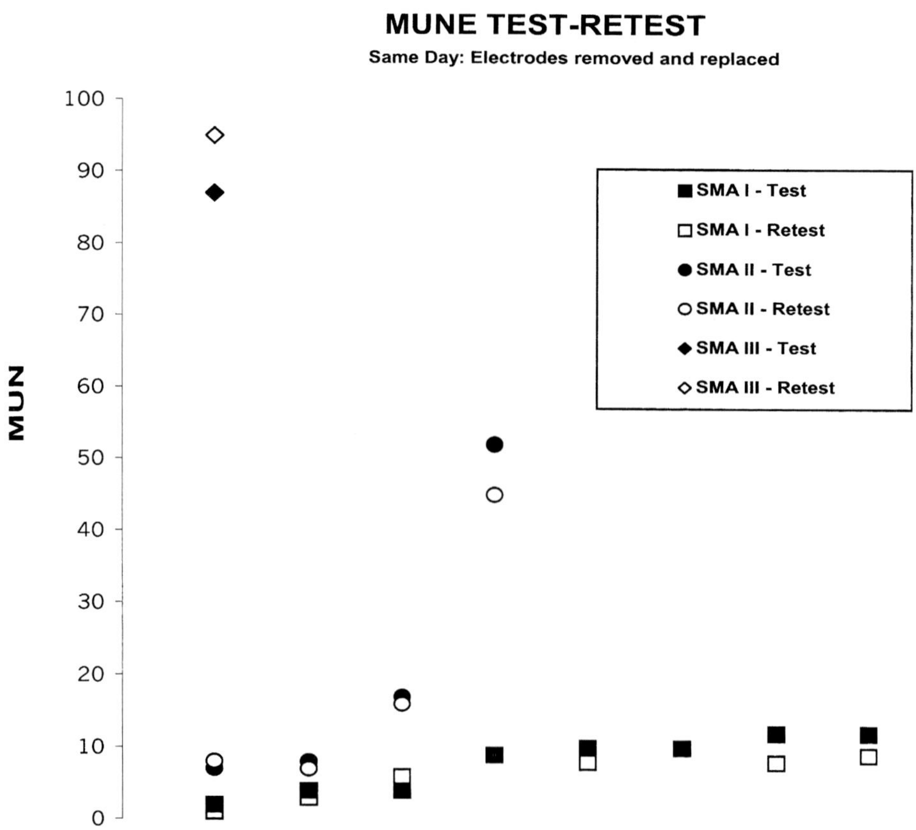

Fig. 2. Plot of MUNE test–retest values in patients with SMA subtypes I, II and III.

References

Bromberg, M.B. and Swoboda, K.J. Motor unit estimation in infants and children with spinal muscular atrophy. *Muscle and Nerve*, 2002, 25: 445–447.

Brown, W. and Milner-Brown, H. Some electrical properties of motor units and their effects on the methods of estimating motor unit numbers. *J. Neurol. Neurosurg. Psychiatry*, 1976, 39: 249–257.

Crawford, T. From enigmatic to problematic: the new molecular genetics of childhood spinal muscular atrophy. *Neurology*, 1996, 46: 335–340.

Doherty, T. and Brown, W. The estimated numbers and relative sizes of thenar units as selected by multiple point stimulation in young and older adults. *Muscle Nerve*, 1993, 16: 355–366.

Hausmanowa-Petrusewicz, I. and Krawanska, A. Electromyographic findings in different forms of infantile and juvenile proximal spinal muscular atrophy. *Muscle Nerve*, 1986, 9: 37–46.

Iannaccone, S.T., Russman, B.S., Browne, R., Buncher, C.R., White, M., Samaha, F.J., Group DSMA. Prospective analysis of strength in spinal muscular atrophy. *J. Child Neurol.*, 2000 15: 97–101.

Lefebvre, S., Bürglen, L., Reboullet, S., Clermont, O., Burlet, P., Viollet, L., Benichou, B., Cruaud, C., Millasseau, P., Zeviani, M., Le Paslier, D., Frézal, J., Cohen, D., Weissenback, J., Munnich, A. and Melki, J. Identification and characterization of a spinal muscular atrophy-determining gene. *Cell*, 1995, 80: 155–165.

McComas, A. Invited review: motor unit estimation: methods, results, and present status. *Muscle Nerve*, 1991, 14: 585–597.

Munsat, T. and Davies, K. In "*Spinal Muscular Atrophy*," 2nd ed. 1997, pp. 37–41. Royal Society of Medicine Press, London.

Russman, B., Melchreit, R. and Drennan, J. Spinal muscular atrophy: the natural course of disease. *Muscle Nerve*, 1983, 6: 179–181.

Slawnych, M., Laszlo, C. and Hershler, C. A review of techniques employed to estimate the number of motor units in a muscle. *Muscle Nerve*, 1990, 13: 1050–1064.

Stålberg, E., Schwartz, M. and Trontelj, J. Single fibre electromyography in various processes affecting the anterior horn cell. *J. Neurol. Sci.*, 1975, 24: 403–415.

Zerres, K and Rudnik-Schöneborn, S. Natural history in proximal spinal muscular atrophy. *Arch. Neurol.*, 1995, 52: 518–523.

Motor Unit Number Estimation (Supplements to Clinical Neurophysiology Vol. 55)
Editor: M.B. Bromberg

Chapter 21

MUNE in prior poliomyelitis and spinal muscular atrophy

Darcy Fehlings[a], Victoria Galea[b], Robert Griggs[c], Susan Kirsch[a], Alan McComas[b,]* and Caroline Quartly[b]

[a]*Bloorview MacMillan Centre, Toronto, ON, Canada*
[b]*Faculty of Health Sciences, McMaster University, Hamilton, ON L8N 3Z5, Canada*
[c]*University of Rochester, New York, NY, USA*

Introduction

Motor unit number estimation (MUNE) is a methodology eminently suited to the study of motoneuron disorders. An account of the findings from our laboratory in ALS is given elsewhere in the Proceedings (Turnbull et al., this volume), and now, for contrast, we present our observations in two slowly developing conditions, the post-polio syndrome and spinal muscular atrophy (SMA), drawing mainly on material in two recent publications (McComas et al., 1997; Galea et al., 2001). In both conditions we wished to document the overall extent of motor unit loss, and to determine if the losses were continuing. We also searched for evidence of differences in the susceptibility of motoneuron pools in each disorder and, in post-poliomyelitis (PP) patients, we looked for any muscle denervation in limbs not thought to have been affected in the initial infection.

**Correspondence to*: Dr. Alan J. McComas, Division of Neurology (4U1), McMaster University Medical Centre, 1200 Main Street West, Hamilton, ON L8N 3Z5, Canada. Tel.: (905) 525-9140x22519, Fax: (905) 521-2656. e-mail: mccomas@fhs.mcmaster.ca

doi:10.1016/S1567-424X(03)00021-7

Methods

Post-polio patients

The post-polio study involved a total of 78 patients with a previous diagnosis of poliomyelitis infection and in all but six of these there had been a recent increase in muscle weakness and fatiguability. Two of the 78 patients were subsequently excluded because, on enquiry and EMG testing, the diagnosis of previous polio seemed unlikely. A further eight patients were over the age of 70 years, and their MUNE values were rejected because of the complication of motor unit losses due to aging. Of the remaining 68 patients, there were 28 men and 40 women, with ages ranging from 29 to 69 years (mean, 53.9 SD $\pm$ 8.9 years). Their mean age at the initial infection was 9.8 $\pm$ 7.8 years, and the mean interval until the development of additional symptoms was 38.1 $\pm$ 10.1 years. Within the total population, there was a group of 22 patients (13 male and 9 female) who participated in a follow-up study at the Strong Memorial Hospital in Rochester, New York State.

SMA patients

The SMA study had two population groups. One of these was the 51 patients, adults and children, aged 6 days to 62 years, who were referred to the EMG clinic at McMaster University Medical Centre because of muscular symptoms and signs, mostly between 1971 and 1985. The second group consisted of 12 children and one young adult, who were volunteers in a recent research study at the Bloorview MacMillan Centre in Toronto. In this last group there were 10 males and three females, and their ages ranged from 5 to 24 years (mean 13.8 ± 6.3 years). In all patients the diagnosis of SMA was consistent with the clinical features, and with the finding of muscle denervation by conventional needle examination as well as by MUNE; in addition, all the children and many of the adults had muscle biopsies, providing further confirmation. There are alternative classifications of patients with SMA and we have adopted one with three types (Tandan, 1989), which might be summarized as follows: *type I.* Infantile severe (Werdnig-Hoffmann); *type II.* Childhood intermediate; *type III.* Adult benign. Of our 64 patients there were 7 type I, 23 type II, and 34 type III.

MUNE

In nearly all cases MUNE was performed using the manual incremental method, as originally described for the extensor digitorum brevis (EDB) muscle by McComas et al. (1971) and for the thenar and hypothenar muscles by Sica et al. (1974). In some patients the plantar muscle group and soleus were also examined, while the biceps brachii was selected for the research study at the Bloorview MacMillan Centre (see above).

Results

Initial MUNEs in PP patients

Figure 1 shows, for the PP patients, the normalized MUNE values in 242 muscles of limbs that were either known to have been affected, or thought not to have been affected, during the original poliomyelitis infection. In the "affected" limbs, 149 of 170 muscles (87%) were found to have reduced MUNEs, and 12 of these muscles were totally denervated. In the supposedly "unaffected" limbs there was a surprisingly high incidence of denervation as well, with 49 of 75 muscles (65%) having diminished MUNE values. In Table 1, the results in the affected and clinically unaffected limbs have been combined and then broken down in terms of the various muscles examined. The most severely affected muscle was the soleus, while in the foot the EDB was more denervated than the plantar muscles, and in the hand the thenar muscles were more involved than the hypothenar ones; these differences were statistically significant.

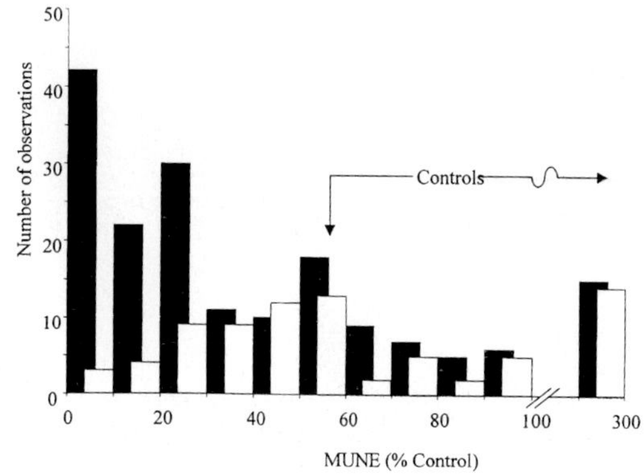

Fig. 1. Normalized MUNEs in 242 muscles of post-polio patients. Filled and open columns indicate values for limbs, respectively known, and not known, to have been affected by the original viral illness. Reproduced with permission from McComas et al. (1997).

TABLE 1

COMPARISON OF MUNEs IN DIFFERENT MUSCLES

Muscle	Observations (*n*)	MUNE	% Control mean
Soleus	38	254 ± 236	26.6 ± 24.7
EDB	86	71 ± 60	34.1 ± 28.6
Thenar	49	145 ± 119	42.3 ± 34.8
Hypothenar	31	269 ± 175	69.6 ± 44.9
Plantar	38	290 ± 254	74.3 ± 65.1

Values are means ± SDs. Reproduced with permission from McComas et al. (1997).

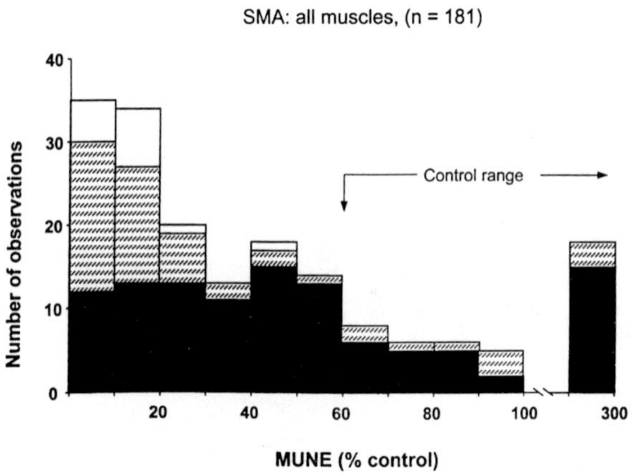

Fig. 2. Normalized MUNEs in 181 muscles of patients considered to have type I (open columns), type II (hatched columns), or type III (filled columns) SMA. As in Fig. 1, 60% has been taken as the lower limit of normal, though there are small differences between muscles.

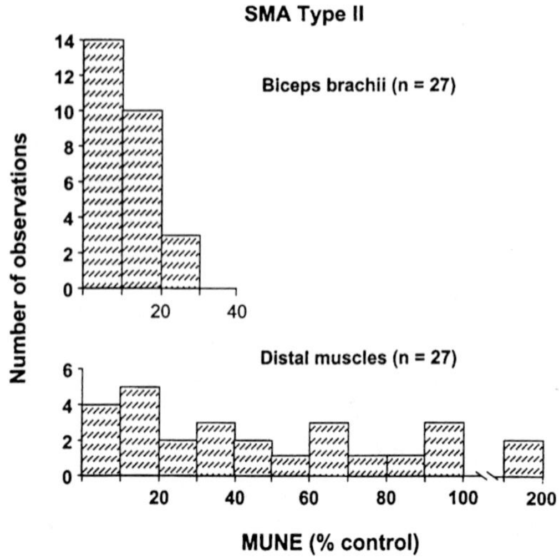

Fig. 3. Normalized MUNEs in biceps brachii muscles (*top*) and small muscles of the hand and foot (*bottom*) in type II SMA.

Initial MUNEs in SMA patients

Figure 2 shows MUNE values for 181 muscles in the total population of 64 SMA patients. As in Fig. 1, the values have been normalized and when serial testing was performed, the values are those for the initial examination. In addition, the sources of the data, in terms of the three types of SMA, have been given. It can be seen that, as for polio, there was a large range of MUNEs, from total denervation in two muscles, to normal innervation, in approximately one quarter of the muscles. As might have been expected, all the type I patients had low MUNEs, as did the majority of type II patients, while the values for the type III patients were more evenly distributed. The results in Fig. 3 carry the analysis further, by comparing the values for a proximal muscle, the biceps brachii, with those for the small muscles of the hand and foot, within type II patients only. Whereas all the biceps muscles had severe denervation, the MUNE values were sometimes normal in the distal muscles. The biceps muscles in the type II patients were also involved in another study, in which their MUNE values were compared with the strength of voluntary elbow flexion in the same arms. It was found that there was no correlation between these two variables (Fig. 4).

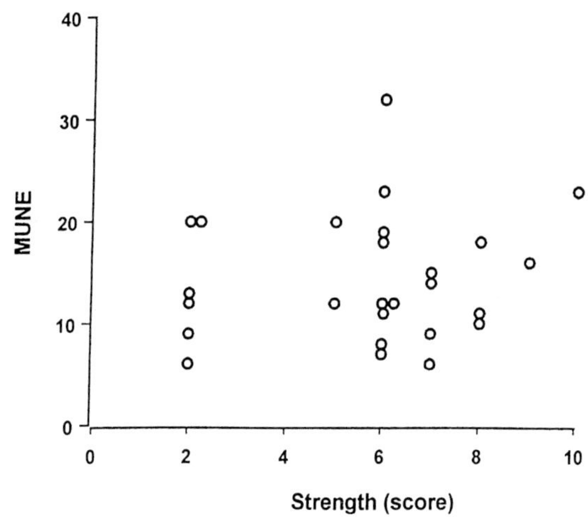

Fig. 4. Comparison of MUNEs in biceps brachii muscles with maximal voluntary elbow flexion in 13 patients with type II SMA. The clinical assessment of strength was made using a scale in which 0 and 10 represent total paralysis and normal strength, respectively (Mendell and Florence, 1990). Reproduced with permission from Galea et al. (2001).

Amplitudes of motor unit potentials in PP and SMA patients

The amplitudes of the motor unit potentials (MUPs) were used as an indication of the relative sizes of the units, and the values for the EDB

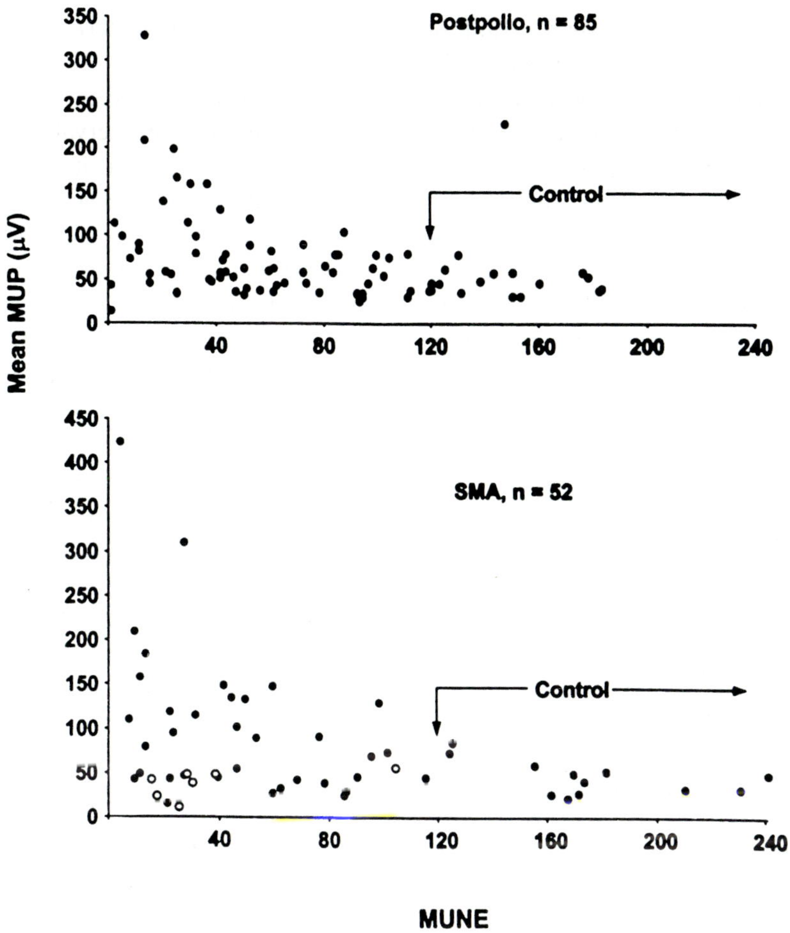

Fig. 5. Mean amplitudes of motor unit potentials for different MUNEs in EDB muscles of post-polio and SMA patients (*top* and *bottom*, respectively). Values for type I SMA shown by open circles and for types II and III SMA by filled circles.

muscles in the two populations of patients have been compared in Fig. 5. In both populations, the mean MUP amplitude for a muscle has been shown against the number of surviving units in that muscle. In the SMA patients age could have been a confounding factor, because the smallest muscle fibers would normally occur in the youngest children and would diminish the MUP amplitude accordingly. For this reason the MUP amplitudes for infants with type I SMA have been identified separately and are seen to be uniformly low; in contrast, the children with type II SMA often had enlarged MUPs in their distal muscles. In both PP and SMA patient groups there was a strong trend for the largest MUP amplitudes to be found in the muscles with greatest denervation, but there were also many normal-sized MUPs in partially denervated muscles.

Follow-up studies in PP patients

Twenty-two PP patients were invited to return after a 2-year interval for a second MUNE assessment, and this proved feasible for 18 of them. In order to minimize the effect of the experimental error inherent in MUNE, six muscles were investigated in each volunteer; these were the EDB and soleus muscles of both legs, and the thenar and hypothenar muscles of one arm. To avoid the distortion that would have occurred if the initial value was adopted as the reference, the first and second values were expressed as percentages of the

voluntary elbow flexion. This surprising result could have been partly due to the unknown degree of pathological involvement of the two other elbow flexors, the brachialis and the brachioradialis. However, the presence of many small MUPs in the biceps, in addition to large ones, suggests that some of the surviving motoneurons are "weakened" in that they are incapable of undertaking axonal branching and enlarging their colonies of muscle fibers. An alternative, but less likely, explanation is that the muscle fibers are not receptive to innervation.

In the types II and III patients, it is not known whether there is a further drop-out of some of the surviving motoneurons innervating proximal muscles such as the biceps, but the present study has clearly shown that, in the case of the distal muscles of types II and III patients, the motoneuron populations may remain stable. Before the cellular basis of SMA was understood, from molecular genetics, we used the non-progressive nature of the MUNE values as an argument that the loss of motoneurons, even in the type III patients, must have occurred in utero (McComas, 1987).

The present study suggests that the sizes of the MUPs may provide one criterion for distinguishing between types I and II SMA infants. Thus, whereas the MUPs were small in all the type I infants examined, some of the type II infants had MUPs which were considerably enlarged. Finally, SMA is the only generalized neuropathic disorder, that we have studied, in which there does not appear greater susceptibility of the thenar muscles, relative to the hypothenar ones, and of the EDB, relative to the plantar group (see McComas, 1977; Turnbull et al., this volume).

Conclusions

MUNE studies have been conducted in two slowly progressive neuropathic disorders, PP and SMA. In PP patients there was often evidence of muscle denervation in limbs not thought to have been affected in the initial viral illness. In some patients the decline of motor unit populations in later life was more rapid than that to be expected from the normal aging process.

In SMA, the losses of motor units were always severe in the type I patients and the MUPs were small. In type II patients, the losses were usually more pronounced in a proximal muscle, the biceps brachii, than in the small muscles of the hand and foot. Unlike the situation in type I patients, in type II children the MUPs were sometimes enlarged in the small muscles of the hand and foot, and this observation, if present, could have predictive value. Also in type II children, there was no correlation between the numbers of surviving units in the biceps and voluntary strength. In the type III patients there was considerable variability in the MUNEs, and approximately one quarter of the estimates in the distal muscles fell within the normal ranges. In both types II and III patients, the motoneuron populations, at least for distal muscles, appeared to be stable. This last finding indicated that the losses of neurons had taken place in utero.

Acknowledgements

We thank Rebecca Newberry and Jane Butler for technical assistance, and the former Leman Brothers Muscular Dystrophy Foundation and the Bloorview Children's Hospital Foundation for financial support.

References

Dalakas, M.C. Pathogenetic mechanisms of post-polio syndrome: morphological, electrophysiological, virological and immunological correlations. *Ann. N.Y. Acad. Sci.*, 1995, 753: 167–185.

Daube, J.R., Windebank, A.J. and Litchy, W.J. Electrophysiologic changes in neuromuscular function over five years in polio survivors. *Ann. N.Y. Acad. Sci.*, 1995, 753: 120–128.

Galea, V., Fehlings, D., Kirsch, S. and McComas, A. Depletion and sizes of motor units in spinal muscular atrophy. *Muscle Nerve*, 2001, 24: 1168–1172.

Harding, A.E. Inherited neuronal atrophy and degeneration predominantly of lower motor neurons. In: *Peripheral Neuropathy* (P.J. Dyck, P.K. Thomas, J.W. Griffin, P. A. Low and J.F. Poduslo, Eds.), 3rd ed. 1993, pp. 1051–1064. W.B. Saunders, Philadelphia.

McComas, A.J. In "*Neuromuscular Function and Disorders*", 1977, pp. 364. Butterworths, London.

McComas, A.J. Motor neurone disorders. *Clinical Electromyography* (W.F. Brown and C.F. Bolton, Eds.), 1987, pp. 431–451. Butterworths, Stoneham, MA.

McComas, A.J., Fawcett, P.R.W., Campbell, M.J. and Sica, R.E.P. Electrophysiological estimation of the number of motor units within a human muscle. *J. Neurol. Neurosurg. Psychiatry*, 1971, 34: 121–131.

McComas, A.J., Quartly, C. and Griggs, R.C. Early and late losses of motor units after poliomyelitis. *Brain*, 1997, 120: 1415–1421.

Mendell, J. and Florence, J. Normal muscle testing. *Muscle Nerve*, 1990, 20, Suppl. S16–S20.

Pezeshkpour, G.H. and Dalakas, M.C. Pathology of spinal cord in post-poliomyelitis muscular atrophy. *Birth Defects*, 1987, 23: 229–236.

Sica, R.E.P., McComas, A.J., Upton, A.R.M. and Longmire, D. Motor unit estimations in small muscles of the hand. *J. Neurol. Neurosurg. Psychiatry*, 1974, 37: 55–67.

Tandan, R. Disorders of the upper and lower motor neurons. *Neurology in Clinical Practice. II. The Neurological Disorders* (W.G. Bradley, R.B. Daroff, G.M. Fenichel and C. D. Marsden, Eds.), 1989, pp. 1687–1717. Butterworth-Heinemann, Boston.

Motor Unit Number Estimation (Supplements to Clinical Neurophysiology Vol. 55)
Editor: M.B. Bromberg

Chapter 22

A longitudinal analysis of MUNE in subjects with a prior paralytic poliomyelitis

E.J. Sorenson*, J.R. Daube and A.J. Windebank

Department of Neurology, Mayo Clinic, Rochester, MN 55905, USA

Introduction

Progressive neurological deficits in patients with prior paralytic poliomyelitis have been reported for over 100 years and has been termed the post-polio syndrome (Mulder et al., 1972; Jublet et al., 1987; Wiechers, 1987). The etiology of this syndrome has been debated. It has been suggested that it is the result of attritional loss of anterior horn cells with aging (Mulder et al., 1972). Others have proposed poor unstable reinnervation from the terminal axonal sprouts in massively reinnervated muscles as the main causative factor (Cashman et al., 1987; Dalakas, 1988). An inflammatory response within the affected muscles has been shown in some instances (Dalakas, 1988). More recently, it has been shown that denervation continues as a late effect and that the large motor units demonstrate ongoing instability (Grimby et al., 1998). Another group has shown that the number of motor units drops with time as well (McComas et al., 1997). It is clear that the syndrome of fatigue, pain and the perceived sensation of progressive weakness is a common feature in patients with remote paralytic poliomyelitis. Previously, a population based, Olmsted County (Minnesota), cohort of patients was studied to assess the natural history of the late effects of paralytic poliomyelitis in a randomly selected and unbiased population (Ivanyi et al., 1999).

At the beginning of the study in 1987, the prevalence of new fatigue, pain and weakness was over 50% (Ivanyi et al., 1999). More recent studies have demonstrated similar findings in populations from The Netherlands and Norway (Windebank et al., 1991; Wekre et al., 1999). This population was followed and re-examined with the same detailed evaluations after a 5-year interval. There was no deterioration in any aspect of nerve or muscle function studied over this time. This included stable strength testing (by manual muscle testing and quantitative maximum voluntary isometric contraction testing) and functional assessments. At the 5-year follow-up period, about 20% of subjects continued to have symptoms of fatigue, weakness and pain. The majority of this group had these symptoms throughout the 5-year study period. For most symptomatic patients, there was an alternative explanation for their symptoms such as degenerative osteoarthritis and other mechanical problems (Windebank et al., 1996). It was concluded as a result of this 5-year detailed study that the symptoms of pain, fatigue, and weakness in this group of post-polio patients were not due to

**Correspondence to*: Dr. Eric J. Sorenson, MD, Department of Neurology, Mayo Clinic, Rochester, MN 55905, USA.
e-mail: Sorenson.Eric@mayo.edu

doi: 10.1016/S1567-424X(03)00022-9

progressive neuromuscular deterioration. For this same population of patients electrophysiological assessments were also performed and assessed as a component of the longitudinal study. These included compound muscle action potential (CMAP) amplitudes and motor unit number estimates (MUNEs) at baseline and at the 5-year follow-up period.

Methods

The demographics of the study population have previously been described in detail (Ivanyi et al., 1999). In the previous studies 50 representative subjects were chosen from 298 patients whom previously had well documented acute paralytic polio (Ivanyi et al., 1999; Windebank et al., 1991). All 50 patients had identical testing performed at the study onset. Forty-six of the 50 were available for follow-up testing at 5 years. Four patients were asymptomatic and declined the follow-up testing.

Electrophysiological testing was performed in all participating subjects. CMAP amplitudes were recorded from bilateral thenar and peroneal motor nerves using standard technique. CMAP amplitudes were recorded from the proximal stimulation sites at the elbows and knees for the median and peroneal nerves, respectively. MUNEs were recorded using the statistical method as originally described by Daube, (1995). These were recorded also from bilateral thenar and peroneal motor nerves.

Analysis of the data was performed by comparing baseline values to the 5-year follow-up values in the following fashion. Thenar and peroneal CMAP amplitudes and MUNE values were compared using a paired *t*-test comparing baseline and 5-year follow-up values. To obtain a global comparison for the individuals, the CMAP amplitudes and MUNE values from all four muscles were summated into a summated CMAP and MUNE and again compared with a paired *t*-test. To further assess the relationship of the MUNE to the CMAP amplitude, for both the thenar muscles and peroneal muscles the CMAP amplitude was plotted against the MUNE values.

Results

The mean thenar and peroneal CMAP amplitudes and summated CMAP amplitudes were unchanged when compared at baseline and 5-year follow-up (Fig. 1). For the MUNE data there was an 18, 17 and an 18% drop in the MUNE values from baseline to 5 years follow-up for the thenar ($P=0.03$), peroneal ($P>0.05$) and summated MUNE ($P=0.05$), respectively (Fig. 2).

Because of the discrepancy between the CMAP amplitude stability and the modest drop in MUNE over time the relationship between MUNE values and CMAP amplitudes was explored further. MUNE data was plotted against CMAP amplitudes to assess for a correlation. Plotting MUNE values (*X*-axis) against the CMAP amplitudes (*Y*-axis) for thenar, peroneal and summated data indicate that the CMAP amplitude is largely independent of the MUNE value above 50 for both thenar and peroneal motor nerves (Fig. 3). Below a MUNE value of 50 there is a precipitous decline in the CMAP amplitude which is directly proportional to the MUNE value.

Discussion

As has been previously shown complaints of fatigue, pain, weakness and sensory loss is quite prevalent with the population of patients with a remote history of paralytic poliomyelitis. In this population however, neuromuscular function has been demonstrated to remain stable, at least over a 5 year period. For the majority of these alternative explanations were identified such as degenerative joint disease (osteoarthritis), tendonitis and other overuse syndromes (Windebank et al., 1996).

In the present analysis, there does appear to be a modest loss of motor neurons as determined by the statistical method of MUNE. This represented a total of approximately 18% over the 5 years and was quite consistent among the different muscles. For the vast majority of muscles this modest loss is of no clinical consequence as the CMAP amplitude and subsequent neuromuscular function is independent of this. For most muscles, even those

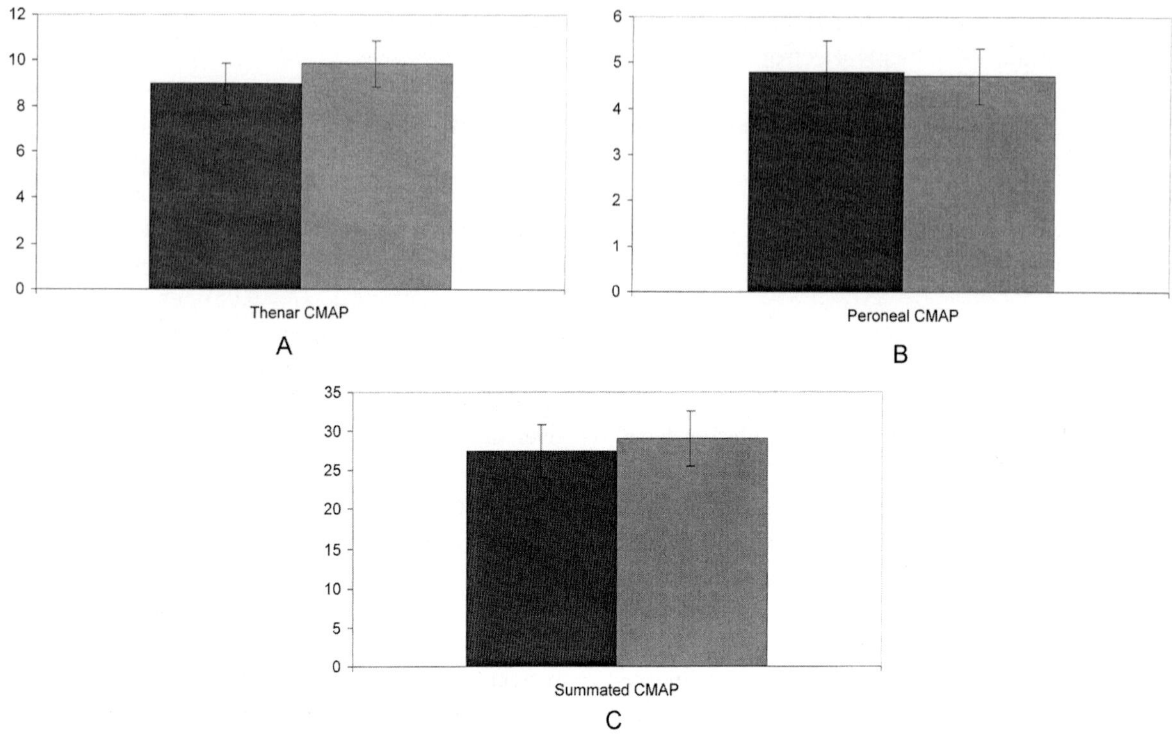

Fig. 1. (A–C) CMAP amplitudes for thenar, peroneal, and summated at baseline (dark bars) and at 5 years follow-up (light bars) demonstrating stability of the CMAP amplitude over time ($P > 0.05$ for all three comparisons).

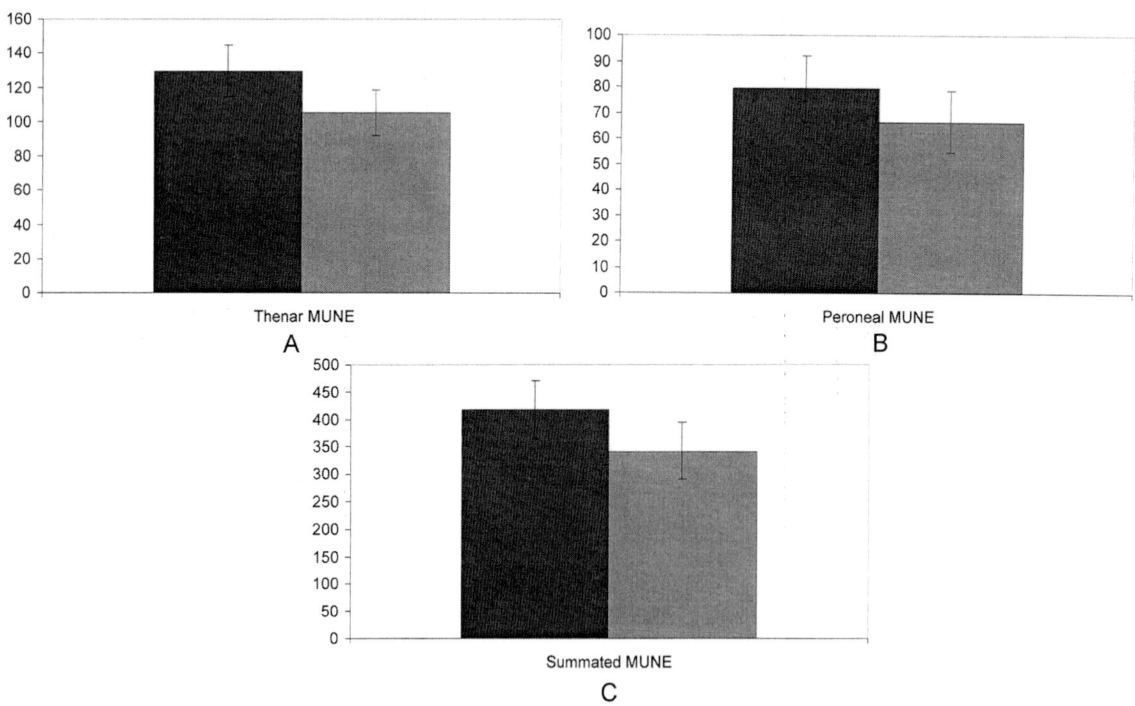

Fig. 2. (A–C) MUNE values for thenar, peroneal, and summated at baseline (dark bars) and at 5 years follow-up (light bars) demonstrating the modest drop in MUNE over the specified time period ($P = 0.03$, > 0.05, and 0.05, respectively).

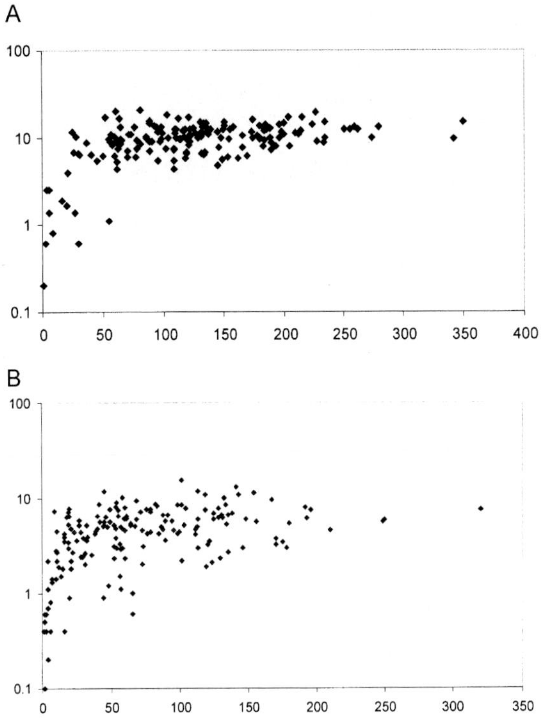

Fig. 3. MUNE values plotted against the CMAP amplitudes for thenar (A) and peroneal (B) demonstrating that the CMAP amplitude is independent of the MUNE value for both thenar and peroneal motor nerves with a MUNE value in excess of 50.

affected remotely by poliomyelitis, the capacity of reinnervation via collateral sprouting exceeds this modest loss of motor neurons. It is likely that there is a very small minority of muscles whose loss of motor neurons is so great that the capacity of reinnervation via collateral sprouting has reached its limits and further attritional loss results in progressive atrophy, weakness and loss of neuromuscular function. While this may occur in a minority, it is clear that the majority of symptoms reported by the post-polio cohort were not on the basis progressive attritional loss of motor neurons with subsequent atrophy, weakness and/or deterioration of neuromuscular function.

References

Cashman, N.R. et al. Late denervation in patients with antecedent paralytic poliomyelitis. *N. Engl. J. Med.*, 1987, 317: 7–12.

Dalakas, M.C. Morphologic changes in the muscles of patients with postpoliomyelitis neuromuscular symptoms. *Neurology*, 1988, 38: 99–104.

Daube, J.R. Estimating the number of motor units in a muscle. *J. Clin. Neurophysiol.*, 1995, 12(6): 585–594.

Grimby, G. et al. An 8-year longitudinal study of muscle strength, muscle fiber size, and dynamic electromyogram in individuals with late polio. *Muscle Nerve*, 1998, 21(11): 1428–1437.

Ivanyi, B. et al. Late onset polio sequelae: disabilities and handicaps in a population-based cohort of the 1956 poliomyelities outbreak in The Netherlands. *Arch. Phys. Med. Rehabil.*, 1999, 80(6): 687–690.

Jublet, B. et al. Neurological manifestations of the post-polio syndrome. *Crit. Rev. Neurobiol.*, 1987, 3: 199–220.

McComas et al. Early and late losses of motor units after poliomyelitis. *Brain*, 1997, 120 (Pt. 8): 1415–1421.

Mulder, D.W. et al. Late progression of poliomyelitis or forme fruste amyotrophic lateral sclerosis. *Mayo Clin. Proc.*, 1972, 47: 756–761.

Wekre, L.L. et al. The Norwegian Polio Study 1994: a nation-wide survey of problems in long standing poliomyelitis. *Spinal Cord*, 1999, 89(4): 183–187.

Wiechers, D.O. Late effects of polio: historical perspectives. *Birth Defects*, 1987, 23: 1–11.

Windebank, A.J., Litchy, W.J., Daube, J.R., Kurland, L.T., Codd, M.B. and Iverson, Rita, Late effects of paralytic poliomyelitis in Olmsted County, Minnesota. *Neurology*, 1991, 41(4): 501–507.

Windebank, A.J., Litchy, William J., Daube, Jasper R. and Iverson, Rita. Lack of progression of neurological deficit in survivors of paralytic polio: a 5-year prospective population-based study. *Neurology*, 1996, 46: 80–84.

Motor Unit Number Estimation (Supplements to Clinical Neurophysiology Vol. 55)
Editor: M.B. Bromberg

Chapter 23

MUNE in Charcot–Marie–Tooth neuropathies

Richard A. Lewis[a,*], Jun Li[a], Michael E. Shy[a,b] and Karen Krajewski[a,b]

[a]*Department of Neurology, Wayne State University School of Medicine, Detroit, MI 48201, USA*
[b]*Center for Molecular Medicine and Genetics, Wayne State University School of Medicine, Detroit, MI 48201, USA*

Introduction

Motor unit number estimation (MUNE) has been shown to be able to detect progressive motor unit loss in amyotrophic lateral sclerosis (ALS) (Olney et al., 2000). ALS is an ideal disorder to evaluate with MUNE because motor unit loss can be profound leading to dramatic changes over a relatively short period of time. It is less clear, however, whether MUNE can also identify progressive motor unit changes in more chronic and insidious disorders such as Charcot–Marie–Tooth disease (CMT).

We have been interested in the factors that cause disability in CMT. There is increasing evidence that in forms of CMT with genetic mutations causing changes in peripheral nerve myelin that slow conduction velocity is not the major determinant of weakness and disability (Dyck et al., 1989; Roy et al., 1989; Krajewski et al., 2000). Rather, functional deficits result from secondary axonal degeneration that occurs gradually. How primary disorders of myelin proteins cause axonal degeneration is not known and is currently under investigation. To understand how weakness develops in CMT, we have been investigating genotype–phenotype correlations for various mutations of peripheral nerve myelin proteins. In particular, we are interested in determining whether rates of progression and patterns of axonal involvement are different in the various forms of CMT.

As part of this endeavor, we have performed a variety of electrophysiologic studies on patients with CMT-1A, CMT-X and CMT-2. This report focuses on studies of the compound motor action potential (CMAP) and MUNE of the abductor digiti minimi (ADM) and of the biceps brachii (BB) muscles. While reductions in CMAP of distal muscles have been shown to correlate with progressive disability in CMT (Roy et al., 1989; Krajewski et al., 2000), we were interested in developing a quantitative method to more precisely measure axonal degeneration in nerves innervating both proximal and distal muscles. We were also interested in developing methods to detect evidence of early denervation in proximal muscles that appeared clinically strong. We hypothesized that CMAP will not be sensitive to early changes, and that MUNE may be a more sensitive measure of motor unit loss in proximal muscles.

A number of different MUNE techniques are available (Doherty et al., 1995; Shefner, 2001), each having advantages and disadvantages. For subjects with CMT, we chose the spike-triggered-averaging (STA) technique because it required less

**Correspondence to*: Dr. Richard A. Lewis, Department of Neurology, Wayne State University School of Medicine, UHC 8D, 4201 St. Antoine, Detroit, MI 48201, USA. Tel.: 313-577-1244, Fax: 313-745-4216. e-mail: RAlewis@med.wayne.edu

doi: 10.1016/S1567-424X(03)00023-0

nerve stimulation, which can be painful and problematic in subjects with CMT-1A, and is the best technique to look at proximal muscles.

Methods

Fifty-three subjects with CMT, including 28 with CMT-1A, 13 with CMT-X, and 12 with CMT-2, along with nine normal controls had routine nerve conduction studies and STA MUNE performed on ADM (53 subjects) and BB (46 subjects) muscles. All CMT subjects were seen in our CMT clinic between 1999 and 2001. Informed consent was obtained from all subjects. CMT-1A and CMT-X was confirmed by genetic testing of the subject or immediate family member. CMT-2 was the presumptive diagnosis in subjects with normal or near normal conduction velocities, evidence of male-to-male transmission and/or negative testing for CMT-1A and CMT-X, and in some instances, point mutations of PMP-22 and P-0.

STA MUNE was performed based on published techniques (Bromberg and Abrams, 1995). A CMAP was obtained from the ADM or BB muscles groups with surface recording electrodes following stimulation of the ulnar nerve at the wrist or the musculocutaneous nerve in the axilla. There were seven subjects with CMT-1A in whom a supra-maximal stimulation of the musculocutaneous nerve could not be accomplished. Peak-to-peak amplitude values were used to calculate the MUNE. A concentric needle electrode was inserted into the ADM or BB muscles and single motor units were identified. These single units were used to trigger and average the surface recording of the same single motor unit (SMUP). We attempted to record at least 10 individual units for each muscle, and with rare exceptions, were able to record at least five different units obtained. Peak-to-peak amplitudes of the SMUPs were averaged to determine the average single motor unit that was then used to calculate the MUNE value.

Clinical strength was graded from 0 to 3 by the following scale: 0 = no movement; 1 = very weak (equivalent to 1–3 on the MRC scale); 2 = mile weakness (equivalent to 4 on the MRC scale); 3 = normal strength. Two neurologists (RAL and MES) independently evaluated each subject, and there was agreement of the ratings in every case. Only 26 subjects had ADM strength assessed, as this was not routinely included until the second year of the study.

Results

Length dependent motor unit loss

MUNE values for control subjects were > 100 in the ulnar-ADM and > 150 in the musculocutaneous-BB muscle groups. There was a large range of normal values, with one subject having an MUNE value greater than 300 in the ulnar-ADM and one subject with a value over 500 in the musculocutaneous-BB muscles. Mean ulnar-ADM and musculocutaneous-BB MUNE values in CMT subjects were significantly reduced compared to controls (Figs. 1 and 2). MUNE values in CMT subjects were < 100 in 96% (51/54) of ulnar-ADM muscles, and < 150 in 57% (26/46) of musculocutaneous-BB muscles. More specifically, the degree of reduction was much greater in ulnar-ADM (MUNE values 14% of control values) than in musculocutaneous-BB (MUNE values 54% of control values). The reduction in musculocutaneous-BB MUNE values was noteworthy given that this muscle was clinically unaffected in all of the subjects. The greater MUNE reduction in the ulnar-ADM compared to the musculocutaneous-BB muscle group is consistent with length dependent axonal degeneration known to occur in CMT-1A. These results also support the notion that MUNE is capable of detecting both clinical and sub-clinical decreases of motor units in our subjects.

Mean SMUP values also showed a distal-to-proximal difference in CMT subjects. The mean SMUP for the ulnar-ADM was 500% higher than in controls subjects while the mean SMUP value for the musculocutaneous-BB was 200% higher than in control subjects, supporting the notion that collateral sprouting and re-innervation were occurring to a much greater extent in distal compared to

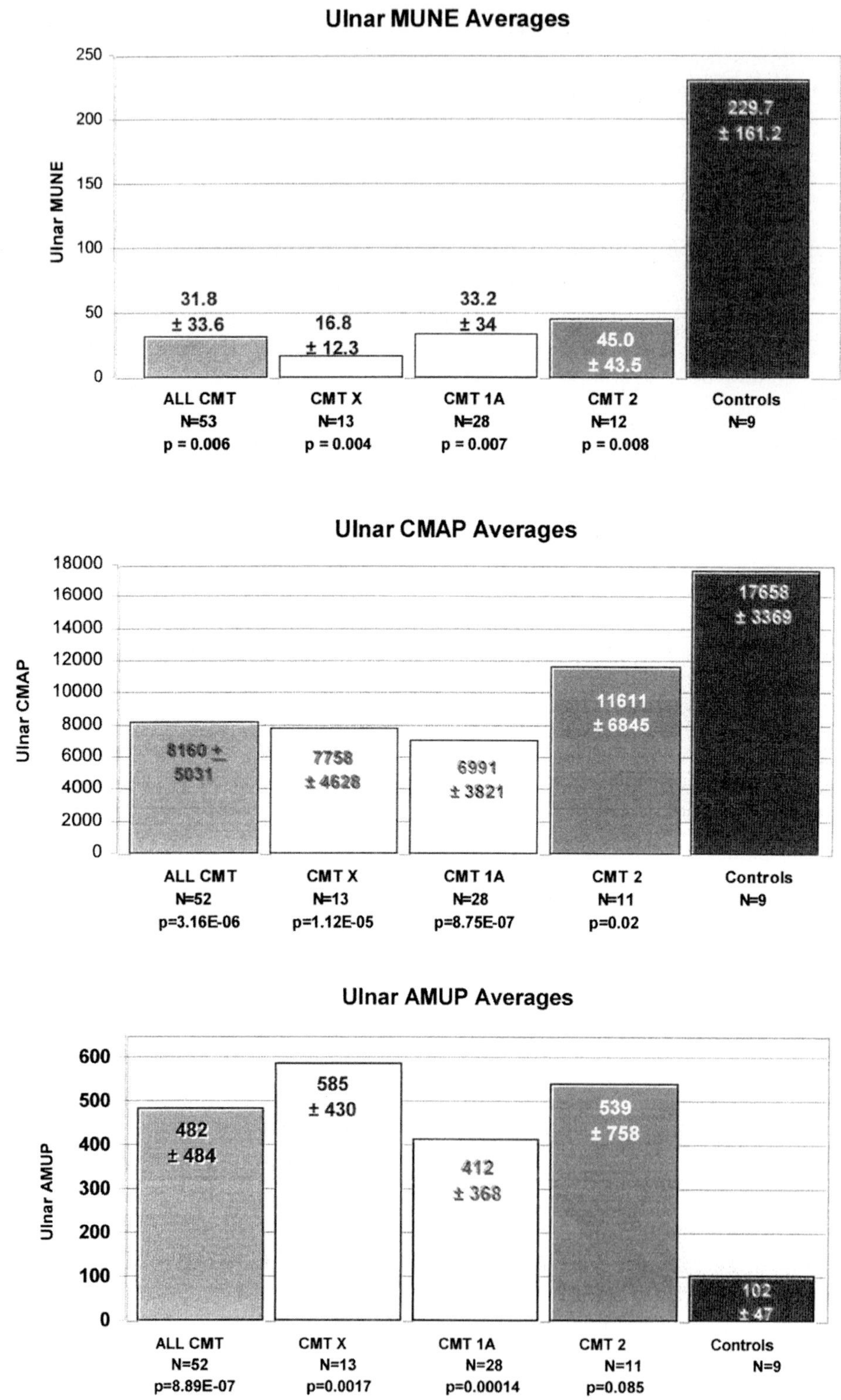

Fig. 1. Bar graphs of ulnar-ADM data for subjects with various forms of CMT and control subjects. Number of subjects and significance levels listed below bar graphs. *Top graph:* MUNE values. *Middle graph:* CMAP amplitude values. *Lower graph:* average single motor units amplitude values.

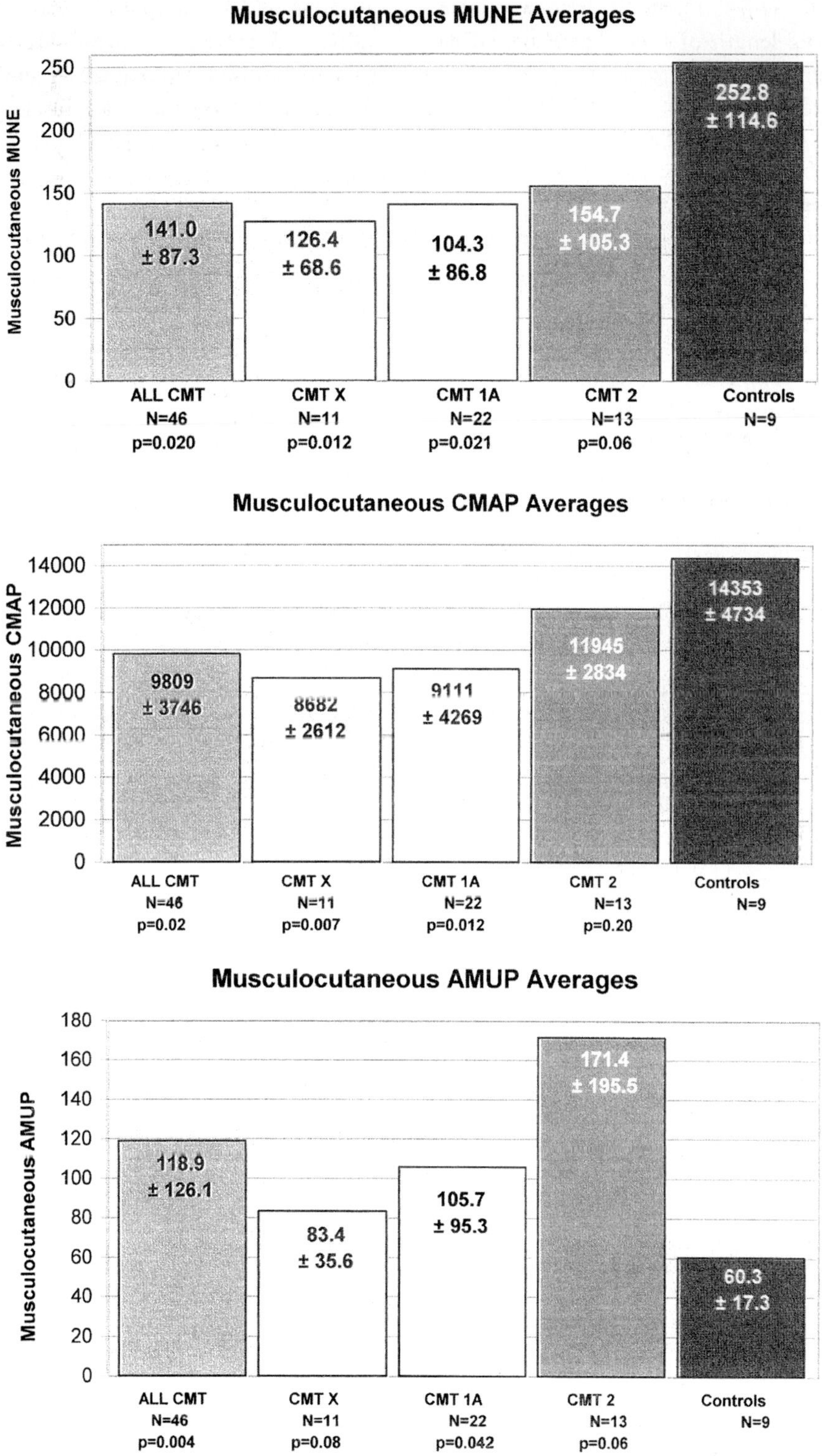

Fig. 2. Bar graphs of musculocutaneous-BB data for subjects with various forms of CMT and control subjects. Number of subjects and significance levels listed below bar graphs. *Top graph:* MUNE values. *Middle graph:* CMAP amplitude values. *Lower graph:* average single motor units amplitude values.

proximal muscles (Figs. 1 and 2). This may also reflect the greater length of time that denervation had been present in distal muscles.

MUNE correlations with CMAP

We analyzed both negative-peak (N-P) and peak-to-peak (P-P) CMAP amplitude values. Although P-P values were 70–100% greater than N-P amplitude values, in every subject correlations with MUNE were virtually identical (data not shown). Since P-P values were used to compute MUNE, we used P-P values in the following analyses. P-P amplitudes in control subject were >10 mV for the ulnar-ADM muscle group and >8 mV for musculocutaneous-BB muscles. CMAP amplitudes was also reduced in distal and proximal muscles in CMT subjects. Comparisons between CMAP and MUNE values showed the following relationships. For the ulnar-ADM muscle group in CMT subjects, CMAP amplitudes were abnormal in 75% (40/53) compared MUNE values that were abnormal in 96% (Fig. 3). Ten subjects had normal CMAP amplitudes but abnormal MUNE values. The average CMAP amplitude was 45% of control values compared to mean MUNE values that were 14% of control values. A similar analysis for the musculocutaneous-BB muscle group in CMT subjects, showed that CMAP amplitude was abnormal in 35% (16/46) compared to abnormal MUNE values in 57% (Fig. 4). Fifteen subjects had normal CMAP amplitudes but abnormal MUNE values. The average CMAP amplitude was 68% of controls compared to MUNE values that were 54% of controls.

Thus, CMAP amplitude reduction was not as impressive as the reduction in MUNE value, particularly for the ulnar-ADM. Both the number of subjects with abnormal MUNE values and the reduction in mean MUNE were greater than the respective changes in CMAP.

MUNE correlations with strength

There were strong correlations between clinical ulnar-ADM strength and MUNE ($r=0.79$) and CMAP amplitude ($r=0.79$). Only one subject had normal strength with a reduced CMAP (8 mV),

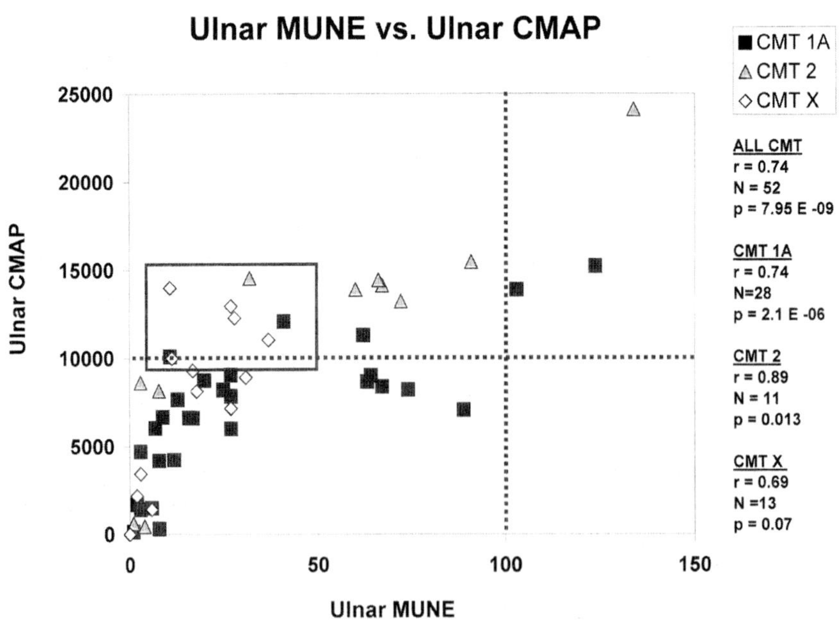

Fig. 3. Plot of unlar-ADM MUNE values versus unlar-ADM CMAP amplitude values for subjects with various forms of CMT (symbol identification, number of subjects, correlation coefficients and significance levels listed along right side of plot). Dotted lines repsenent lowest MUNE and CMAP amplitude values recorded from normal subjects. Boxed area represents CMT subjects who have very low MUNE values but normal CMAP amplitudes.

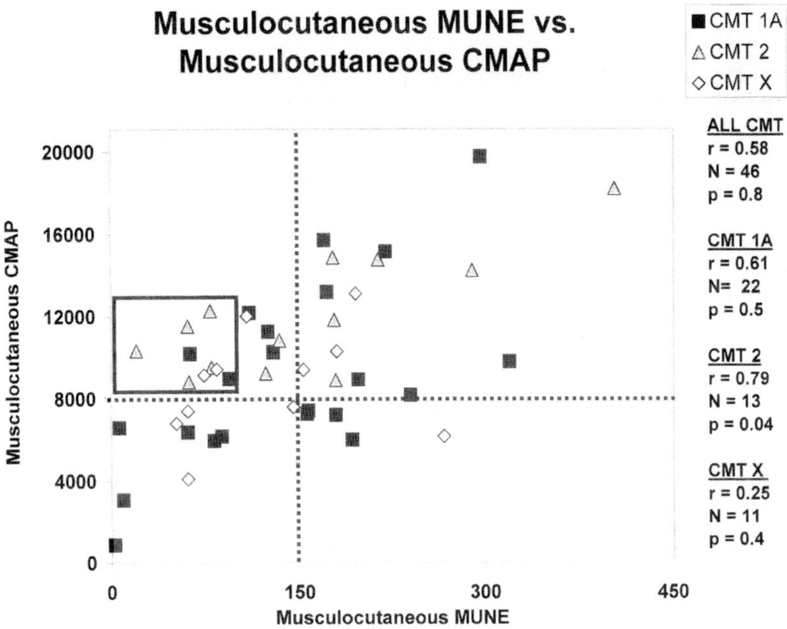

Fig. 4. Plot of musculocutaneous-BB MUNE values versus musculocutaneous-BB CMAP amplitude values for subjects with various forms of CMT (symbol identification, number of subjects, correlation coefficients and significance levels listed along right side of plot). Dotted lines repsenent lowest MUNE and CMAP amplitude values recorded from normal subjects. Boxed area represents CMT subjects who have very low MUNE values but normal CMAP amplitudes.

while 12% (3/26) of subjects had normal clinical strength but reduced MUNE values (55, 65, 90). This is consistent with the hypothesis that MUNE, more than CMAP, can detect sub-clinical axon loss even in distal muscles.

This hypothesis was more evident in the musculocutaneous-BB muscle group. Although we could not perform clinical correlation between MUNE and strength in proximal muscles because all subjects were graded as having normal biceps strength, 57% of subjects had reduced MUNE values compared to 35% with reduced CMAP values.

MUNE correlations in CMTX

We compared our findings in subjects with CMT-1A ($n=28$), CMT-X ($n=13$) and CMT-2 ($n=13$) to determine whether there were differences in MUNE values in subjects with different forms of CMT. MUNE values were decreased in distal and proximal muscles in each CMT groups (Tables 1). However, the ratio of distal-to-proximal MUNE values was only 0.13 in CMT-X compared to a ratio of 0.31 in CMT-1A suggesting that the distal reductions are more pronounced in CMT-X. Distal-to-proximal ratios for CMT-2 (0.29) were similar to that found for CMT-1A, but inferences from these subjects are tentative because of the small numbers and heterogenous genetic CMT-2 population.

MUNE correlations with age and gender

We determined if MUNE values decrease with age in CMT-1A subjects (Table 1). Both MUNE values from the musculocutaneous-BB muscles ($r=0.67$) and from ulnar-ADM muscles ($r=0.64$) decreased with age, consistent with the hypothesis that disease progression correlates with axonal loss in CMT-1A (Krajewski et al., 2000). A similar analysis for CMT-X showed no statistically significant decreases in MUNE values with age. With the possibility that differences between males and females might this analysis, we repeated the analysis according to sex. These data demonstrated a strong correlation between MUNE values in ADM muscles with age ($r=0.9$) for men but not for women. Interestingly, MUNE musculocutaneous-BB values for men did not correlate with age. The significance

TABLE 1

CORRELATION OF MUNE AND CMAP AMPLITUDE WITH SUBJECT AGE

	N	Correlation coefficient (r)	P-value
All CMT	52		
CMAP		−0.06	< 0.00013
MUNE		−0.22	< 0.0003
CMT-1A	29		
CMAP		−0.49	< 0.0000006
MUNE		−0.64	< 0.0000012
CMT-X	13		
CMAP		0.06	< 0.09
MUNE		0.05	< 0.16
CMT-2	11		
CMAP		0.25	< 0.6
MUNE		0.36	< 0.94
Control	9		
CMAP		0.34	< 0.049
MUNE		−0.49	< 0.024

of this finding will need to be addressed with larger numbers of subjects of both genders with CMT-X analyzed.

Discussion

This study demonstrates that the STA MUNE technique can be used to investigate the degree of motor unit loss in CMT. The major findings are: (1) In CMT, MUNE values are reduced in ulnar-ADM to a greater degree than in musculocutaneous-BB muscles, consistent with the concept that axon loss occurs in a length dependent fashion. (2) While MUNE and CMAP values correlate well in both ulnar-ADM and musculocutaneous-BB muscles, there are subjects in whom the CMAP amplitude may not reflect the full extent of motor unit loss, particularly in ulnar-ADM muscles. The marked increase in the average SMUP amplitude for the ulnar-ADM shows the extent that collateral re-innervation may preserve a relatively normal CMAP amplitude despite severe motor unit loss. (3) In the ulnar-ADM muscle group, MUNE and CMAP values correlate with ADM strength, but there are subjects who have normal clinical strength but mild to moderate reductions in MUNE values. Better correlations between strength and electrodiagnostic metrics are likely if quantitative measurements of strength are used, and we are currently developing a strain gauge to assess the ADM muscle strength. (4) There is a suggestion that motor unit loss in CMT-X may not be the same as in other forms of CMT that have a greater degree of distal motor unit loss in comparison to proximal reductions. This is consistent with clinical observations (Hahn et al., 1999) in which distal hand muscles were severely weak and atrophied even in younger patients, and may reflect the particular function of connexin-32. (5) Correlations between MUNE and age point to the progressive nature of the motor unit loss. It is still not known whether the majority of motor unit loss occurs in the first few decades of life and then plateaus, or whether motor unit loss is more linear and extends throughout life. Clinically, most patients have marked atrophy and weakness of distal limbs prior to the age of 20, but describe progressive weakness throughout their adult years. To answer to this question we investigating whether the STA MUNE technique can reliably track progressive motor unit loss over time.

There are challenges for the use of the STA MUNE technique, in particular in longitudinal studies. MUNE remains an estimate with a variability that ranges from 8 to 15% (Shefner, 2001; Simmons et al., 2001). Thus, small changes in motor unit numbers will be difficult to measure precisely in longitudinal studies. The STA technique tends to have a sampling bias towards smaller motor units that are recruited early with minimal effort (Bromberg, 1993). This potentially alters the average SMUP value, skewing the MUNE to a higher number. However, new techniques have been developed for isolating single motor units during moderate contractions that may reduce sampling bias and reduce the variability of the technique (Stashuk, 2001). In our studies, we experienced difficulty obtaining a maximal CMAP from the BB muscle group. This is a concern in CMT-1A and obese subjects where stimulation thresholds can be very high. While we did not analyze subjects in whom we felt a maximal CMAP could not be obtained, this problem may account, in part, for the subjects who had normal BB MUNE values but low CMAP values. While an artifactually low CMAP amplitude would result in a lower MUNE value, we are confident that our findings remain valid. Support comes from the high average SMUP amplitude values that are independent of whether a supramaximal CMAP was obtained.

Acknowledgements

This study was supported by grants from the Muscular Dystrophy Association and Charcot Marie Tooth Association.

References

Bromberg, M.B. Motor unit estimation: reproducibility of the spike-triggered averaging technique in normal and ALS subjects. *Muscle Nerve*, 1993, 16: 466–471.

Bromberg, M.B. and Abrams, J.L. Sources of error in the spike-triggered averaging method of motor unit number estimation (MUNE). *Muscle Nerve*, 1995, 18: 1139–1146.

Doherty, T., Simmons, Z., O'Connell, B., Felice, K.J., Conwit, R., Chan, K.M., Komori, T., Brown, T., Stashuk, D.W. and Brwon, W.F. Methods for estimating the numbers of motor units in human muscles. *J. Clin. Neurophysiol.*, 1995, 12: 565–584.

Dyck, P.J., Karnes, J.L. and Lambert, E.H. Longitudinal study of neuropathic deficit and nerve conduction abnormalities in hereditary motor and sensory neuropathy type 1. *Neurology*, 1989, 39: 1302–1308.

Hahn, A.F., Bolton, C.F., White, C.M., Brown, W.F., Tuuha, S. E., Tan, C.C. and Ainsworth, P.J. Genotype/phenotype correlations in X-linked dominant Charcot–Marie–Tooth disease. *Ann. N.Y. Acad. Sci.*, 1999, 883: 366–382.

Krajewski, K., Lewis, R.A., Fuerst, D., Turansky, C., Hinderer, S., Garbern, J., Kamholz, J. and Shy, M.E. Neurological dysfunction and axonal degeneration in CMT 1A. *Brain*, 2000, 123: 1516–1527.

Olney, R.K., Yuen, E.C. and Engstrom, J.W. Statistical motor unit number estimation: reproducibility and sources of error in patients with amyotrophic lateral sclerosis. *Muscle Nerve*, 2000, 23: 193–197.

Roy, E.P., Gutmann, L. and Riggs, J.E. Longitudinal conduction studies in hereditary motor and sensory neuropathy type 1. *Muscle Nerve*, 1989, 12: 52–55.

Shefner, J.M. Motor unit number estimation in human neurological diseases and animal models. *Clin. Neurophysiol.*, 2001, 12: 955–964.

Simmons, Z., Epstein, D.K., Borg, B., Mauger, D.T., Kothari, M.J. and Shefner, J.M. Reproducibility of motor unit number estimation in individual subjects. *Muscle Nerve*, 2001, 24: 467–473.

Stashuk, D. EMG signal decomposition: how it can be accomplished and used? *J. Electromyogr. Kinesiol.*, 2001, 11: 151–173.

Discussion after Section VI

Eric Sorensen, Rochester, Minnesota

I have a question for Ken Arasaki. You concluded after you compared MUNE data with the Appel score, that early in the disease, MUNE values were more sensitive to change or are a better outcome measure. However, you really cannot compare rates of change of these outcome measures because they have different units and measure different functions. In fact, what you really need to compare is the variance in the population rather than the absolute rate of change. I was wondering if you have any data based on this for the Appel score versus the MUNE values.

Ken Arasaki, Tokyo, Japan

The only subset that I looked into was pinch force, and differences in MUNE compared to this small component of Appel score were small.

Gordon Smith, Salt Lake City, Utah

I have a question for Rich. Have you tried using near-nerve stimulation of the musculocutaneous nerve to obtain your biceps CMAP as a means of reducing stimulating current intensities?

Richard Lewis, Detroit, Michigan

I have not. It is not clear that near-nerve stimulation would reduce tissue impedance in CMT 1A patients; I have tried this in the past and even then it can still be fairly painful and difficult. It may be that studying the biceps in CMT 1A patients is not the right thing to do, and maybe these are not the patients we are going to follow in the long run. We do need to look at better ways to get reproducible CMAPs from the biceps. Maybe motor point stimulation, or near-nerve stimulation. Do you have any experience with near-nerve stimulation?

Gordon Smith, Salt Lake City, Utah

Not in the biceps muscle. I tried it in distal nerves and the subjects, including those with CMT 1, and they found it very uncomfortable. What is the experience with the femoral nerve?

Richard Lewis, Detroit, Michigan

No, I have stayed away from the femoral nerve. My patients have thanked me, by the way, for that.

Jack Petajan, Salt Lake City, Utah

I think we need to make clear distinctions between different techniques for different purposes. We are considering six or seven different MUNE techniques. Among us we are interested in different aspects of the motor unit; physiology, function, reinnervation, longitudinal changes, etc. I think somewhere in this report we need to have a review of MUNE techniques in terms of what kind of questions they are designed to answer. We cannot expect a person with ALS to spend an hour or more in a laboratory every month or two to get a complete evaluation with comparisons of clinical scores with motor unit number and so on. Many of these things are in different domains. We really need to direct some attention to the application of these techniques.

Jasper Daube, Rochester, Minnesota

I have a question for Rich Lewis. In patients with CMT, there is usually a fair bit of muscle atrophy compared with normal muscles. When you use the needle to find motor units for the spike triggered averaging technique, you are more likely to record from deeper units, but the surface representation may be different just because of atrophy. Have you given that any consideration to where you put your intramuscular needle electrode and the effect of atrophy?

Richard Lewis, Detroit, Michigan

I have noticed some things about the intramuscular and surface motor units in atrophied hand muscle. The biceps is not atrophied in CMT, so it is really only the abductor digiti minimi where atrophy is a factor. The area of the motor unit is larger than I expected; when I move the needle to another area I move it as far away as I can, and the intramuscular motor unit seen by the needle looks entirely different, yet the surface motor unit seems to be the same. So there is a problem finding new motor units because the size of each motor unit is large. I have seen some motor units that do not have large intramuscular potentials yet have large surface motor units. So I am not sure that atrophy is affecting the surface potential per se.

Mark Bromberg, Salt Lake City, Utah

At least in the biceps in ALS subjects, when I was using the spike triggered averaging technique, I moved the intramuscular trigger electrode to three different positions and at varying depths. There were areas where I got many trigger units and areas where there were almost no units even though the patient was vigorously contracting the muscle. I interpreted this as moving the needle from one fascicular area to another. I believe that what limits the geographic area over which collateral sprouting can cover is dependent upon fascicular boundaries. I am a little surprised that in the hand muscles you found that the territories could be large because Erik Stålberg and others have shown that the motor unit territory becomes denser but does not appreciably enlarge in area.

Richard Lewis, Detroit, Michigan

Well, it is a relatively small muscle to begin with, so when I say it is large, it is only relatively large. I have not seen enlargement to the same extent in the biceps, but they are not as denervated. We are going to look at fiber density to get a better feel for the territory of the motor units; we have studied one patient and the fiber density was clearly increased, as would be expected.

Jasper Daube, Rochester, Minnesota

I have another question for Rich that others will want to comment on. You made a comment that you have been using peak-to-peak amplitude and you want to shift to using the negative peak amplitude. A number of other speakers have talked about using negative peak amplitude while others have used peak-to-peak amplitude in assessing the motor unit potentials either on the surface or in the muscle. This might be a point about which we should reach some consensus. Clearly, when you are summating, you are ideally summating the entire waveform, where you include the latency and the positive components. Should we be doing what Rich suggested, getting away from peak-to-peak amplitude and moving toward negative peak amplitude?

Richard Lewis, Detroit, Michigan

I have always been concerned about using peak-to-peak amplitude because physiologically I knew that we are going to deal with the phase cancellation issues. But since Mark Bromberg had done most of his work using peak-to-peak amplitude, I did not want to make any changes given the fact that I did not know what I was doing. My problem with going back is that I have done a fair number of patients, so if I want to follow them longitudinally, I am clearly going to have to analyze with both measures because I do not want to lose the data I already have. I think physiologically we should look at the negative peak amplitude and area.

Timothy Doherty, London, Ontario

I have experience with the spike triggered averaging technique both with the traditional method and now with the decomposition method. In theory, we would like to use negative peak areas for those reasons that you mentioned. However, there are challenge that you will see in the demonstration that there are units that probably represent a reasonable average but it is difficult to determine the true onset, and the area measurement will be potentially difficult to determine. I think that is part of the reason why in Bill Brown's original work and Mark Bromberg's work, that the negative peak or peak-to-peak amplitude was used, but with the proviso that it may not be the theoretically best measurement.

Richard Lewis, Detroit, Michigan

I would like to ask Mark whether MUNE values changed much when using peak-to-peak or negative peak amplitude values.

Mark Bromberg, Salt Lake City, Utah

My impression is that differences were not greater than what I consider to be the experimental error of the test. There were two reasons why I used peak-to-peak amplitude for my earlier work. One is that Bill Brown's initial study used it. The second is that the software I had at that time, the original Viking EMG machine, did not allow me to measure anything other than peak-to-peak amplitude automatically. The newer Vikings allow one to gather other measures. A related issue that was mentioned earlier is that it can be difficult to determine the onset for measuring negative peak amplitude or area in the averaged surface waveforms. Peak-to-peak amplitude may be more accurate to measure.

Let me ask a question about old polio. I recall a study by Marinas Dalakas looking at old polio (*N. Engl. J. Med.*, 1986, 314: 959–963), and I think he found, using quantitative isometric strength testing, that patients lost only 1% a year in objective strength testing. I think that would fit with what Eric talked about or what he found with his data.

Timothy Doherty, London, Ontario

I have a question for Eric. Is there a concern that you are studying predominantly distal muscles and much of the functional complaint may be related to more proximal muscles?

Eric Sorenson, Rochester, Minnesota

It can be an issue looking at one or two muscles and translating that information into what is happening globally with the individual. At least with the statistical MUNE technique that we use there really is no way of looking at proximal muscles. With polio in general, even though it is a diffuse disease, it is very patchy and multifocal, and what is happening in one muscle is not necessarily reflective of what is happening in other muscles.

Benn Smith, Scottsdale, Arizona

Eric, to that point, you said that you determined the neuropathy impairment score in the subjects. That score incorporates measures of proximal muscle strength. Was there any decline in proximal muscles by that measure?

Eric Sorenson, Rochester, Minnesota

No.

Richard Lewis, Detroit, Michigan

Can I ask how large was the size of single motor units? If the MUNE value dropped and the CMAP stayed the same, there must be collateral sprouting and single motor units are getting larger.

Eric Sorenson, Rochester, Minnesota

Presumably, that is what is happening. There was a wide range in the size of single motor unit potentials; some muscles showed no effect at all and other muscles were severely affected.

Gordon Smith, Salt Lake City, Utah

Eric, we heard earlier this morning about motor unit decline with aging. What were the age of your polio patients, and do you think you are seeing age-related declines or is this related directly to the old polio?

Eric Sorensen, Rochester, Minnesota

We do not really know the answer to that issue. The mean age of subjects at the beginning of the study was the low 50s, and they are now in the low 60s, and we are now studying them again. We have only recently had a control population for comparison. My suspicion is that it is an age-related change and that there is nothing unique about polio patients to make them lose their motor neurons faster.

Ming Chan, Edmonton, Alberta

I have a question for Alan McComas. Eric has presented a mean decline of about 18% in the motor unit number estimate, a percentage that is fairly similar to what you found in your study. But, your conclusion was that this was not necessarily a significant decline. Can you explain that discrepancy between the conclusions of the two different studies?

Alan McComas, Hamilton, Ontario

You make a good point. Our study was based on a 2-year interval, as opposed to the 5-year interval of Eric Sorenson. I think it really comes down to sampling. Of our 20 subjects, there were two or three who showed major changes over that 2-year period.

Clifton Gooch, New York, New York

I have questions for Kathy Swoboda. I assume you used the international collaborative criteria for your classification of SMA types 1, 2, and 3. Have you been able to sort out in any way, using electrophysiologic data any pattern of degeneration related to the survival motor neuron (SMN) genes 1 and 2?

Kathryn Swoboda, Salt Lake City, Utah

I think that the SMN 2 copy number is going to be a small part of the story. There are lots of genes that could be interacting in both ALS and SMA. I do not think we have enough patients yet, and we need more longitudinal data. Surrogate markers such as the level of SMN protein expressed (from fibroblasts) can be correlated with MUNE values. I do not think we will be able to use MUNE number per se across the whole group. We will have to follow MUNE values longitudinally because some motor unit numbers in SMA 2s and 3s overlap.

Mark Bromberg, Salt Lake City, Utah

I want to make one other point. We agree with Alan that there are probably some people with SMA 2 and 3 who have only a few motor neurons that tend to survive indefinitely, as the 45-year-old gentleman who only has four or five motor units in his hands, probably for many, many years.

Kathryn Swoboda, Salt Lake City, Utah

I think there is something special about those last few motor units; they stay alive. SMA 1 babies do not die because they lose their last motor units. They die because they get pneumonia. So, maybe there is something special about those last few units, and I think you are seeing them in the older SMA 2s and 3s. I do not personally believe that the 45-year-old patient we tested has had three or four motor units for a long time. I think he probably had five or six for a very long time and now has only three or four. He has lost hand function over the last year and he is not able to write anymore. That is why I think we are going to have to follow individual patients.

Jasper Daube, Rochester, Minnesota

I think the issue just raised is important, and I would like to ask those people who are tracking motor units whether they have been able to see physiologic differences between motor units that are lost early compared to those that last a long time in ALS?

Ming Chan, Edmonton, Alberta

From the limited data we have from the two last remaining motor units in two different subjects, they behaved very differently, suggesting that there may not be a homogeneous pattern of how these motor units change with the disease. I do not have any data from the earlier stages when the motor pool is larger.

Clifton Gooch, New York, New York

I might speculate without hard data that motor units that very rapidly expand by collateral reinnervation to form a large motor unit may, in effect, contribute to their own demise by overextending their resources too rapidly. Motor units that reinnervate more slowly tend to be more stable. If this is true, are there specific electrophysiologic parameters that we can look at? For example, a motor unit that has a higher rate of decrement with repetitive stimulation, may be less likely to survive for longer periods of time, but this is highly speculative.

Richard Olney, San Francisco, California

The expansion of a motor unit's territory may have a long-term detrimental effect for some, but not all, motor units. François Wang hinted at this by showing that several patients who had the largest motor units progress slowly; and might live the longest.

Clifton Gooch, New York, New York

I would say that the rate of expansion is a key factor. With rapid denervation motor units are rapidly expanding to try to keep up, and these patients may have a worse disease to begin with. As an example, in polio you can get very large motor units that develop very slowly over time and that tend to be extremely stable.

Richard Finkelstein, Philadelphia, Pennsylvania

I have been trying to correlate in SMA with what you see in a muscle biopsy with the change from the random checkerboard pattern to grouped atrophy. From the early studies of Betty Banker in the 1960s, it seems that there are different populations of motor neurons. From some of the data presented here, there is a suggestion that there are motor neurons of different subtypes that we are dealing with, a group that are lost early on and another group that tends to be relatively preserved. I think we are seeing physiologically what we have seen both pathologically.

Jasper Daube, Rochester, Minnesota

I would like to come back to Cliff's speculation, and I will speculate to the contrary. I say this based on data we have collected which reproduced what Bill Brown and Alan McComas have collected. There is rapid loss of a significant number of units early in the disease, at different times in different muscle groups, corresponding to the clinical picture. However, there are some lasting large units regardless of the rate of progression. There are some characteristics of the unit, no matter how quickly they expand and how much they expand, that allows them to survive. Is there something different about that type of motor unit? During the tracking process, is there anything to do to try to define which motor unit is more likely to survive, are they fast or slow motor units that live longer?

Clifton Gooch, New York, New York

Clearly, correlations between strength and survival in ALS patients are not just keyed to motor unit number. I think it is important to recognize that there is a dynamic process between motor unit size and motor unit number, and survival is a product not only of the degree and rate of motor unit loss but also the degree and rate of motor unit expansion to compensate for loss. I also agree that probably there are types of motor neurons that have different properties at the beginning that may affect their long-term survival in progressive denervating disease like ALS. And it may be possible to identify electrophysiologic features of different types of motor units so we can better identify them and longitudinally track them to see if in fact this is the case. But, I still maintain that there may be a role for a threshold at which collateral reinnervation becomes too much and becomes deleterious.

Benn Smith, Scottsdale, Arizona

One brief comment. We have been talking about differences in motor units in particular muscles. There are recognized regional differences in muscles, for example, the nucleus of Onofrowicz. In the CNTF trial, we performed serial MUNE studies and found that MUNE values in the abductor hallucis muscle declined at a rate that was 10 times slower than that in the intrinsic hand muscles. So there is something different about these muscles and their anterior horn cells.

Section VII

MUNE Correlations with Other Metrics

Motor Unit Number Estimation (Supplements to Clinical Neurophysiology Vol. 55)
Editor: M.B. Bromberg

Chapter 24

Relationships between motor unit activation and muscle force generation

R.A. Conwit[a,]*, D.W. Stashuk[b] and E.J. Metter[c]

[a]*Department of Neurology, Johns Hopkins Bayview Medical Center, Baltimore, MD 21224, USA*
[b]*Department of Systems Design Engineering, University of Waterloo, Waterloo, ON, Canada*
[c]*National Institute on Aging, Gerontology Research Center, Baltimore, MD, USA*

Introduction

Clinical techniques are now available that allow for the study of motor unit activity during muscle activation (Doherty et al., 1995; McComas, 1995). These techniques have lead to methods to estimate the number of motor units in a muscle (motor unit number estimation, MUNE) that have proven useful in monitoring the progression of motor neuron diseases, where the anatomical changes are of foremost importance.

In a number of diseases and health-related processes, the activation pattern of motor units rather than the number of motor units may be the critical issue. For example, increasing age in adults is associated with progressive losses of muscle mass and strength, called sarcopenia. This process has a major impact on the elderly by contributing to frailty and disability. Previous work (Doherty, 1993; Doherty and Brown, 1997) has shown a decline in the number of motor units with age that could have a negative impact on physical function. However, the way in which motor units are activated by an aging nervous system has not been clarified. Perhaps critically important for physical functioning are alterations in the pattern of motor unit activation in response to the loss of motor units. Similarly, for some diseases, abnormalities in motor unit activation may be an important part of the pathophysiology, particularly in relationship to fatigue.

We have been interested in understanding how motor unit activation is related to force generation across the full range of a muscle's activity, and in the degree to which motor unit size and firing rate (FR) are related to muscle force. Specifically, we have been interested in developing a method that can be applied clinically to populations of motor units across many subjects.

Motor unit activation: an orderly process

Henneman (1980) observed that motor unit recruitment follows an orderly sequence according to size, such that smaller type I "slow twitch" motor units are activated before larger type II "fast twitch" units. As more motor units are progressively recruited within a muscle, the force of the contraction increases. Conversely, contraction force is reduced by deactivating motor units,

**Correspondence to*: Dr. Robin A. Conwit, Department of Neurology, Johns Hopkins Bayview Medical Center, 4940 Eastern Avenue, Baltimore, MD 21224, USA.
e-mail: rconwit@jhmi.edu

doi: 10.1016/S1567-424X(03)00024-2

usually in the reverse order of their recruitment. The size and tension produced by a single motor unit is dependent on the cross-sectional area and specific tension of its muscle fibers, and its innervation ratio (Burke et al., 1974). Thus larger motor units tend to produce greater force. By the Henneman principle, as more motor units are recruited the total force generated by the muscle will progressively increase, and this increase may not be linear, because larger units will progressively contribute a greater force than will smaller units.

The second way by which the force of contraction is modulated is by changing the FRs of motor neurons, a mechanism termed 'rate coding'. Recruitment and rate coding are not independent, and the relationship between these two mechanisms differs depending on the character of the contraction and the size of the muscle. For example, in larger muscles, such as the biceps brachii, motor unit recruitment continues over the entire force range and rate coding tends to play a significant role only towards the high end of the force spectrum (Kukulka and Clamann, 1981; DeLuca et al., 1996). By contrast, in smaller muscles such as the first dorsal interosseous, recruitment is usually complete by the time the muscle contraction reaches 30% of maximal voluntary contraction (MVC), beyond which further increases in force are mediated entirely by rate coding.

Furthermore, it has been suggested that there is a 'muscle wisdom', with fine adjustment of motor unit firing rates to take advantage of muscle fiber contraction properties (Marsden et al., 1983). For example, the instantaneous FR (iFR) at the start of a contraction may be very high to 'jump start' the contraction. As the contraction increases, iFR falls to minimize the impact of fatigue on the motor unit and to take advantage of the accompanying increases in the contraction times of the unit as it continues to fire.

Twitch contractile properties of single human motor units have been studied using carefully graded percutaneous electrical stimuli (Doherty and Brown, 1997) or intraneural stimulation (Thomas et al., 1990) to activate single units. Little research has addressed the progressive contribution of individual motor units to force production across a range of voluntarily produced force levels.

Motor unit activation: force production

The two most basic factors determining the amount of force produced by a motor unit are its size and firing rate. Motor unit size can be assessed by measuring the average force, in Newtons [N], produced by a motor unit, and this may be estimated by multiplying the area under the unit's twitch profile [Ns] by its average firing rate [l/s]. The twitch profile is dependent on specific muscle-fiber contraction and activation characteristics, and the accuracy of such an estimate will be affected by twitch potentiation, non-linear summation, and fatigue. The size of a motor unit can also be estimated by the size of its surface-detected motor unit potential (SMUP). SMUP size can be measured by peak to peak voltage or negative peak area, and both measures correlate approximately with the motor unit twitch tension (Doherty, 1993). Although direct measurements of the force produced by individual motor units during voluntary contractions are difficult, the firing patterns and rates of individual motor units can be easily determined using techniques that decompose the needle-EMG signal into individual motor unit potentials. The decomposed needle-detected EMG signals can be combined with surface EMG signals to estimate SMUPs using spike-triggered averaging (STA) techniques (Doherty et al., 1995). A motor unit's SMUP size, measured as area [μV s], multiplied by its average firing rate [l/s] might be used to estimate its contribution to average muscle force.

Factors determining the amount of force produced by a whole muscle at a point in time are the number of active motor units, the size of the active motor units, and their firing rates. The average force produced by a muscle can be approximated by the product of the mean SMUP (mSMUP) area and mean FR (mFR) of a representative sample of motor units. The units of the product of mSMUP area times mFR are microvolts $[(\mu V\, s)(1/s) = \mu V]$, and this product is called the 'mean motor unit mean voltage' (mMUmV). Similarly, the product of SMUP area times FR for a motor unit becomes the motor unit mean voltage (MUmV).

A similar relationship, expressing motor unit size in terms of intramuscular macro EMG amplitude, has been discussed by Jabre and coworkers. Their findings indicate that the product of the iFR of a motor unit times the area of its macro EMG potential (Mar), which they termed the "electrotwitch" (iFR×Mar = "electrotwitch"), is correlated with the instantaneous force produced by the muscle (Jabre and Salzsieder, 1993, 1997 and 1999). The MUmV used in the current study is directly related to electrotwitch, but differs in that an average firing rate rather than an iFR is used.

The product of mFR and mSMUP size (represented by area) differs from electrotwitch in that it is defined using average values calculated from a sample of 15–20 active motor units rather than the instantaneous values of individual units. Both approaches have merit for examining the FR and SMUP size of a sample of active motor units. Using a large sample of MUs may provide a more comprehensive view of the overall average of a pool of motor units and their effects on average muscle force production than can be obtained from studies of single motor units. Using measurements from individual units, the distributional characteristics of motor unit activity can be explored as muscle force is increased.

Methods

Subjects sat on an equipment bed with a dynamometer (Kin-Com 125E, Chattecx, Chattanooga, TN) set to measure force production of the quadriceps femoris muscle group at a knee angle of 120° (180° = full extension). Three efforts of maximal exertion were performed with vocal encouragement, and each lasted 3 s with at least a 1-min rest between efforts. The average of the two highest peak force readings was considered the maximum voluntary contraction (MVC).

Recording electrodes were placed on the thigh. The active surface electrode was placed over the motor point of the vastus medialis muscle which was identified by repositioning the surface electrode to obtain a compound muscle action potential (CMAP) of maximum amplitude and minimum rise time in response to supramaximal stimulation of the femoral nerve in the groin. The inactive surface electrode was placed on the patellar tendon, and the ground on the lateral thigh between the stimulation and recording sites.

Subjects were asked to generate specific levels of force at different percentages of MVC. Each contraction was held for 20–30 s while EMG data were collected. There were 5 min of rest between contractions. Before each submaximal isometric contraction, a concentric needle electrode inserted in the vastus medialis muscle was positioned to maximize the amplitude of motor unit potentials (MUP) generated by motor units recruited during the contraction. Typically, 3–5 motor units (range 1–10) were sampled with each contraction. After all force levels were studied, the needle was repositioned and data collection was repeated at each force level. This resulted in 15–20 motor units for each force level. We previously determined that sampling 15–20 motor units was necessary in order to obtain a coefficient of variation of approximately 10% (Conwit et al., 1997). The level of pain reported was mild and in no case necessitated stopping a study.

During each sustained contraction, needle- and surface-detected signals were acquired using sampling rates of 25 and 2.5 kHz, respectively. EMG signal decomposition and firing rate software developed by Stashuk and coworkers (Stashuk and Qu, 1996a,b; Stashuk and Paoli, 1998) was used for analysis. The needle-detected signal was decomposed using algorithms designed to distinguish different MUPs. The surface-detected signal and decomposition results were then used to estimate a SMUP for each motor unit tracked by the decomposition algorithms using spike triggered averaging techniques.

Data analysis

The average firing rate of an individual motor unit during a constant contraction was calculated using the inverse of the mean value of the main component of the MUP interdischarge interval

(IDI) histogram. The main component was identified using a robust technique which discards erroneous IDI information which may exist in a train of MUPs (Stashuk and Qu, 1996a). The size of a motor unit was represented by SMUP amplitude or area, and was calculated for each SMUP.

Muscle force was represented in two ways, as a percentage of MVC, or in terms of absolute force. Percentage MVC adjusts for individual differences in absolute strength and presents a relative expression of muscle exertion. Absolute force is dependent on muscle mass and overall strength. Both measures have physiological importance and were examined.

Data analysis followed several strategies. To examine the relationship between motor unit activation and muscle force generation, the mFR was calculated as the mean of the individual FRs of the 15–20 motor units sampled from a subject at a given force level. A similar calculation was made for motor unit size, mSMUP amplitude or area, and for the product of mFR and mSMUP area. An ANOVA design with repeated measures using a mixed-effects model was used to test whether mFR, mSMUP area, mSMUP amplitude and mMUmV were the same across percentage of MVC as shown in Table 1. To examine the relationship between motor unit properties and force levels, muscle force was regressed on mSMUP area, mFR and mMUmV using a mixed-effects model to account for the repeated measures.

The analysis for the resistive training study used the individual motor units (FR, SMUP area, MUmV) rather than the means across a percentage MVC. The subsequent analyses included ANOVA mixed-effects models to examine motor unit differences at different percentages of MVC and mixed-effects regression models to examine the relationship of the force levels to motor unit measures.

Motor unit activation and muscle force generation

Table 1 shows the overall mSMUP amplitude and area and mFR characteristics across all subjects for different levels of effort expressed as a percentage of MVC. Both mSMUP area and mSMUP amplitude increase with increasing force generation (Conwit et al., 1997). The correlation between negative peak amplitude and negative peak area was high for both average or individual SMUPs, suggesting that either area or amplitude could be used to represent mSMUP or SMUP size (Table 2).

TABLE 1

SMUP SIZE, MEAN FIRING RATE, AND FORCE GENERATION AT DIFFERENT PERCENTAGES OF MAXIMAL VOLUNTARY CONTRACTIONS

Percent MVC	Samples	Force [N]	Std. error	Mean firing rate[a] [Hz]	Std. error	mSMUP area[a] [μV s]	Std. error	mSMUP amplitude[a] [μV]	Std. error	MUmV [μV]	Std. error
5	8	27.7	6.1	10.1	0.7	323.6	198.0	43.2	27.1	32.2	19.6
10	78	50.7	15.4	10.0	1.2	305.9	149.0	48.0	23.3	29.3	14.6
20	20	112.1	29.3	10.7	1.4	599.1	325.4	87.8	42.8	63.6	40.4
30	78	152.0	46.0	10.8	1.6	657.1	309.8	102.2	44.3	69.1	37.8
50	17	268.6	61.4	12.5	2.5	1156.6	448.6	160.6	46.7	147.5	71.5
75	5	418.5	105.2	13.7	2.3	1955.3	658.9	270.5	57.4	259.7	111.6
100	2	470.3	170.1	16.0	1.3	2332.5	0.9	321.3	5.3	351.3	44.4
Entire population	208	124.4	96.3	10.7	1.8	595.1	463.1	89.2	62.2	65.9	64.9

Samples included 78 individuals who were tested at one or more force levels.

[a] Mean firing rate and mean SMUP area and amplitude represent average firing rate and SMUP size parameters across all of the subjects. All variables differ at $P < 0.001$ by MVC with $r^2 = 0.31$ for mean firing rate, $r^2 = 0.54$ for MS-MUP area, $r^2 = 0.52$ for M-MUP amplitude, $r^2 = 0.50$ for MUmV.

In the past, we reported data for both SMUP negative peak amplitude and peak to peak amplitude (Conwit et al., 1997). Subsequently, we began to use SMUP macro area, which includes integrated signal from onset to endpoint, and found it highly correlated with negative peak amplitude (correlation coefficient = 0.96) and with negative peak area (correlation coefficient = 0.86).

Absolute average force, like percentage of MVC, increased linearly with mSMUP area (Fig. 1) ($r^2 = 0.67$, $P < 0.001$). At force levels of 30% MVC or below, mFR showed little change with overall mFR, going from 10.1 to 10.8 Hz (Table 1). At higher percentages of MVC, the overall mFR progressively increased, suggesting a quadratic relationship.

The mMUmV is likely to be a better single representation of motor unit activity as it indicates the average contribution of a motor unit to the surface potential (last column of Table 1). The mMUmV increased with increasing percentage MVC. A large increase was observed in mMUmV particularly between 10 and 20% MVC, and at levels higher than 30%. However, Fig. 1 suggests an overall

TABLE 2

STATISTICAL CORRELATIONS FOR SMUP SIZE USING DE-STA

	Average	All units
Peak to peak SMUP amplitude vs negative peak area	0.90	0.63
Peak to peak SMUP amplitude vs negative peak amplitude	0.98	0.92
Negative peak SMUP area vs negative peak amplitude	0.96	0.83

Average: mean motor unit size for 15–20 MU at a given force level. All units. each motor unit at a given force level

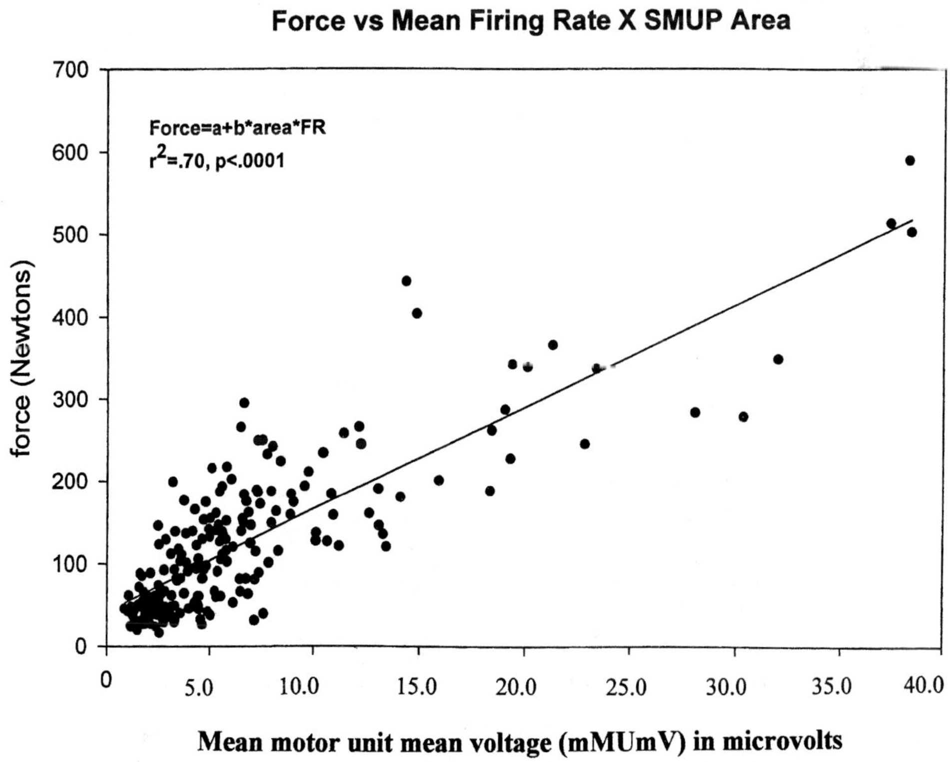

Fig. 1. Muscle force in Newtons vs mean motor unit mean voltage in microvolts.

strong relationship between mMUmV and actual force levels.

Motor unit activation and resistive strength training

To further illustrate the potential of these methods, they were applied in a study of the effects of unilateral leg extension exercise in 48 community dwelling sedentary subjects. The exercise program consisted of training knee extensor muscles of the dominant leg. Training occurred three times per week for approximately 9 weeks. The training was performed on a Keiser K-300 air powered knee extension machine.

Strength was measured in two ways. One measurement was 1 RM strength, which corresponded closely to the training paradigm and represents the maximal expected improvement in strength. The second strength measurement was maximal isometric strength measured using the Kin-Com 125E isokinetic dynamometer (Chattecx Corp., Chattanooga, TN). Motor unit activation measurements were obtained during isometric contraction levels of 10 and 30% of a subject's MVC measured during the initial baseline phase of the study.

After resistive training, 1 RM strength measurements increased significantly by 27–39.1% ($P < 0.001$), while maximal isometric strength showed a small increase after training < 10% (Fig. 2). A significant decline relative to the baseline values in the SMUP area was seen in the motor units active following training and after detraining. Figure 3 shows the average motor unit amplitude for all measured units at 10 and 30% MVC. No change was observed in FR. Thus, smaller units were generating a fixed percentage of MVC for post-training, and perhaps more interestingly 6 months post training.

Contractions performed at baseline required larger motor units that had higher levels of MUmV than similar contractions performed following training or detraining. This can be seen in Fig. 4 where the value of MUmV is plotted against the absolute level of force for contractions performed at baseline and after training and detraining. The pattern indicated that at low force levels similar sized units were responsible for the force, while at higher forces larger units were required at baseline. Overall, the motor units that were active and

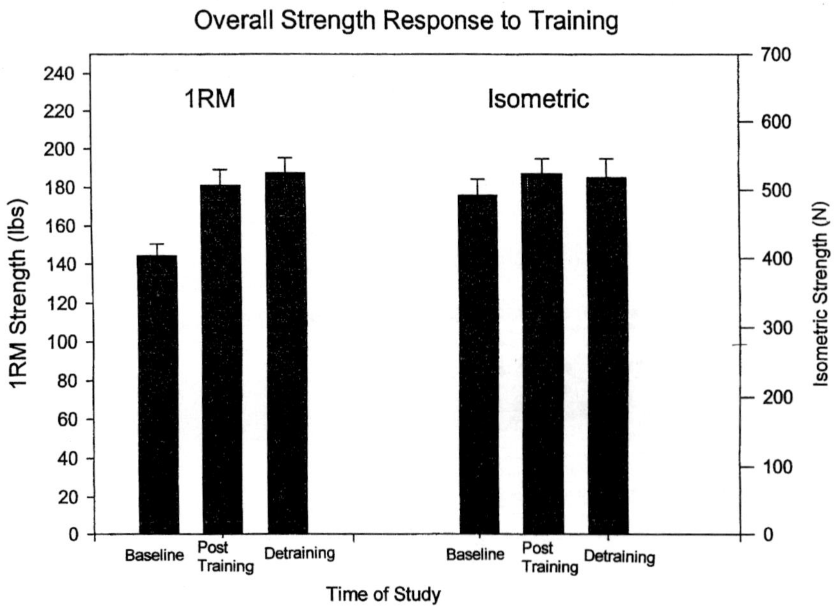

Fig. 2. One RM force production and isometric strength at: (1) baseline; (2) after 16 weeks of training; and (3) after up to 20 weeks of detraining.

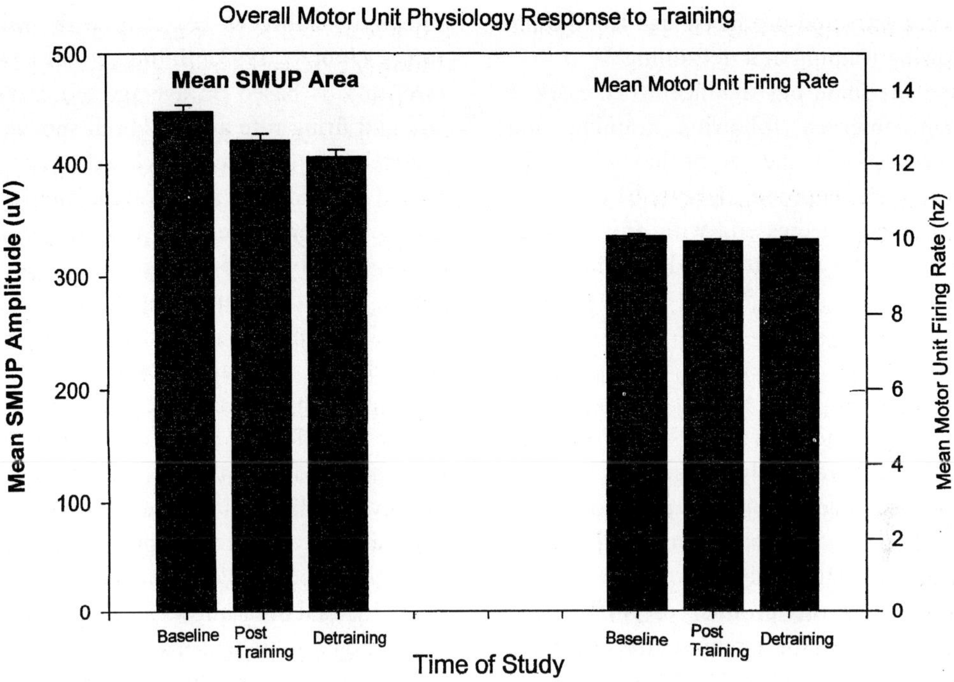

Fig. 3. Overall motor unit physiology response to training: SMUP size and motor unit firing rate after training and detraining.

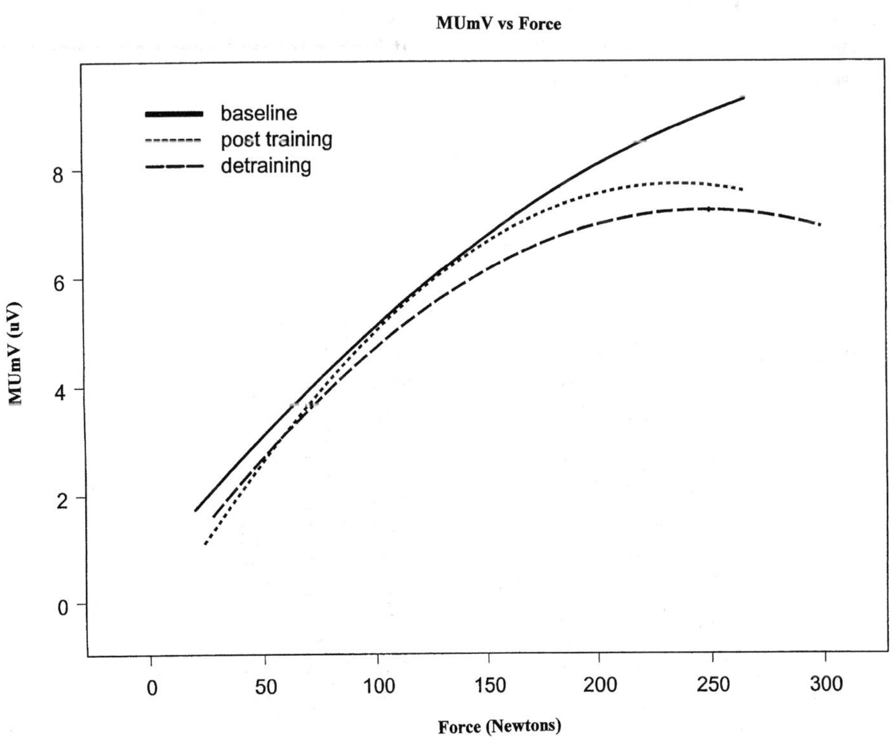

Fig. 4. Motor unit mean voltage in microvolts vs muscle force production in Newtons; at baseline, and post-training and detraining.

how they were activated produced smaller MUmV values following training and detraining.

Therefore, the small but significant decreases in SMUP area observed following training and detraining suggests that the size of the motor units active during the generation of both 10 and 30% MVC contractions decreased, with the changes most prominent after 6 months of detraining.

Discussion

The methodology used in these studies expands upon relationships previously determined between motor unit physiological properties and motor unit force production that was based on smaller numbers of motor units. Our study demonstrates that in the vastus medialis the product of SMUP size and average firing rate of a representative sample of a muscle's motor unit pool (MUmV and/or mMUmV) is strongly related to force generation. Furthermore, motor unit size in the vastus medialis appears to be more important to this relationship than mFR, as the linear relationships between mSMUP size and force and mMUmV and force explained 67 and 70% of the force variance respectively, while mFR alone accounted for only 38%. Mean FR of the sampled units, in contrast to mSMUP area or amplitude, showed little change until at least 30% MVC (Table 1). The vastus medialis is a large muscle with many motor units. The findings presented are consistent with observations that large muscles rely heavily on recruitment for increases in force (Kukulka and Clamann, 1981). This, combined with Henneman's size principle (Henneman, 1980), supports the strong relationship between mSMUP size and force.

The difference in behavior between size (recruitment) and rate coding has been previously described (Kukulka and Clamann, 1981). Our results are consistent with prior work by Marsden, Brown and others (Burke et al., 1974; Henneman 1980; Kukulka and Clamann, 1981; Marsden et al., 1983; Jabre and Salzsieder, 1993, 1997 and 1999; DeLuca et al., 1996; Doherty and Brown, 1997). Unlike the product of instantaneous motor unit firing rate and macro MUP area, that has been shown by Jabre to correlate with instantaneous force (Jabre, 1993; Jabre et al., 1993), the mMUmV is based on average motor unit SMUP size and firing rate and has been shown to be linearly related to muscle force. Although individual motor unit SMUP size is significantly related to motor unit twitch tension, the relationship can be confounded by deep-lying motor units. For example, a large deep unit may have a small SMUP whereas a small shallow motor unit may have a large SMUP. Averaging over a sample of motor units or sampling a large number of units can reduce the effect of depth of the individual motor units and produce a more consistent relationship. However, individual units were used in the exercise analysis and yielded very similar conclusions as the averaging model. The main advantage is that using the individual units allows for modeling the increasing variance at higher force levels. Furthermore, the methods used in this study can be implemented in a clinical EMG laboratory.

The results presented are based on the study of a large group of subjects. What is striking is that force production is strongly related to data on SMUP size and motor unit firing rate. Twitch potentiation and non-linear summation no doubt affect this relationship, as do many other factors which affect force generation, including muscle mass, gender, age and physical fitness level of the subject. These studies so far have been done in healthy subjects. Healthy muscles, depending both on the number of motor units and their motor unit size distribution, use different strategies (i.e. relative number of motor units recruited and their firing rates) to vary the level of force produced (Kukulka and Clamann, 1981). Nonetheless, mMUmV and MUmV should still be related to average muscle force. Indeed, the individual components of this product of SMUP size and FR could be used to characterize the various muscles based on their control strategies. As neuromuscular morphology changes as a result of pathological motor neuronopathies and axonopathies or myopathies, MUmV and/or mMUmV might provide some clinically useful information. For example, when motor unit number is reduced, firing rate and size of individual motor units may increase, while force production may decrease.

Likewise, when average motor unit size decreases, such as with small muscles or in muscles affected by myopathy, the effect of firing rate on force production becomes more important. Changes in the relationship between motor unit size, FR and force may occur with pathology and the ability to track such changes may be clinically useful, however, this is yet to be established and requires further study.

The observations from the exercise intervention argue that motor unit physiology is pliable, and changes in response to new demands and presumably to disease. Changes were observed in motor unit activation during isometric contractions following resistive training with little increase in isometric strength. The changes argue for a reorganization in motor unit activation that leads to the utilization of smaller units at higher force levels as functional performance of the muscle improves. This suggests an improved efficiency with conservation of the largest, most fatigable units. The question becomes whether this efficiency leads to a more capable muscle, which shows less fatigability and a greater range of force levels where optimal work can proceed. Likewise, in the presence of disease, is the opposite pattern observed, where there is less efficiency at higher force levels that reduces the functional capability of the muscle? This alteration, if present, is likely to depend on the physiology, but may or may not be reflected in the number of units present. As when performing MUNE, the sample used to predict average force must be large enough and suitably representative of the underlying motor unit population. Considering the high percentage of force variance accounted for in this study, the sample sizes chosen (15–20) and the decomposition techniques used results in suitable motor unit samples consistent with our previous work (Conwit et al., 1997).

It was observed in pilot studies (Conwit et al., 1997, 1998) that populations of SMUPs sampled during higher force levels consist of a greater percentage of larger SMUPs. Specifically, the distributions of SMUP sizes tend to broaden and shift to higher SMUP size as the force level increases. The larger mean SMUP sizes observed during stronger contractions may reflect an inherent bias in the signal analysis technique. However, when the data collected at 75 and 100% MVC were excluded, the analysis results did not change. On the other hand, the sample size at 75 and 100% MVC was small because of difficulty obtaining and processing data at these high levels. Therefore, the increase in SMUP size with level of contraction may be a combination of the inability to consistently sample smaller SMUPs at higher force levels, because of the complexity of the interference pattern and the recruitment of larger motor units with increasing force (Conwit et al., 1997).

The advantages of the methods used in this study are the ability to follow a large group of subjects in a clinical setting over a range of force levels in large muscles. The disadvantages include the inability to reliably follow a fixed sample of motor units over time. Instead, statistical trends in the population of motor units must be inferred from the data supplied from studying various samples including different individual motor units. Using these methods, motor unit physiology can be assessed during muscle activity. Potentially, the methods may prove useful in understanding the consequences of pathology, aging or fatigue on the neuromuscular system.

Future directions

The focus of research in MUNE has been on direct clinical applications, with a major emphasis on motor neuron diseases. The impact of the motor unit on health and disease should be far greater than considered currently. The examination of motor unit physiology in an exercise intervention as shown here is one example. The work by Chan et al. (1998) examining the response of individual motor units to an exercise load lead to the important observation that a given work load, while beneficial for one motor unit, actually degraded the performance of another unit.

The impact of the motor unit on non-neuromyopathic processes has been largely ignored. On the other hand, it is now well understood that many major disease processes cause significant changes in muscle. The focus on muscle is based in part on the concept of sarcopenia (i.e. age associated loss of muscle mass and strength), which has been associated with a variety of conditions including aging, frailty, congestive heart failure, cachexia and osteoarthritis. These areas generate research monies that can include both epidemiological and intervention studies. Although muscle related questions permeate many of these studies, little interest has been directed toward the motor unit.

There are a number of important areas for future research.

Aging

The approach so far with MUNE has focused on a comparison between young and old in reference to sarcopenia. Older subjects have fewer motor units than young subjects. However, aging changes actually begin during middle age. The loss of motor units in older subjects may be a cause or an effect of the age-associated changes that lead to sarcopenia. If motor unit loss is only an effect of other processes, then the work may not be important. However, if the loss of motor units is a cause, then greater emphasis on what is occurring becomes important. If the motor unit losses are a cause, they need to precede or co-occur with the loss of muscle mass and strength. There is very limited information showing this relationship.

We published a study of the impact of nerve conduction velocity on muscle strength and power (Metter et al., 1998). Nerve conduction velocity accounted for 10% of the variance in strength in subjects aged from 20 to 90 years. When considered in relation to age and muscle mass, nerve conduction velocity had an independent contribution of 4% of the variance. This does not sound like much, however, age independently accounted for only 10% and muscle mass 12% of the variance. Combined, the three measures account for approximately 50% of the variance in strength. The level of independent variance explained by the motor unit is equivalent to that found for serum testosterone, a hormone that is being intensely studied to intervene in the process of sarcopenia. While nerve conduction velocity is a crude measure of nerve function, we were able to show that it had independent importance on strength levels.

The study of the motor unit is a promising area with a large potential for impact on the aging process, if the role can be defined and potential interventions developed. The current limitations relate to intervention. This has not been the case for muscle, where exercise intervention clearly can improve strength and muscle mass.

Osteoarthritis

Osteoarthritis is a major contributor to disability in the elderly and affects several million individuals in the U.S. Muscle weakness is a frequent finding in these subjects. One current hypothesis is that muscle weakness may precede and be an important contributor to the development of the disease. There is research underway examining the impact of sarcopenia on osteoarthritis. Yet there appears to be little understanding of the process that occurs in the motor unit. The muscle is clearly important as seen by increasing interest on the use of exercise in treating osteoarthritis. The exercise concepts are associated primarily with muscle function and not with the nerve. However, exercise physiologists have long noted that with an exercise intervention, there is an early change in strength that precedes muscle hypertrophy. These early increases in strength are attributed to "neural" factors, an undefined concept that includes changes in the central nervous system, spinal cord, and peripheral nerve. If the nervous system is important for these early changes, does it also have a later role? Do changes in the nervous system and the expression of any changes through the motor nerve have an impact on hypertrophy? Specifically related to osteoarthritis, if changes in muscle are important, are the changes in the muscle secondary to changes in motor unit physiology?

Congestive heart failure

Congestive heart failure is a major complication of coronary heart disease, and has become a major health care problem. As part of the process, weakness frequently becomes the limiting factor in treatment and recovery. Recently, there has been increasing interest in the role of exercise training therapy. Again the focus of the studies are on the muscle. Does the motor unit have a contribution to the problem? Is there intermittent neural dysfunction, as shown by McComas (1995) that may impact on the process? Are there independent treatments that can improve the problem?

Cachexia

In addition to its relevance in ALS, cachexia is a major problem that is associated with AIDS and cancer. Cachexia is believed to be an inflammatory process that leads to muscle wasting and involves the interaction of a number of cytokines and other circulating hormones. What is the role of the nerve? Research focuses on the issue of the presence of and characterization of associated neuropathies. Is there a more general role for the nerve that is not exactly pathological? Are motor units lost in association with these processes, does less efficient use lead to greater fatigability (ala Marsden's muscle wisdom)? A number of questions can be raised where MUNE and motor unit activation techniques could be applied to obtain important insight to a devastating and common problem.

In closing

There are a number of potential areas of interest where the study of motor unit physiology may add important information to the general medical and scientific community. The EMG community should do a better job in demonstrating the importance of studying the peripheral nerve and motor units in a broader context. Currently, for example, concepts of sarcopenia mention the importance of the nervous system, but typically do not consider it further. Improving the general understanding of the importance of motor unit homeostasis can increase the number of opportunities for applying clinical neurophysiology methodologies for the diagnosis and treatment of the most compelling disease processes such as ALS. The methodology discussed here offers one potential approach to study motor unit physiology in these and other situations where muscle force generation is important to health.

References

Burke, R.E., Levine, D.N., Saloman, M. and Tsairis, P. Motor units in cat soleus muscle: physiological, histochemical and morphological characteristics. *J. Physiol. (Lond.)*, 1974, 238: 503–514.

Chan, K.M., Doherty, T.M., Andres, L.P., Porter, M.M., Brown, T. and Brown, W.F. Longitudinal study of the contractile and electrical properties of single human thenar motor units. *Muscle Nerve*, 1998, 21: 839–849.

Conwit, R.A., Tracy, B., Jamison, C., McHugh, M., Stashuk, D., Brown, W.F. and Metter, E.J. Decomposition-enhanced spike-triggered averaging: contraction level effects. *Muscle Nerve*, 1997, 20: 976–982.

Conwit, R.A., Tracy, B., Cowl, A., McHugh, M., Stashuk, D., Brown, W.F. and Metter, E.J. Firing rate analysis using decomposition-enhanced spike triggered averaging in the quadriceps femoris. *Muscle Nerve*, 1998, 21: 1338–1340.

DeLuca, C.J., Foley, P.J. and Erim, Z. Motor unit control properties in constant-force isometric contractions. *J. Neurophysiol*, 1996, 76: 1503–1516.

Doherty, T. Age-related Changes in the Numbers and Physiological Properties of Human Motor Units, PHD Thesis, University of Western Ontario, 1993.

Doherty, T. and Brown, W.F. Age-related changes in the twitch contractile properties of human thenar motor units. *J. Appl. Physiol.*, 1997, 82(1): 93–101.

Doherty, T., Simmons, Z., O'Connell, B., Felice, K.J., Conwit, R., Chan, K.M., Komori, T., Brown, T., Stashuk, D.W. and Brown, W.F. Methods for estimating the numbers of motor units in human muscles. *J. Clin. Neurophysiol.*, 1995, 12(6): 565–584.

Henneman, E. Skeletal muscle: the servant of the nervous system. "*Medical Physiology*" (V.B. Mountcastle, Ed.), Medical Physiology, 14th ed., 1980, pp. 674–702.

Jabre, J.F. New insights into motor neuron firing behavior and the generation of force. Fifth International Conference on Computerized and Quantitative EMG, Hamilton, ON 1993, p. 25.

Jabre, J.F. and Salzsieder, B.T. The study of upper and lower motor neuronal firing behavior and the generation of force. *Muscle Nerve*, 1993, 16(10): 1085A.

Jabre, J.F. and Salzsieder, B.T. The volitional unit: a functional concept in cortico-motoneuronal connections in humans. *EEG Clin. Neurophysiol.*, 1997, 105: 365–369.

Jabre, J.F. and Salzsieder, B.T. An EMG study of functional cortico-motoneuronal connections in humans. *J. Physiol. (Paris.)*, 1999, 93: 147–154.

Kukulka, C.G. and Clamann, H.P. Comparison of the recruitment and discharge properties of motor units in human brachial biceps and adductor pollicis during isometric contractions. *Brain Res.*, 1981, 219: 45–55.

Marsden, C.D., Meadows, J.C. and Merton, P.A. "Muscular Wisdom" that minimizes fatigue during prolonged effort in man: peak rates of motoneuron discharge and slowing of discharge during fatigue. *Motor Control Mechanisms in Health and Disease*, 1983, 169–211.

McComas, A.J. Motor unit estimation: anxieties and achievements. *Muscle Nerve*, 1995, 18: 369–379.

Metter, E.J., Conwit, R., Metter, B., Pacheco, T. and Tobin, J. The relationship of peripheral motor nerve conduction velocity to age-associated loss of grip strength. *Aging Clin. Exp. Res.*, 1998, 10: 471–478.

Stashuk, D.W. and Paoli, G. Robust supervised classification of motor unit action potentials. *Med. Biol. Eng. Comput.*, 1998, 36: 75–82.

Stashuk, D.W. and Qu, Y. A robust method for estimating motor unit firing pattern statistics. *Med. Biol. Eng. Comput.*, 1996a, 34: 50–57.

Stashuk, D.W. and Qu, Y. Adaptive motor unit action potential clustering using shape and temporal information. *Med. Biol. Eng. Comput.*, 1996b, 34: 41–49.

Thomas, C.G., Bigland-Ritchie, B., Westling, G. and Johansson, R.S. A comparison of human thenar motor-unit properties studied by intraneural motor-axon stimulation and spike-triggered averaging. *J. Neurophysiol.*, 1990, 64: 1347–1351.

Motor Unit Number Estimation (Supplements to Clinical Neurophysiology Vol. 55)
Editor: M.B. Bromberg

Chapter 25

Longitudinal tracking of contractile properties of human motor units by the multiple point stimulation technique

K. Ming Chan[a,*] and William F. Brown[b]

[a]*Division of Physical Medicine and Rehabilitation, University of Alberta, Edmonton, AB T6J 2S2, Canada*
[b]*Department of Neurology, Tufts University, Boston, MA, USA*

Introduction

Serial motor unit number estimates (MUNE) provide specific information about the numbers and rates of losses of motor unit (MU) in motoneuron diseases. However, knowing the numbers of surviving motoneurons alone provides little information about the health of surviving motoneurons or the responses of affected motoneurons to treatment. Several techniques for measuring single human MU contractile and electrical properties exist (Stein et al., 1972; Taylor and Stephens, 1976; Westling et al., 1990), but none lend themselves to serial tracking the same MUs. The physiological properties of normal and diseased motoneurons span a wide range, and comparisons of the physiological properties in samples of MUs drawn at various stages in a progressive motoneuron disease are an indirect means of determining the survival times and adaptive responses of individual motoneurons. Further, sampling errors are likely unless a large number of MUs are studied.

Almost three decades ago, Bergmans (1970) showed that it was possible to find the same motor axon in repeated studies in humans using surface stimulating electrodes placed over a motor nerve. Later, Doherty and Brown (1994), Chan et al. (1998a) confirmed and extended Bergmans' finding by showing that the same single MUs could be repeatedly studied weeks and even months apart. These studies also showed that the electrical properties of the same MUs in healthy subjects, including stimulus thresholds relative to those of their neighbors and their conduction velocities (CV) were remarkably stable in serial studies. To test the clinical utility of the technique, it was applied to patients with amyotrophic lateral sclerosis (ALS) and also to evaluate the adaptive capacity of normal MUs in healthy individuals to 'training' using an electrical stimulation paradigm.

We will describe the methods used to longitudinally track the contractile properties of MUs in the median-innervated thenar muscles. Findings from MUs in healthy individuals and the adaptive capacity of a subset of these MUs to an electrical stimulation program will be summarized. Finally, the temporal evolution of two MUs in patients with ALS will be presented.

**Correspondence to*: Dr. K. Ming Chan, 513 Heritage Medical Research Center, University of Alberta, Edmonton, AB T6G 2S2, Canada. Tel.: (780) 492-1614, Fax: (780) 492-1617.
e-mail: ming.chan@ualberta.ca

doi: 10.1016/S1567-424X(03)00025-4

Methods

Subject lay comfortably in a semi-supine position. The forearm and hand were fitted with a custom made splint, open on the ventral aspect of the wrist and forearm to allow access to the median nerve. The splint was secured firmly to a platform on which the force transducers were mounted. This arrangement was designed to ensure that the arm, hand and thumb were positioned in a similar manner and orientation with respect to the strain gauges for each study.

Electrical recording

Hand temperature was checked with a thermister to ensure that it was 30–32 °C. Surface electrodes were used to detect both the thenar maximum compound muscle action potential (CMAP) and single motor unit action potentials (MUAPs). The active electrode was positioned over the innervation zone of the thenar muscles, and the reference electrode over the first metacarpophalangeal joint. A metal strap embedded within a saline-soaked Velcro band wrapped around the forearm served as the ground electrode. Surface EMG signals were acquired with a bandwidth of 5 Hz to 5 kHz (3 dB down). The following EMG parameters were measured: (1) terminal motor latency (time from onset of the stimulus artifact to onset of the MUAP); (2) MUAP size defined by negative peak-amplitude (from the baseline to the negative peak), negative-peak area (area between the negative phase and the baseline) and peak-to-peak amplitude (between the negative and positive peaks); (3) F-wave latency (time from onset of the stimulus artifact to onset of the F-response).

Electrical stimuli were delivered through a stimulus isolation unit connected to a Grass S48 stimulator. During the search for suitable single thenar motor axons, stimuli with a duration of 10–25 μs were delivered at 1 Hz. Once a MU was found which met criteria for a single thenar motor axon, the position of the active recording electrode was adjusted to find the site at which the MUAP waveform showed the shortest rise time and maximal amplitude. The optimal recording site usually coincided with the site where visible dimpling of the skin was observed when the MU was stimulated at 10–20 Hz. Following the initial studies, the position of the active recording electrode was noted and the hand with the electrodes attached was photocopied. The photocopy made it much easier to return to the same recording sites in subsequent studies. In addition, the distance between the stimulation electrode site and the distal wrist crease was measured and was used in subsequent studies. In general, the length of the median nerve over which a given thenar motor axon could be found varied from 5 to 30 mm, but there was usually one 'preferred' site where the threshold of the axon was most widely separated from its neighboring thenar motor axons.

Selection of single MUs

The first step was to find thenar motor axons meeting criteria for serial studies of single MUs. This initially involved exploring the median nerve at various sites between the motor point and the axilla using finely graded electrical stimuli delivered through a bipolar electrode applied to the skin overlying the median nerve. The median nerve lay too deep in the mid and proximal forearm to be accessible to surface stimulation of single thenar motor axons without requiring uncomfortably high stimulus intensities or causing unwanted direct or indirect stimulation of forearm muscles.

Criteria for activation of a single motor axon included two obligatory criteria (1 and 2) and a third criterion (3) sometimes found with MUs whose contractions deformed the overlying skin:

1. The putative single MUAP and associated twitch appeared in an 'all-or-nothing' manner in response to finely graded electrical stimuli without evidence of fractionation of the response such as might indicate the presence of two or more thenar motor axons with overlapping thresholds.
2. When a late F-response was observed, the shape and size of the latter was identical to the earlier 'direct' response for the putative single MUAP (Fig. 1A).

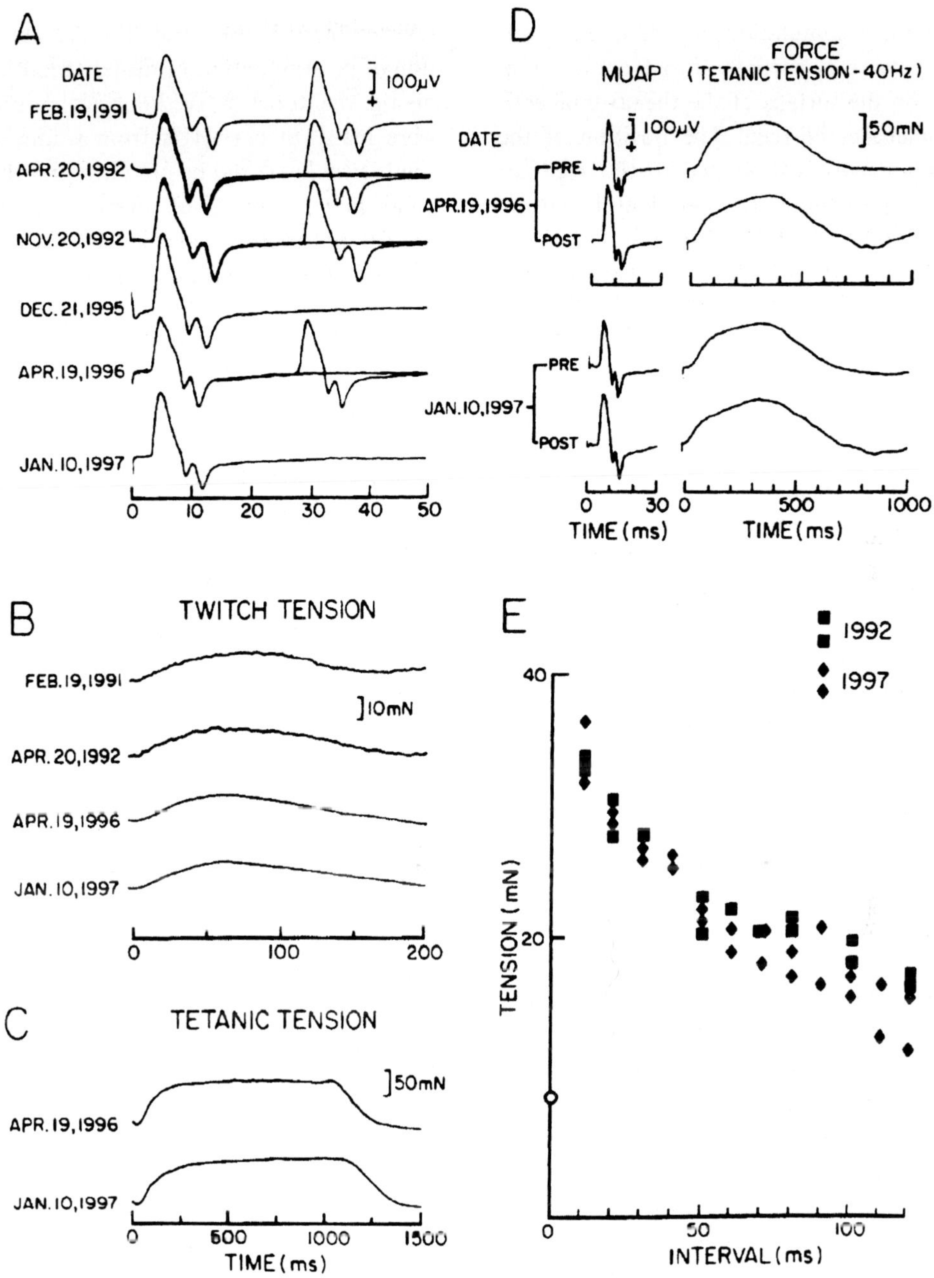

Fig. 1. Panel A illustrates the highly reproducible shapes and sizes of surface detected MUAPs in the direct and late F-responses for motor unit (MU) 'O'. The 'preferred' stimulation site for this MU was 35–49 mm proximal to the distal wrist crease along the median nerve. Panel B illustrates the nearly identical single twitch tensions for MU 'O' in four separate test sessions spread over 6 years. Panel C illustrates the consistency of the maximal tetanic tensions when tested almost a year apart. Tetanic and fatigue stimulations were not performed prior to 1996. Panel D illustrates the changes in tetanic tensions for MU 'O' pre- and post-fatigue stimulation, induced by the 'Burke' protocol (Burke et al., 1973). Panel E illustrates differences in peak tension produced by a pair of stimuli, the so called 'catch' response, delivered at inter-pulse intervals of 10–120 ms in studies carried out twice in 1992 and twice again in 1997. The single twitch tension is represented by an open circle on the *y*-axis. In the 1992 studies, the full range of inter-pulse intervals was not assessed. For all of the above studies there was a remarkable similarity in the contractile properties, shape and size of the MUAPs as well as the conduction velocities (58 m/s in 1992, and 57 m/s in 1997). From Chan et al. (1998a).

3. With repetitive stimulation at a frequency sufficient to evoke a partially fused contraction, dimpling on the surface of the thenar eminence could sometimes be seen. The position of the dimpling usually corresponded to the approximate location of the MU as determined by surface mapping of the MUAP.

To be accepted for longitudinal studies, suitable thenar MUs had to meet the following additional criteria:

1. The shape and size of the MUAPs were very similar in repeated studies.
2. The site along the median nerve at which the putative single thenar motor axon was found was within 5–10 mm of the original 'preferred' site for stimulation of the associated motor axon.
3. The contractile characteristics including the twitch and tetanic tensions, contractile speeds and resistance to fatigue were similar in serial studies.
4. The latencies of the direct and F-responses, were very similar in repeated studies.
5. The threshold for the associated motor axon at its 'preferred' site for stimulation had to be widely separated from those of other thenar motor axons at the same site.

Although the size indices (amplitude and area) were useful general guides, the shape of the MUAP waveform was more specific to each MU and could be readily recognized. From our experience with the multiple point stimulation technique, it was very uncommon for surface detected MUAPs generated by stimulating neighboring motor axons at the same site to be so similar in shape that they could not be distinguished from each other. Through careful surface mapping, differentiation from other neighboring MUs was further facilitated by placing the active recording electrode at the most optimal location for the chosen MU. The last stipulation was necessary if the chosen motor axon was to be stimulated over a broad enough range of frequencies to fully explore the force–frequency relationships and fatigue index (FI) of the associated MU without the risk of stimulating other neighboring thenar motor axons. MUs were rejected from further study if there was any indication of co-stimulation of median motor axons supplying the forearm or lumbrical muscles. There were many thenar MUs from whom satisfactory single twitches could be obtained, but the threshold separation of most of them from neighboring thenar motor axons at the same stimulation site was insufficient to allow them to be stimulated at suitably high frequencies to determine their tetanic tensions or fatigue indices. This rendered them unacceptable for longitudinal studies.

Motor unit latencies and conduction velocities

F-wave latencies, when present, and motor terminal latencies were measured for each MU at each study. Motor axon conduction velocity could be determined from these latencies by the following equation:

$$\text{Conduction velocity} = \frac{\text{distance between the cathode and C7 spinous process (mm)}}{(\text{F latency} - \text{MTL} - 1)/2\ (\text{ms})},$$

where MTL is motor terminal latency.

Force detection system

At the outset, the prime vector for each thenar MU is unknown. Therefore, a two-axis force collection system was used to determine the resultant force and prime vector. It consists of two force transducers (Grass FT10) arranged at right angles to one another in the flexion and abduction axes of the thumb. Once the prime vector had been determined, a single axis force collection system was substituted with the axis of the transducer aligned with the thumb at that angle. This step simplified the set up and improved the signal-to-noise ratio for the force measurement, and was especially important for smaller MUs generating twitch forces of 1–5 mN. A passive preload tension of 300 mN was applied to the thumb. To minimize movement artifact, activity in the thumb muscles was monitored with surface EMG. Cardiac pulse artifact was avoided, at least until the following heartbeat, by employing a cardiac monitor and delivering the stimulus to the nerve 150 ms following the heart beat. Additionally, to avoid respiratory artifact, the subjects were instructed to hold their breath for the duration of each trial.

Contractile parameters for each MU were measured in the following order: twitch tension, tetanic tensions at 10, 20, 30, 40, 50 and 100 Hz, and fatigue index. The contraction time (time from onset to peak tension) and half relaxation time (time to decline from peak to 50% of peak) were also measured from the twitch tension records. The number of stimuli was kept to a minimum to reduce the influence of the activation history of a MU on the contractile characteristics of some MUs. Twitch tensions were unpotentiated and the single shocks were delivered at a frequency of less than 0.3 Hz to avoid the 'staircase' phenomenon. The duration of the stimulus train was set at 2 s for 10 Hz tetanic stimulation and 1 s for all other frequencies. A minimum of 3 min of rest was given between successive trains of stimuli at different frequencies and prior to fatigue studies.

The fatigue profile was determined by stimulating the motor axon with trains at 40 Hz, each lasting 330 ms, and repeated every second for a total of 2 min (Burke et al., 1973). The fatigue index was defined as the ratio of tetanic tension from the last train at 2 min to the tension from the initial train.

The 'catch' property is a term describing the marked increase in force output of a MU, over and above what might be expected from the simple addition of two successive single twitches. This was examined in 2 MUs by delivering a second stimulus at various intervals (from 10 to 120 ms in 10 ms increments).

Results in healthy young subjects

Five healthy subjects between 28 and 55 years of age were studied. Ten MUs meet criteria for longitudinal studies. A high degree of test–retest reproducibility was found (Fig. 1). Six of the 10 motor axons were found near the elbow and the remainder near the wrist. The distributions of contraction times, half relaxation times, twitch tensions, maximal tetanic tensions and fatigue indices of these 10 units (Fig. 2) were similar to larger samples of thenar MUs reported by others (Thomas et al., 1990, 1991; Doherty and Brown, 1997).

Electrical properties

Peak-to-peak MUAP amplitudes of the 10 longitudinally tracked MUs ranged from 152 to 821 μV (mean ± SD = 391 ± 207 μV). Coefficients of variation for peak-to-peak and negative-peak amplitudes and negative-peak areas were less than 10% of the mean in serial studies. For seven of 10 MUs from whom F-responses could be elicited, the calculated conduction velocity ranged from 49 to 70 m/s. For each MU, the motor terminal latencies and F-wave latencies in serial studies differed by less than 0.6 ms in the case of the former and 1.1 ms in the case of the latter. Conduction velocities for the MUs were remarkably similar in repeated studies, and the highest coefficient of variation for any one MU was less than 2% of the mean. For example, the conduction velocity values for MU 'O', measured over a 6-year time period, were 58, 57, 57, 57, 59 and 57 m/s.

Contractile properties

The distributions of contraction time, maximal tetanic tension and fatigue index of the 10 MUs studied is shown in Fig. 3. There was a significant positive correlation between contraction time and fatigue index ($r = 0.72$; $P > 0.05$) and a negative correlation between maximal tetanic tension and fatigue index ($r = -0.84$; $P > 0.05$). Although not statistically significant, there appears to be a tendency for a negative correlation between contraction time and maximal tetanic tension. There was no correlation between axonal conduction velocity and contractile tension.

Single twitches

The prime vectors for the 10 MUs were evenly spread between full flexion and full abduction. The mean twitch tensions of the group of MUs ranged

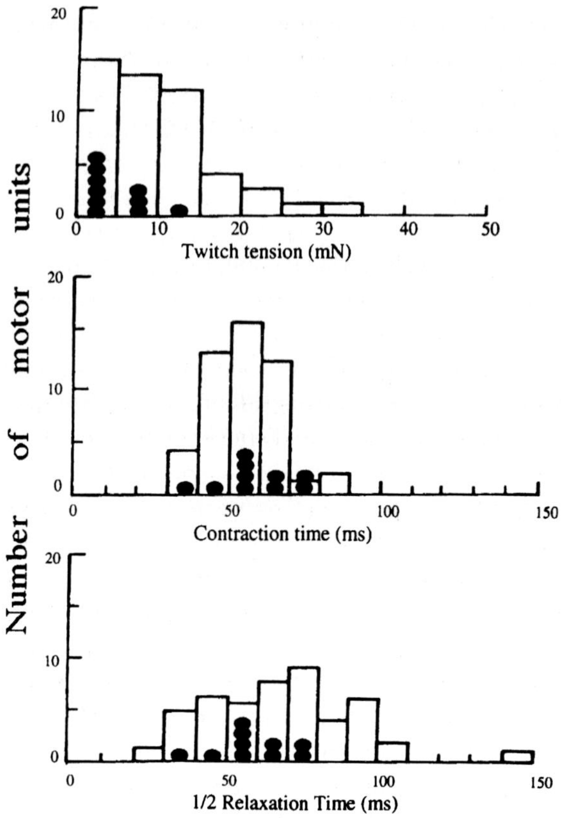

Fig. 2. Figure shows the distribution of the twitch tensions, contraction times, and half relaxation times for 48 thenar MUs from younger subjects in a previous study (Doherty and Brown, 1997) and the corresponding values for the 10 longitudinally tracked thenar MUs in the current study (denoted by filled circles). These longitudinally studied MUs were representative of the distribution of contractile properties drawn from the larger sample of MUs in the earlier study. Their maximal tetanic tensions, fatigue indices (shown in Fig. 3), not studied by Doherty and Brown, were very similar to the sample of thenar MUs studied by Thomas et al. (1990, 1991). From Chan et al. (1998a).

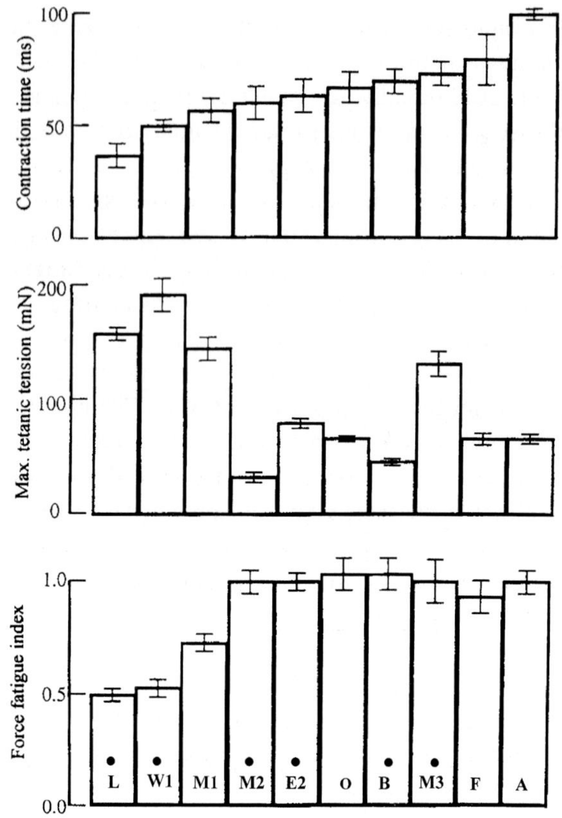

Fig. 3. Ten motor units are ranked by their mean contraction times in an ascending order in the top panel, and the mean maximal tetanic tensions and force fatigue profiles of the corresponding MUs are shown in the lower two panels. Bars above and below the means indicate ± 1 SD MUs marked with a black dot underwent an electrical stimulation 'training' program. From Chan et al. (1998a).

from 1.4 to 10.3 mN (mean $\pm$ SD $= 5.2 \pm 2.9$ mN). The highest coefficient of variation between sessions for twitch tension of any of the 10 MUs was less than 27% of the mean, with one exception. The mean twitch tension of the smallest MU, 'M2', was less than 1.5 mN, which approached the limit of resolution of our force measurement system. The high coefficient of variation for M2 at 50% of the mean was not surprisingly large. The greater variability in twitch tensions compared to the electrical and other contractile properties was in part due to the susceptibility of these minute forces to distortion from many potential sources such as respiration, anxiety, movements, cardiac impulses or even floor vibration. Although efforts were used to minimize them, they could not always be entirely eliminated. Contraction times for the 10 MUs ranged from 37 to 99 ms, and half relaxation times ranged from 31 to 84 ms. The highest coefficient of variation for any single MU between sessions was 18% of the mean for the contraction time and 21% of the mean for the half relaxation time. This variability probably reflects the difficulty of accurately determining the times of the peak tensions and half relaxation times from some single twitches.

Maximal tetanic tensions

Mean tetanic tension for the 10 MUs ranged from 29 to 194 mN (mean ± SD = 98 ± 56 mN). Tetanic tensions were highly reproducible for each of the MU and exhibited much lower coefficients of variation between sessions (< 15% of the mean) than the corresponding twitch tensions. All MUs reached their maximal tetanic tensions between stimulus frequencies of 30 and 50 Hz.

Fatigue indices

Force fatigue indices in the 10 MUs ranged from 0.50 to 1.07 (mean ± SD = 0.89 ± 0.21 mN). The variability between test sessions was very small and the highest coefficient of variation was less than 10% of the mean.

Adaptive capacity of normal MUs to 'training' through an electrical stimulation program

We sought to determine the effect of a stimulus-based training program on the properties of single motor neurons.

Methods

Six thenar MUs in two young healthy subjects were studied (Fig. 3) (Chan et al., 1999).

Baseline studies

Each MU was studied at least three or more times, several days apart to establish the variance for each of the contractile and electrical properties of the MU.

Training

All MUs were 'trained' by electrical stimulation three times a week for 7 weeks, except MU 'W1' which was trained for 11 weeks. The following intermittent, high frequency stimulation protocol was used to train all MUs. Each stimulation cycle was 15 s long with a duty cycle of 33% (5 s on/10 s off), and each MU received 24,000 stimuli per session. The stimulus frequency was specifically set for each MU according to its force frequency response, specifically, the stimulus frequency used was 10 Hz above the minimum stimulation frequency required to elicit 90% of the maximum tetanic tension. For this sample of MUs, stimulus frequencies ranged from 30 to 50 Hz, and the duration of stimulation was between 24 and 40 min, depending on the stimulus frequency used. This step was necessary because the stimulus frequency required to achieve the maximal tetanic tension varied between MUs.

During each training session, the specific MU to be trained was isolated by finely graded threshold stimulation in the same manner as described above. The MU was trained isometrically with the thumb securely fixed in a fully adducted position. The electrical signature of the specific MU being trained was closely monitored at all time throughout the session. Position of the stimulator and the stimulus intensity were adjusted whenever necessary to ensure that the MU was fully activated without co-activation of other neighboring MUs.

Periodic assessments of MUs

MUs were tested once a week during the training period, and at weekly intervals for 5 weeks following training to monitor their recovery. This re-evaluation schedule was designed to identify and track any changes in electrical and contractile characteristics in response to the training program.

Results

For each MU, 15–17 test sessions and 21 training sessions (33 sessions in the case of 'W1') were required. Each test or training session took 1 h or more to complete. All MUs were successfully tracked and studied throughout the training and subsequent recovery periods. Figure 4 illustrates

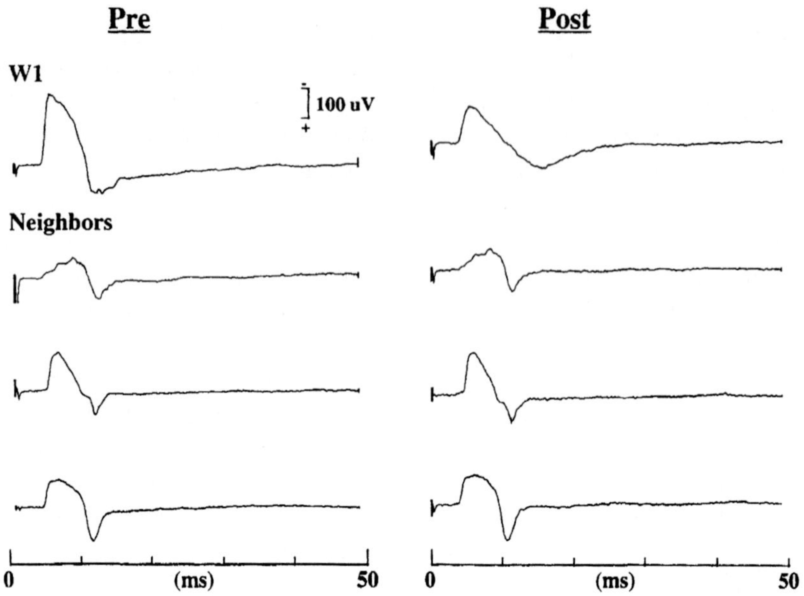

Fig. 4. Motor unit action potentials associated with 'W1', the lowest threshold MU, and three other neighboring MUs with successively higher stimulus thresholds. Peak-to-peak amplitude of the MUAPs associated with 'W1' dropped markedly after selective stimulation for 24 min. MUAPs associated with the neighboring MUs, which were not selected, remained the same. From Chan et al. (1999).

the security with which these single axons could be selectively stimulated without stimulating higher threshold motor axons. In this example, MUAP 'W1' declined in amplitude by more than 30% after a 24-min session of stimulation, while MUAPs of the neighboring MUs, which were not stimulated, remained unchanged.

Contractile characteristics of the MUs at baseline

The sample of MUs in this study was small, but the ranges and distributions of their twitch and tetanic tensions, contractile speeds and fatigue indices were similar to those in larger samples of thenar MUs using intraneural microstimulation and surface stimulation (Thomas et al., 1990; Doherty and Brown, 1997). Twitch tensions in the six MUs in this study ranged from 1.4 to 7.1 mN, the maximum tetanic tensions ranged from 29 to 194 mN, the contraction times ranged from 37 to 70 ms, half relaxation times ranged from 33 to 84 ms, and the fatigue indices from 0.50 to 1.07.

Responses of MUs of differing contractile characteristics to training

Throughout the course of training, the twitch and tetanic tensions of the slower, non-fatiguing MUs ('M3', 'E2' and 'B') showed gradual increases (Fig. 5). Following 7 weeks of training, increases of their twitch tensions ranged from 25 to 54%, and their maximum tetanic tensions increased from 23 to 49%. In spite of these changes in tensions, contractile speeds and fatigue indices remained within the baseline range. The original records in one example, MU 'M3', are illustrated in Fig. 6A.

At the other end of the spectrum, changes in the two faster and more fatigable MUs, 'W1' and 'L' were very different. Their fatigue resistance increased by 36 and 68%, respectively, at the end of the stimulation program. For 'W1', whose contractile speeds remained unchanged, there was a concomitant reduction in its twitch (by up to 75%) and tetanic tensions (by up to 52%) which continued until training was stopped (Fig. 6B). Although the twitch and maximum tetanic tensions of MU 'L' also fell initially, they gradually

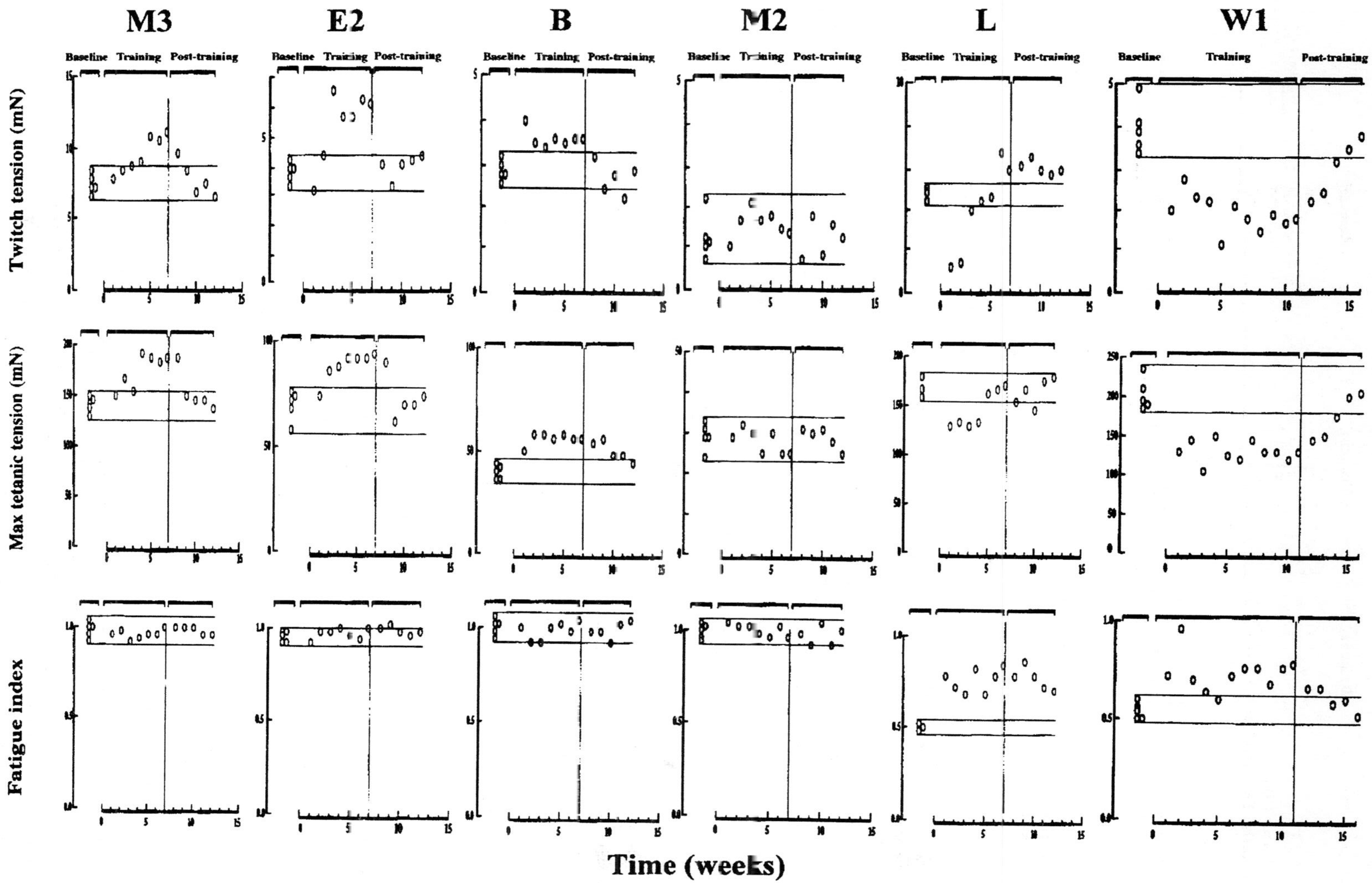

Fig. 5. Composite figure showing changes in force fatigue indices, twitch and tetanic tensions of six MUs that underwent training. Horizontal lines on each plot represent upper and lower limits of the baseline values. Twitch and tetanic tensions of the three slower non-fatiguing MUs on the left improved, and their fatigue indices remained within the baseline range. Tensions of the two fast and more fatigable MUs, shown on the right declined but their fatigue resistance improved. A full description of all the contractile and electrical changes is given in the text. From Chan et al. (1999).

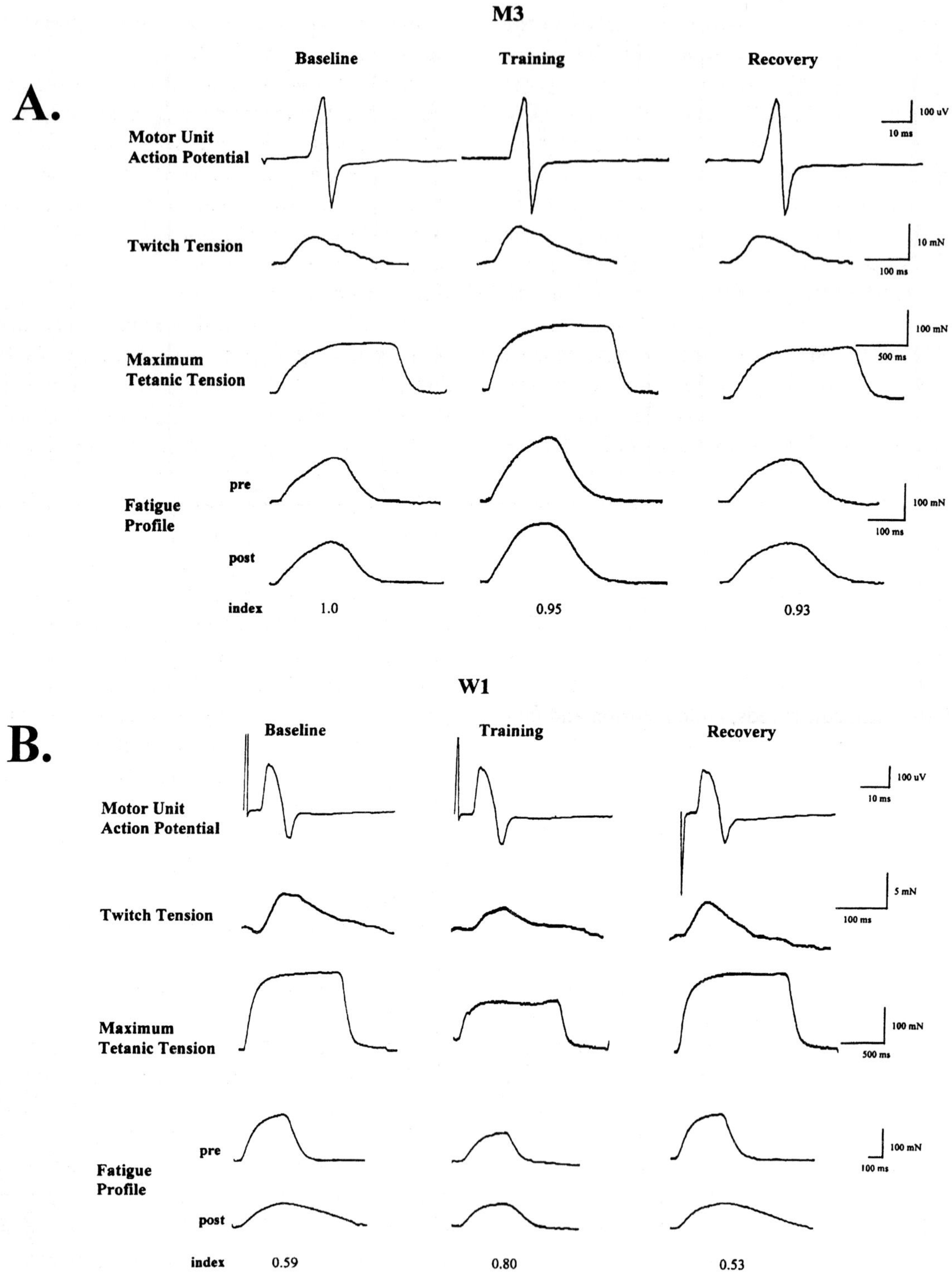

Fig. 6. Part A shows original records of MU 'M3' to illustrate the extent of changes of its physiological properties after 7 weeks of training and their subsequent recovery 5 weeks after training was stopped. Part B shows original records of MU 'W1' to illustrate the vastly different physiological responses compared with those of MU 'M3'. The middle column shows electrical and mechanical records of 'W1' after 11 weeks of training. The records in the right hand column were obtained after 5 weeks of de-training. From Chan et al. (1999).

recovered toward their baseline range later in the course of training. Twitch tension, in fact, eventually rose above the baseline range after 6 weeks of training, accompanied by a concomitant slowing of their contractile speeds (contraction time increased from 37 to 58 ms and half relaxation time from 31 to 55 ms). The greater increase in twitch tension, compared with the maximal tetanic tension, was most likely due to prolongation of the 'active state' of the innervated muscle fibers as reflected by the increase in the contraction time.

The contractile properties of the remaining MU, 'M2', whose baseline contractile speeds and fatigue index lay between the three MUs 'M3', 'B' and 'E2' and the two MUs 'W1' and 'L', remained within the baseline range throughout training.

Post-training changes in MUs

For all MUs except MU 'L', contractile changes returned to baseline levels within 5 weeks after training (Fig. 5). Although the maximum tetanic tension of MU 'L' also returned to its pre-training level, its contractile speeds, twitch tension and fatigue resistance had not yet returned to the baseline within that time.

Changes in the electrical characteristics of MUs in response to training

No changes were observed in any of the MUs throughout the training or post-training periods in the shapes or sizes of the MUAPs, the motor terminal latencies, the F-wave latencies or the axonal conduction velocities. Although intermittent high frequency trains, e.g. those used to determine the fatigue index, were frequently associated with temporary changes in the sizes and durations of the MUAPs, they always returned to baseline values within a short time following each study.

Changes in temporal MU profile in amyotrophic lateral sclerosis subjects

Due to the time required for each study and the necessity of examining each subject repeatedly over a long period of time, only two subjects were studied (Chan et al., 1998b).

Subject A was a right handed 47-year-old female with definite limb onset ALS diagnosed in 1995 without evidence of any other systemic or neurologic disease. Marked weakness and atrophy of the thenar muscles were already present at the time of initial diagnosis. MU 'S', the MU tracked, was one of three remaining MUs in the subject's right thenar muscles.

Subject B was a 65-year-old male with diagnostically definite limb-onset ALS diagnosed in 1996. At the time of study he had marked atrophy of the thenar muscles, and MU 'J', the most extensively studied MU, was one of the four remaining MUs in right thenar muscles.

The objective of this study was to examine the feasibility of tracking pathophysiological changes in single MUs in a rapidly progressive disease. We concentrated on one MU per subject to allow comprehensive evaluation of a wide range of physiological functions during serial studies.

As a result of the greatly depleted motoneuron pools in these two subjects, the task of finding readily trackable single MUs was much easier than in healthy subjects who have many more motor axons with closely overlapping stimulus thresholds. By the use of a decomposition routine, the recruitment threshold and firing rates of these ALS MUs during voluntary contractions could be determined and their central motor drive thereby assessed.

Description of single MU changes

At the time of initial study, MU 'S' was already markedly expanded and had a relatively high fatigue resistance (fatigue index = 0.84) (Fig. 7). Over the 2 years of tracking, its MUAP size, axonal conduction velocity and motor terminal latency remained remarkably stable. At the outset the patient could readily recruit this MU and F-wave responses could be readily elicited (F-persistence > 20%). However, during the 2nd year, the patient experienced increasing difficulty in voluntarily recruiting this MU (Fig. 7F) which was accompanied by a marked reduction of the occurrence of F-wave responses (F-persistence < 0.5%). Concomitantly,

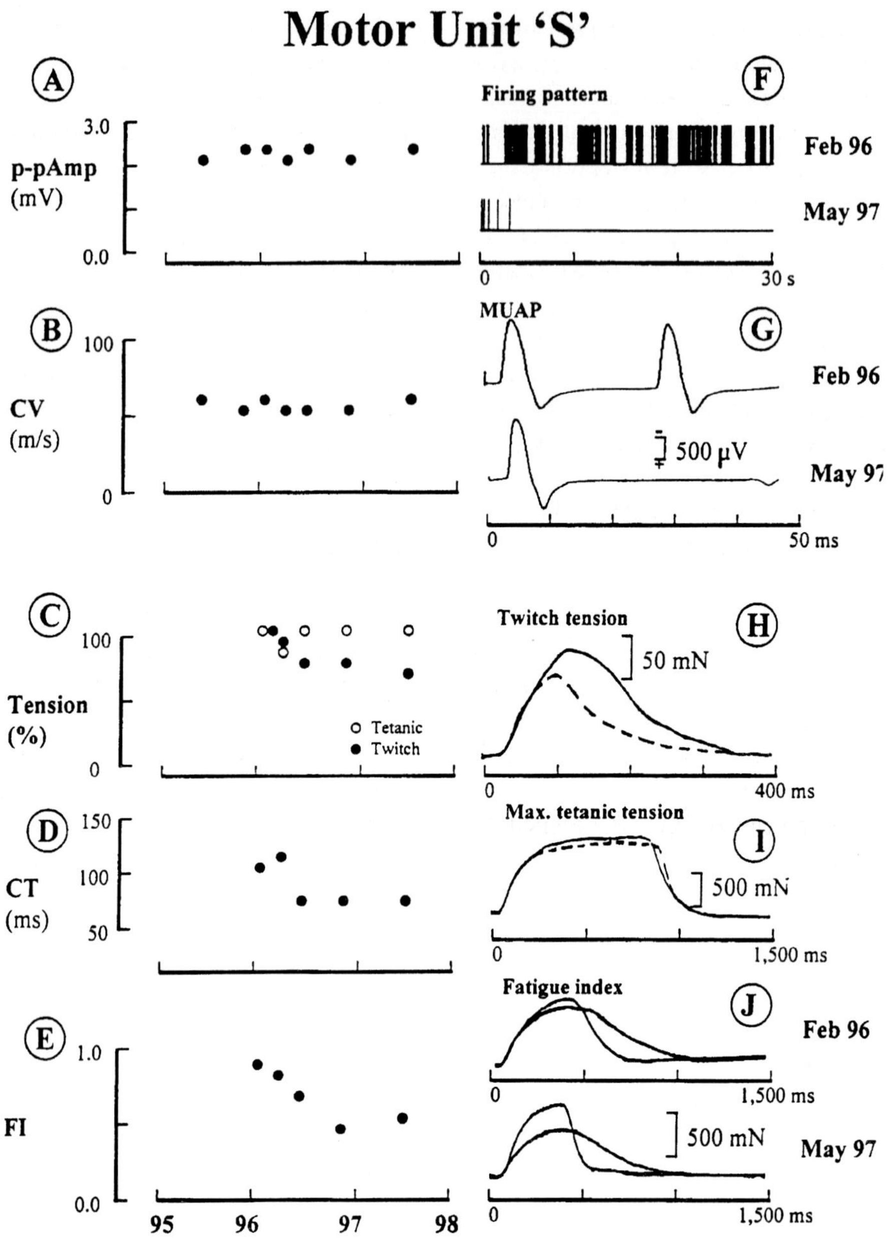

Fig. 7. Temporal profile of pathophysiological changes in MU 'S'. Changes in electrical and contractile properties over a 2-year period are shown in the plots on the left (A–E), some are illustrated by original records on the right (F–J). The electrical properties including peak-to-peak amplitudes (p–p Amp) of the MUAPs and axonal conduction velocities (CV) (A and B) remained stable but the contractile properties, including contraction time (CT) (D) and force fatigue index (FI) (F), both decreased. The apparent decline in twitch tension (shown in C and illustrated in H), even though the maximal tetanic tension remained unchanged (I), was due to shortening of the 'active state'. Note that tracking of the contractile properties only began in 1996. The firing rate plot in 1996 (F) shows the onset firing rate, at about 8 Hz, obtained at recruitment threshold. The firing rate plot in 1997 was obtained with the patient exerting maximal efforts but the MU was only recruited five times in total. F-responses were frequently elicited initially (the late response in G) but later became much more difficult to elicit. The twitch and maximal tetanic tensions obtained in early 1996 (solid line) and mid 1997 (dash line) are shown superimposed (in H and I) to contrast their differences (see text for details). The tetanic tensions of MU 'S' before and after a standard fatigue protocol (Burke et al., 1973) are shown superimposed. From Chan et al. (1998a,b).

the fatigue resistance of this MU progressively declined and the contractile speeds became more rapid. Although the twitch tension declined, the maximal tetanic tension was well maintained throughout. Preservation of the maximal tetanic tension in the face of a decline in the twitch tension suggests that the latter is due to shortening of the 'active state' associated with the more rapid contractile speeds.

MU 'J' was also an enlarged MU at the time of initial study (Fig. 8). However, compared with MU 'S', this unit's initial contractile speeds were more rapid and the unit more fatigable (fatigue index = 0.64). This MU could be readily recruited by weak voluntary contractions (< 10% MVC) and remained the case throughout the 5 months of study. In contrast, the physiological properties of this MU declined rapidly during the period of the study. For example, the conduction velocity slowed by 29% and the motor terminal latency increased by 34%. These changes were accompanied by a decline of the maximal tetanic tensions (by 29% over a 3-month period) and the peak-to-peak amplitude of the associated MUAP declined by 58%. Paradoxically, the twitch tension increased from 13 to 21 mN, possibly as a result of prolongation of the 'active state' associated with slowing of the contraction time of the MU from 68 to 100 ms. The fatigue index increased modestly from 0.64 to 0.71. An interesting observation was that tetanic tensions of MU "J" declined during tetanic stimulation, first observed at the 4-month point when it was stimulated at 100 Hz. This behavior is not seen in healthy MUs whose tetanic tensions in response to short trains of high frequency stimulation reach a plateau that is maintained until stimulation is stopped. Arguably, stimulation at 100 Hz is well beyond the physiological firing rates during sustained contractions. However, this abnormal feature rapidly progressed so that within a month, the decrement appeared at frequencies as low as 20 Hz (Fig. 9). This decrement could be circumvented by either reducing the stimulus frequency or reducing the stimulus intensity to the point when the motor axon failed to fire intermittently. Under these circumstances, tetanic tension was surprisingly well sustained despite the reduction in the number of discharges of the MU (Fig. 10). Accompanying the force decrements in response to high frequency stimulation were decrements in the sizes of the associated MUAPs. At lower stimulation frequencies (1, 3 and 10 Hz), however, no decrement in force or MUAP size was observed. The decrements in the tetanic tension at higher frequencies were paralleled by progressive reductions in the maximal firing rates at which this unit could be voluntarily driven (from 34 to 19 Hz).

Discussion

How practical are longitudinal studies of single MUs for clinical studies? The number of MUs meeting our requirements for tracking is small, on the order of 1–3 MUs per subject. An implication is that when pooling data from different subjects in a clinical study, measures to ensure homogeneity of the population characteristics will be necessary to provide sufficient statistical power. However, the relatively small numbers of MUs and the effort required to measure their contractile properties are offset by the amount of information the assessments can bring to the study of motoneuronal function.

But what of the difficulties of tracking single MUs in diseases where changes in some of the electrical and contractile properties might be expected to occur? For example, motor terminal latencies and F latencies might increase and the conduction velocities correspondingly be reduced, perhaps in association with changes in the shape and 'signature' of surface detected MUAPs in neuronal and other disorders of the neuromuscular system. The foregoing changes in the electrical characteristics of MUs are probably accompanied by changes in their contractile characteristics as MUs respond to the losses of neighboring units or as themselves are affected and become increasingly dysfunctional. Some or all the above are possible and are indeed anticipated outcomes of longitudinal studies of diseased single MUs. However, it is unlikely that the electrical and contractile properties will change so rapidly or in concert with one another that there will be any case of mistaken identity. In particular, it is highly unlikely that the position of the MU, its

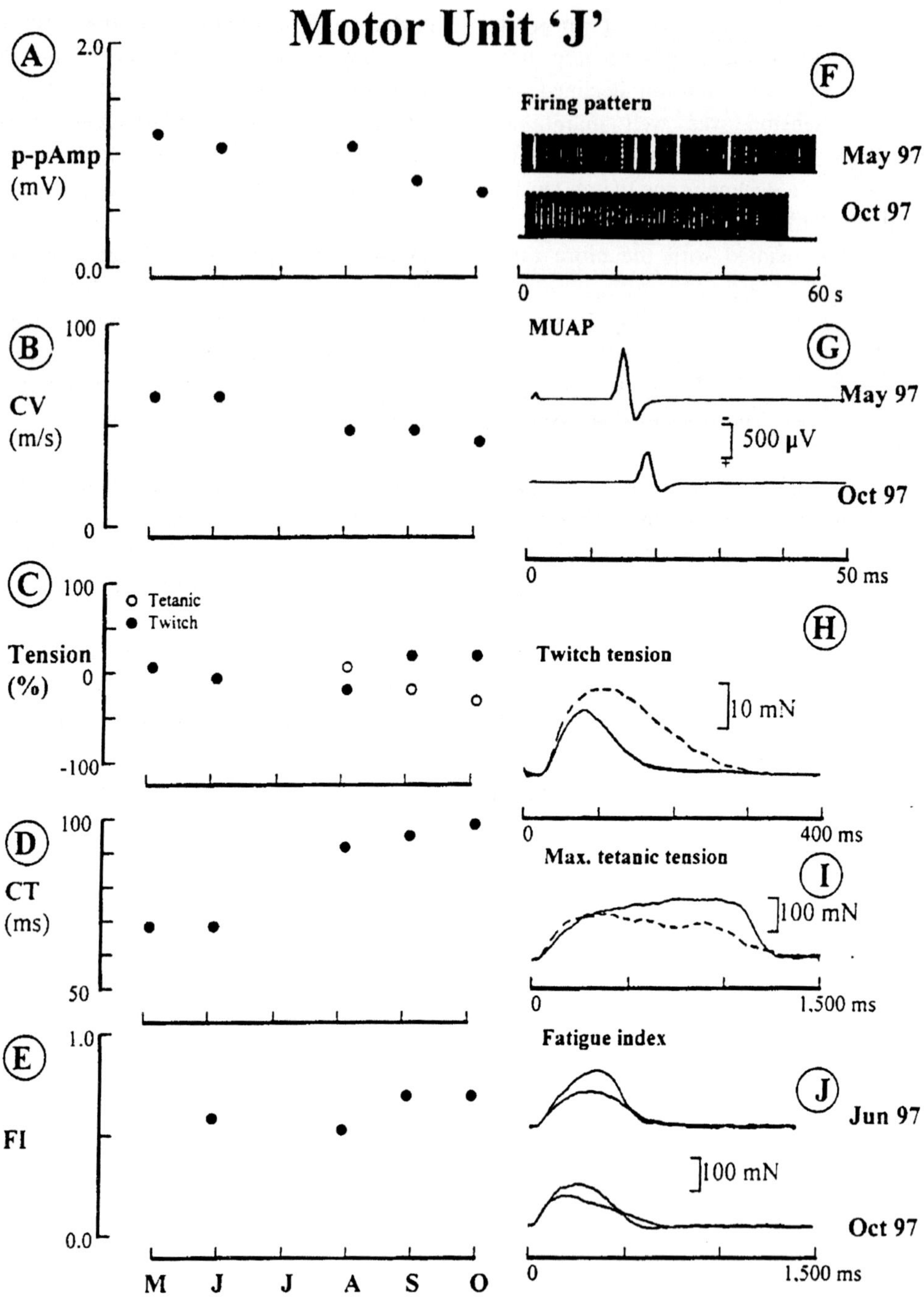

Fig. 8. Temporal profile of pathophysiological changes in MU 'J'. The scheme of presentation is identical to Fig. 7. Over the 5-month period (from May to October, 1997), the peak-to-peak amplitude of the MUAP (A and G), axonal conduction velocities (B) and maximal tetanic tension (C) progressively fell (note that maximal tetanic tension was not tested in the first two studies). In H and I, the dash lines represent twitch and maximal tetanic tension records obtained in October. The earlier (solid lines) twitch tension record was obtained in May while the earlier maximal tetanic record was obtained in August. In contrast to MU 'S', the twitch tension of MU 'J' showed an apparent increase (H) due to a lengthening of the 'active state' as reflected by the prolongation in its contraction time (D). Both firing rate plots in F represent the maximal firing rates. From Chan et al. (1998b).

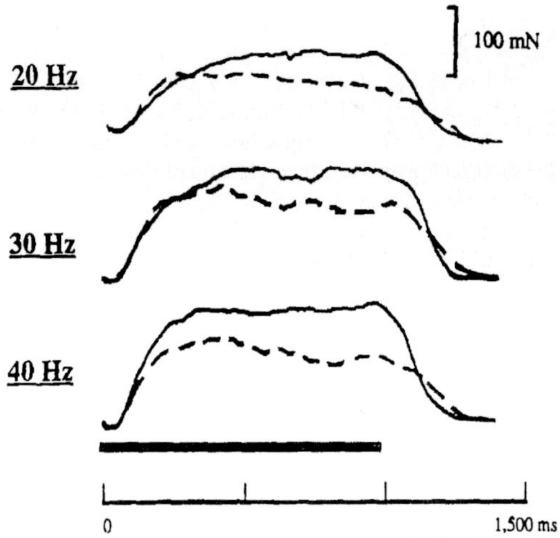

Fig. 9. Tetanic failure of MU 'J' in the last 2 months of the studies are shown. In September 1997, tetanic tensions were well maintained (solid lines) in response to 20, 30 and 40 Hz train of stimuli, each lasting 1 s (represented by the horizontal bar). However, 1 month later, tetanic tensions at these frequencies fell ('tetanic failure') during stimulation (dash lines). From Chan et al. (1998b).

prime vector or the preferred site for stimulation of its axon will change. Of course the more rapidly evolving the changes, the shorter the intervals between studies have to be in order to capture any trends in any of the properties as the disease progresses or responds to treatment. Based on our experience in the longitudinally studied MUs in ALS, it seems that intervals between studies of the order of 1–2 months should suffice to recognize any changes in the MUs. Of course there is the added advantage in ALS and some peripheral neuropathies that losses of motor axons (units) so depletes the available number of MUs as to make the finding and selection of suitable MUs for longitudinal studies easier than in healthy subjects.

How useful is the information gained by studying individual MUs? As illustrated by the adaptive capacity of normal MUs to an electrical stimulation program, the response of individual MUs with different physiological characteristics can range widely. These changes cannot be readily appreciated by studying the contractile properties of the

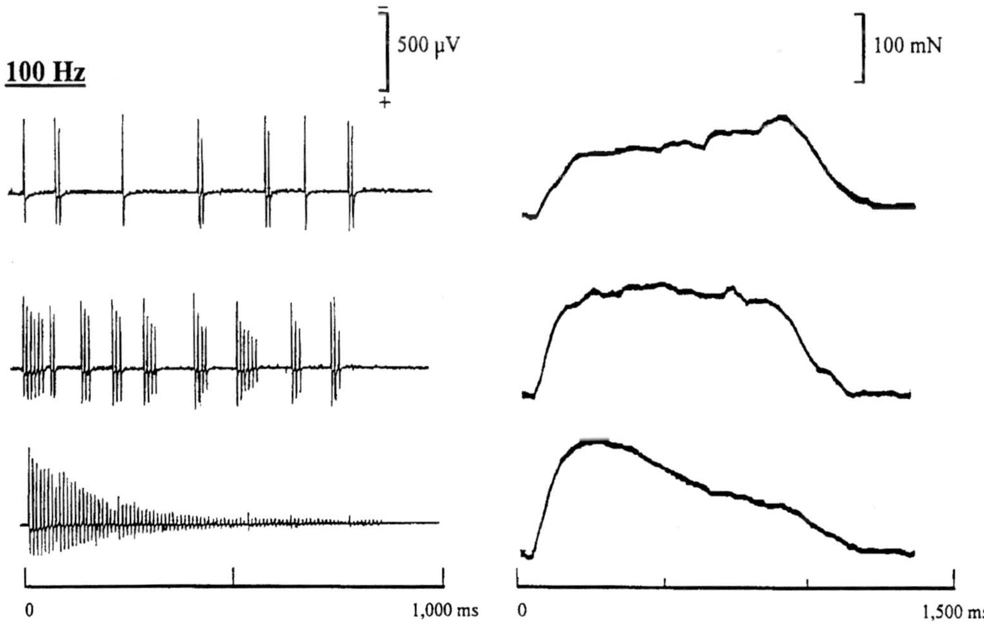

Fig. 10. Motor unit 'J' from October, 1997. Decrement of tetanic tension in response to a 1 s 100 Hz train of stimuli was observed (bottom row), similar to those seen at lower frequencies in Fig. 9. However, when the stimulus intensity was deliberately decreased so that the MU only fired intermittently (middle row), the tetanic failure largely disappeared while a similar peak tension was maintained. When the stimulus intensity was decreased still further so that the MU only fired 11 out of 100 times (top row), the tetanic tension was still surprisingly well preserved. Note that along with the tension decrements, the MUAPs also progressively decremented within the train. When the MU only fired intermittently, the MUAPs had a chance to recovered to its original size. From Chan et al. (1998b).

whole muscle which represents an 'average' response of all the constituent MUs. Furthermore, an understanding of individual MU differences could be of practical importance, especially in diseases in which different muscle fibre types are differentially affected. The differences we found in MUs in ALS subjects are another striking example. The remarkably different pattern of natural progression demonstrated suggests that different MUs could well show very different treatment responses. Based on these observations, we believe that the technique could offer potentially useful insight into MU functions and their adaptive capacity to treatment – information that is otherwise difficult to gain. However, even though the initial data seems to offer an enticing prospect, whether the technique will realize its full potential still needs to be established. Further studies will need to establish the feasibility of using this technique in large-scale clinical studies.

Acknowledgements

KMC receives salary support from the Alberta Heritage Foundation for Medical Research.

References

Bergmans, J. *The physiology of single human nerve fibres* [Ph.D. thesis]. Vander, Belgium: Louvain University, 1970.

Burke, R.E., Levine, D.N., Tsaris, P. and Zajac, F.E. Physiological types and histochemical profiles in motor units of the cat gastrocnemius. *J. Physiol.*, 1973, 234: 723–748.

Chan, K.M., Doherty, T.J., Andres, L.P., Porter, M.M., Brown, T. and Brown, W.F. Longitudinal study of the contractile and electrical properties of single human thenar motor units. *Muscle Nerve*, 1998a, 21: 839–849.

Chan, K.M., Stashuk, D.W. and Brown, W.F. A longitudinal study of the pathophysiological changes in single human thenar motor units in amyotrophic lateral sclerosis. *Muscle Nerve*, 1998b, 21: 1714–1723.

Chan, K.M., Andres, L.P., Polykovskaya, Y. and Brown, W.F. The effects of training through high-frequency electrical stimulation on the physiological properties of single human thenar motor units. *Muscle Nerve*, 1999, 22: 186–195.

Doherty, T.J. and Brown, W.F. A method for the longitudinal study of human thenar motor units. *Muscle Nerve*, 1994, 17: 1029–1036.

Doherty, T.J. and Brown, W.F. Age related changes in human thenar motor unit twitch contractile properties. *J. Appl. Physiol.*, 1997, 82: 93–101.

Stein, R.B., French, A.S., Mannard, A. and Yemm, R. New methods for analysing motor function in man and animals. *Brain. Res.*, 1972, 40: 187–192.

Taylor, A. and Stephens, J.A. Study of human motor unit contractions by controlled intramuscular microstimulation. *Brain. Res.*, 1976, 117: 331–335.

Thomas, C.K., Johansson, R.S., Westling, G. and Bigland-Ritchie, B. Twitch properties of human thenar motor units measured in response to intraneural axon stimulation. *J. Neurophysiol.*, 1990, 64: 1339–1346.

Thomas, C.K., Johansson, R.S. and Bigland-Ritchie, B. Attempts to physiologically classify human thenar motor units. *J. Neurophysiol.*, 1991, 65: 1501–1508.

Westling, G., Johansson, R.S., Thomas, C.K. and Bigland-Ritchie, B. Measurement of contractile and electrical properties of single human thenar motor units in response to intraneural motor axon stimulation. *J. Neurophysiol.*, 1990, 64: 1331–1338.

Motor Unit Number Estimation (Supplements to Clinical Neurophysiology Vol. 55)
Editor: M.B. Bromberg

Chapter 26

Longitudinal tracking of single motor units: techniques and applications

Clifton L. Gooch*

Department of Neurology, Columbia Presbyterian Medical Center, 710 West 168th Street, New York, NY 10032, USA

Introduction

The ability to isolate and reproducibly track single motor unit action potentials (S-MUAP) in human subjects provides unique longitudinal data regarding motor unit function. Motor unit tracking represents an expansion of the multiple point stimulation (MPS) technique of motor unit number estimation (MUNE) where S-MUAPs are activated by transcutaneous stimulation of a motor nerve (Kadrie et al., 1976; Doherty and Brown, 1993). Criteria for recognition of the same S-MUAP waveform over separate study sessions have been described (Doherty and Brown, 1994). Longitudinal tracking has been successfully applied to patients with amyotrophic lateral sclerosis (ALS) (Gooch and Harati, 1997). Single motor unit tracking has been extended in several ways. In addition to recording S-MUAPs, single motor unit twitch data can be recorded to assess contractile properties, and has been used to study changes in ALS patients (Chan et al., 1998a,b, 1999). Repetitive stimulation of single motor units has used to assess motor unit function in ALS subjects (Gooch, 1998). A technique combining MPS MUNE and S-MUAP tracking has also been developed and tested in control and ALS subjects (Gooch and Wagner, 1998; Gooch et al., 2001). This article reviews our work in S-MUAP tracking, detailing our techniques and results in control and ALS subjects. Our combined MPS MUNE and S-MUAP tracking method is detailed elsewhere in this volume, as are the studies of our colleagues in this area.

*Correspondence to: Dr. Clifton Gooch, Department of Neurology, Columbia Presbyterian Medical Center, 710 West 168th Street, New York, NY 10032, USA.
e-mail: CLG33@columbia.edu

doi:10.1016/S1567-424X(03)00026-6

Methods

We have used an adapted method to identify and tract S-MUAPs in ALS patients with rapidly progressive disease. Motor units were studied at three to four separate sessions over an 8–12-week period (Gooch and Harati, 1997).

Subjects

Three sporadic ALS patients with significant and active involvement of the thenar musculature were studied to assess the technique.

Patient A was a 60-year-old male with a 5-month history of symptoms. Left thumb abduction was MRC grade 3− to 2+ that worsened during recording sessions.

Patient B was a 53-year-old male with 3–4 months of symptoms. Left thumb abduction strength was grade 2+ to 3− with no change over the study period.

Patient C was a 35-year-old male with a 6-month history of symptoms. Left thumb abduction was 3+ to 4+ and remained unchanged throughout the study.

Single motor unit studies

Our recording and stimulating techniques have been previously reported (Gooch and Harati, 1997). Recording electrodes were disposable 8 × 30 mm adhesive strips (TECA Co., Pleasantville, NY) placed transversely over the thenar eminence in close approximation to the end-plate zone of the abductor and flexor pollicis muscles. Reference electrodes were placed over the distal interphalangeal joint of the thumb, and ground electrodes were placed over the ulnar surface of the palm. The thumb was taped to the lateral surface of the hand to reduce movement artifact (Kelkar and Ross, 1993). The recording electrode position was noted using anatomical surface landmarks for future reference. Median nerve stimulation was performed with a hand-held bipolar electrode (Nicolet Biomedical, Madison WI) through saline-soaked felt pads (5 mm diameter, 30 mm apart, cathode distal). S-MUAPs and compound motor action potentials (CMAPs) were recorded from the thenar musculature on an Advantage EMG system (Advantage Medical, London, Canada) at a band-pass of 2 Hz to 2 kHz (12 bit resolution). S-MUAPs were activated by 0.05 ms square wave pulses at various intensities, from 5 to 50 mA. A surface map of the median nerve was made noting anodal and cathodal positions and current levels that produced a given S-MUAP.

Single motor units were identified using previously published criteria (Doherty and Brown, 1994). (1) Each S-MUAP demonstrated an "all-or-nothing" response with no fractionation. Specifically, stimuli near threshold produced either a MUAP with consistent morphology and latency, or no response. (2) The threshold for eliciting a given S-MUAP was distinctly different from that eliciting the next highest motor axon at a specific stimulation site. Repeat excitation of the same baseline S-MUAP during sequential sessions was assumed when the potential fulfilled the above criteria, more closely resembled its predecessor than any other potential elicited from other stimulation sites, and was activated from the same anodal and cathodal coordinates and similar stimulus strengths as at baseline (Fig. 1). MUNE by the F-wave method (Stashuk et al., 1994) was also performed at each session, utilizing the same electrode array, with an inter-electrode distance of 6.5 cm between the stimulating cathode and active recording electrode.

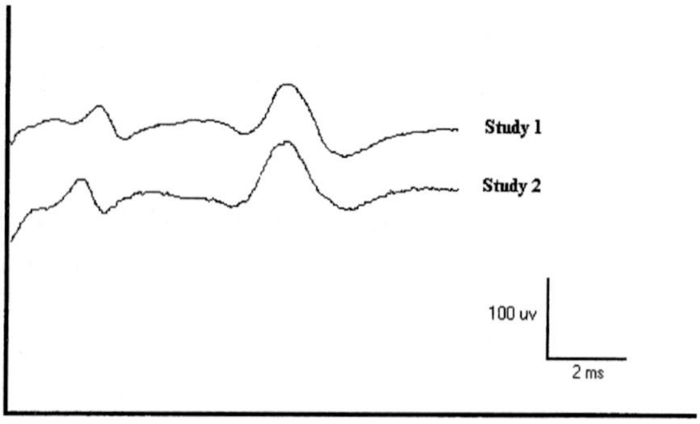

Fig. 1. Longitudinal tracking of the same S-MUAP waveform over two separate consecutive sessions (rastered and superimposed). The smaller, earlier waveform is the incidentally recorded median sensory nerve action potential (SNAP) at the base of the first digit.

Results

MUNE was also performed in the thenar muscle group, utilizing the F-wave method. Baseline MUNE values were initially low, and showed slight declines in Patients A and B, while remaining relatively constant in patient C. The F-wave MUNE technique is not sufficiently sensitive to reliably detect the loss of five to 15 motor units during the course of a 12-week longitudinal study.

At least three S-MUAPs which had similar latencies, negative peak amplitudes and waveform morphologies following stimulation at the same coordinates and amperage levels were tracked in three separate sessions in each patient over 8–12 weeks. We also recorded a consistent waveform in all subjects attributed to the median sensory response at the first digit (3) (Fig. 1).

S-MUAP latency, amplitude, morphology, stimulation current and MUNE for each session are summarized in Table 1. The latencies of each S-MUAP remained relatively constant throughout the study, with less than 0.3 ms or less variation from session to session, possibly due to minor temperature changes over the 45–60 min course of each session. The negative peak amplitudes of each S-MUAP also remained relatively constant from session to session in most cases, with less than 30% variation between the highest and lowest values. Those demonstrating greater variation typically showed a trend towards decreasing amplitudes throughout the course of the study despite consistent latency and morphology (motor units B2 and C2). Motor unit C2 demonstrated very low baseline amplitude with significant decline throughout the three sessions, and could no longer be elicited at a fourth session. Waveform morphology remained consistent from session to session for all patients in all recordings, with one exception. The morphology of waveform C1 was constant in sessions one and two but was altered in session three, becoming more complex without significant changes in amplitude or latency. Changes in waveform morphology might accompany terminal reinnervation, though this remains speculative. Other motor units were recorded with waveforms that changed over the course of the study but were not included.

Summary

The longitudinal tracking of S-MUAPs is possible in ALS patients. We choose patients with an advanced degree of baseline hand involvement and a history of rapid progression to test this technique. We did not use computerized subtraction or decomposition algorithms (which extract reconstituted additional S-MUAPs from their summated compound motor unit action potentials after baseline S-MUAPs are obtained) (Doherty and Brown, 1993; McComas, 1995), but relied solely upon acquiring direct, unreconstituted, S-MUAPs. Although subtraction algorithms may speed waveform acquisition, we were uncertain of the precise effect of such processing on S-MUAP waveform morphology and other parameters critical to longitudinal study. Since no special software is necessary for this basic MPS-based technique, longitudinal S-MUAP studies can be performed on virtually any EMG machine after suitable training and experience. F-wave MUNE, however, does require specific software programming, but is rapid and easy to perform.

Longitudinal S-MUP tracking with repetitive nerve stimulation

Repetitive whole nerve stimulation is widely utilized in electrodiagnostic medicine, but repetitive stimulation of single motor axons (repetitive axonal stimulation or RAS) has not been widely used (Kadrie and Brown, 1978a,b). This technique provides a unique assessment of neuromuscular junction functioning within an individual motor unit, but is of even greater value when single motor unit responses can be tracked over time. We have devised and assessed the feasibility of tracking the responses to RAS of the same S-MUAP over two recording sessions. Three S-MUAPs over two separate sessions in three healthy control subjects.

Methods

Three control subjects with a normal neurologic examination were selected.

Repetitive nerve and repetitive axonal stimulation and tracking

Standard repetitive nerve stimulation was performed (Stålberg and Sanders, 1981), with trains of 10 supramaximal stimuli delivered at 3 Hz. Trains were delivered immediately before exercise, immediately after 30 s of maximal voluntary contraction, and at 60 and 120 s following the contraction.

S-MUAP identification, recording and tracking was performed as described above (Gooch and Harati, 1997). RAS was performed for each tracked S-MUAP during each session. Trains of 10 stimuli

TABLE 1

SUMMARY OF WAVEFORM PARAMETERS TRACKED OVER THREE SESSIONS IN THREE PATIENTS WITH ALS

Patient A				Patient B				Patient C			
S-MUAP A1	Latency (ms)	Amplitude (μV)	Stimulus (mA)	S-MUAP A1	Latency (ms)	Amplitude (μV)	Stimulus (mA)	S-MUAP A1	Latency (ms)	Amplitude (μV)	Stimulus (mA)
Study 1	3.4	37.6	15	Study 1	3.6	64.5	27	Study 1	4.2	53.0	15
Study 2	3.3	38.8	15	Study 2	3.6	50.8	21	Study 2	4.2	65.0	13
Study 3	3.3	37.9	15	Study 3	3.4	37.4	16	Study 3	4.5	47.9	15
S-MUAP A2											
Study 1	6.5	24.2	15	Study 1	4.3	48.6	41	Study 1	1.5	10.5	11
Study 2	6.3	18.1	15	Study 2	4.6	32.0	16	Study 2	1.4	6.3	20
Study 3	6.6	25.2	19	Study 3	4.4	25.9	25	Study 3	1.2	1.7	21
S-MUAP A3											
Study 1	12.5	35.7	18	Study 1	5.8	80.3	21	Study 1	7.3	170	27
Study 2	12.7	25.0	18	Study 2	6.1	62.5	11	Study 2	7.0	164	26
Study 3	12.8	34.7	16	Study 3	6.1	80.3	17	Study 3	7.2	234	23
MUNE	Value										
Study 1	19			Study 1	15			Study 1	6		
Study 2	18			Study 2	11			Study 2	9		
Study 3	15			Study 3	6			Study 3	8		

Motor unit number estimates were simultaneously recorded utilizing the F-wave technique during each session (see text).

were delivered at 3 Hz, paralleling the repetitive nerve stimulation protocol described above. The position, angle and pressure of the stimulating anode and cathode were carefully maintained and the amperage level was held constant throughout RAS acquisition. Each subject was studied at two separate sessions, from 1 day to 1 week apart. Facilitation and decrement were calculated by comparing the first to the fourth waveform within each S-MUAP and CMAP train.

Results

Three S-MUAPs were successfully identified, tracked and subjected to RAS in each subject (Fig. 2; Table 2). Five of the nine S-MUAP trains obtained during session 1 demonstrated no decrement or increment and remained unchanged at session 2. Of the remaining S-MUAP trains, two demonstrated decrement (varying less than 5% between sessions 1 and 2) and two demonstrated

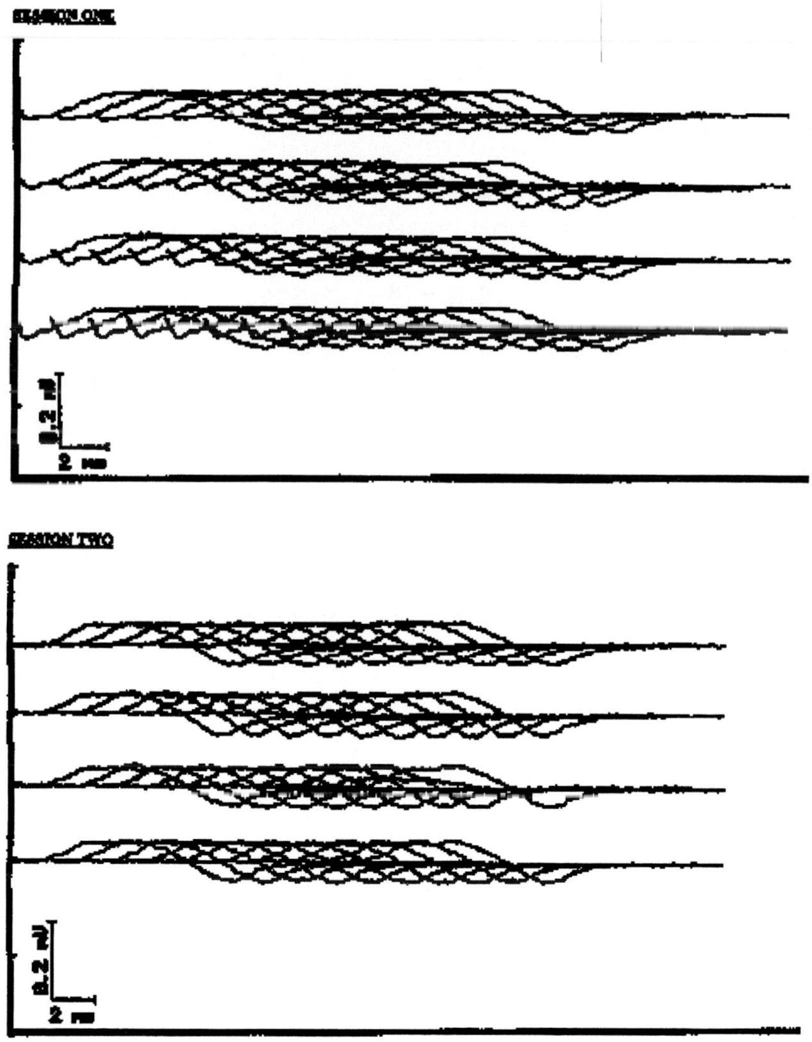

Fig. 2. RAS of the same single motor unit, tracked over two separate sessions. During each session, a baseline, pre-exercise train of 10 waveforms was recorded, followed by 30 s of maximal volitional contraction, an immediate post-exercise train and two additional trains at 60 and 120 s following relaxation, as illustrated in rastered mode here. Note the highly reproducible morphology from train to train, within each train and from session to session, with minimal increment or decrement.

TABLE 2

SUMMARY OF PARAMETERS FOR CMAP AND S-MUAP WAVEFORM TRAINS, INCREMENT AND DECREMENT RECORDED BY REPETITIVE NERVE AND RAS IN FIVE NORMAL CONTROL SUBJECTS

Subject A					Subject B					Subject C				
	Amp 1	Amp 2	Percent Amp 1	Percent Amp 2		Amp 1	Amp 2	Percent Amp 1	Percent Amp 2		Amp 1	Amp 2	Percent Amp 1	Percent Amp 2
S-MUAP 1														
Train 1	66	58	0	0	Train 1	115	91	0	0	Train 1	85	79	−16	−15
Train 2	66	58	0	0	Train 2	108	91	0	0	Train 2	100	100	−18	−15
Train 3	66	50	0	0	Train 3	108	91	0	0	Train 3	88	84	−10	−12
Train 4	66	50	0	0	Train 4	115	91	0	0	Train 4	88	84	−8	−11
S-MUAP 2														
Train 1	410	410	−1	−1	Train 1	59	66.4	14	14	Train 1	67	83	0	0
Train 2	410	410	−1	−1	Train 2	59	74.4	10	13	Train 2	76	91.3	0	0
Train 3	410	410	0	−2	Train 3	51	65	6	6	Train 3	67	91.3	0	0
Train 4	410	410	0	0	Train 4	51	65	6	6	Train 4	67	91.3	0	0
S-MUAP 3														
Train 1	83	75	0	0	Train 1	56	62.2	8	7	Train 1	50	55	0	0
Train 2	83	75	0	0	Train 2	50	58.1	14	10	Train 2	50	58	0	0
Train 3	83	67	0	0	Train 3	56	58	14	14	Train 3	50	66.4	0	0
Train 4	83	67	0	0	Train 4	50	62.3	11	13	Train 4	50	58.1	0	0
CMAP														
Train 1	10,700	10,300	−2	−1	Train 1	5500	6500	−1	−2	Train 1	13,300	12,700	0	−2
Train 2	10,400	10,200	0	−2	Train 2	6000	6800	−1	−3	Train 2	12,400	12,200	6	1
Train 3	10,600	10,600	−1	−1	Train 3	5800	6700	0	−2	Train 3	13,100	12,400	2	0
Train 4	10,700	10,700	−2	−1	Train 4	5700	6500	−1	−2	Train 4	13,500	12,600	1	−2

Individual S-MUAP waveforms and their responses were tracked over two separate sessions (see text). S-MUAP: Single motor unit action potential. CMAP: compound muscle action potential. Amp 1: amplitude of first waveform in train during session 1. Amp 2: amplitude of first waveform in train during session 2. Percent Amp 1: percent change in amplitude 1st waveform versus 4th in each train (1st session). Percent Amp 2: percent change in amplitude 1st waveform versus 4th in each train (2nd session). Train 1: immediate pre-exercise. Train 2: immediate post-exercise. Train 3: 60 s post-exercise. Train 4: 120 s post-exercise.

increment (varying less than 5%). Of the 72 total S-MUAP trains recorded, 40 (56%) showed no increment or decrement. Sixteen trains (22%) demonstrated decrement, eight trains (11%) showed decrements of less than 3%, and eight trains (11%) showed decrements of 8% or greater (absolute range 0–18%). Conversely, 16 trains (22%) demonstrated increments, with six trains (8%) showing increments of less than 10%, and 10 trains (14%) showing increments of 10% or greater (absolute range 0–14%). The majority of S-MUAP trains with increments in excess of 10% also demonstrated concurrent shortening of the negative peak duration, suggesting pseudofacilitation. No consistent S-MUAP post-exercise facilitation was observed. All 36 S-MUAP trains showing decrement and increment at session 1 varied less than 5% on repeat testing at session 2. The percentage difference in amplitude between the first and fourth response in the train (decrement or increment) was highly reproducible on repeat testing, with a test–retest correlation coefficient of 0.98.

Among the 24 CMAP trains recorded, 16 trains (67%) showed a decrement of less than 4%, three trains (13%) an increment of less than 3%, and one train (4%) an increment of 6%. No increment or decrement was observed in the remaining four trains (16%). Mild post-exercise CMAP amplitude facilitation of 9 and 4% (in two different sessions) was noted in one subject. No correlations were observed between CMAP decrement or increment and S-MUAP decrement or increment. Successful S-MUAP elicitation and subsequent RAS were highly dependent on finding and maintaining proper stimulating electrode position and pressure, and tracking was most easily and rapidly performed in the thinnest of the three subjects.

Summary

RAS of the same single motor unit can be performed over at least two sessions in control subjects with reproducible results and a limited range of variation. S-MUAP increments and decrements, when present, were also reproducible during separate sessions. The occasional S-MUAP increments are likely due to pseudofacilitation within the single motor unit, as they were usually accompanied by shortening of S-MUAP duration. The one waveform demonstrating decrement in excess of 10% may represent an outlying unit, although the number of trains reported here is not adequate to establish a normal range for the RAS technique, which may be somewhat different than that derived from whole nerve stimulation studies. As with S-MUAP tracking, this technique can be performed on virtually any commercial device capable of repetitive nerve stimulation and recording by an examiner with experience with the technique. Further studies are needed to provide more normative data and to establish patterns of abnormality in patients with neuromuscular disease.

Techniques for single motor unit tracking, have become increasingly sophisticated over the last 5 years, and are now being applied to an ever more detailed exploration of motor unit physiology in the living human subject. These methods provide unique electrophysiologic information, unobtainable by any other method, and are even more powerful when combined with MUNE data. The extension of S-MUAP tracking methods to the contractile physiology of the motor unit, and to further studies in the natural history of ALS and in treatment trials of motor neuron disease are detailed elsewhere in volume.

References

Chan, K.M., Doherty, T.J., Andres, L.P., Porter, M.M., Brown, T. and Brown, W.F. Longitudinal study of the contractile and electrical properties of single human thenar motor units. *Muscle Nerve*, 1998a, 21: 839–849.

Chan, K.M., Stashuk, D. and Brown, W.F. A longitudinal study of the pathophysiological changes in single human thenar motor units in ALS. *Muscle Nerve*, 1998b, 21: 1714–1723.

Chan, K.M., Andres, L.P., Polykovskaya, Y. and Brown, W.F. The effects of training through high-frequency electrical stimulation on the physiological properties of single human thenar motor units. *Muscle Nerve*, 1999, 22: 1–10.

Doherty, T.J. and Brown, W.F. The estimated numbers and relative sizes of thenar motor units as selected by multiple point stimulation in young and older adults. *Muscle Nerve*, 1993, 16: 355–366.

Doherty, T.J. and Brown, W.F. A method for the longitudinal study of human thenar motor units. *Muscle Nerve*, 1994, 17: 1029–1036.

Gooch, C.L. Repetitive axonal stimulation of the same single motor unit: a longitudinal tracking study. *Muscle Nerve*, 1998, 12: 1537–1539.

Gooch, C.L. and Harati, Y. Longitudinal tracking of the same single motor unit in amyotrophic lateral sclerosis. *Muscle Nerve*, 1997, 20: 511–513.

Gooch, C.L. and Wagner, T. Longitudinal S-MUAP tracking and MUNE: validity of a combined method. *Muscle Nerve*, 1998, 21: 1601.

Gooch, C., Pleitez, M., Ciabarra, T., Kaufmann, P., and Harati, Y. Motor unit survival in a controlled trial of Xaliproden, for the treatment of amyotrophic lateral sclerosis. *Ann. Neurol.*, 2001, 50: 523.

Kadrie, H.A. and Brown, W.F. Neuromuscular transmission in human single motor units. *J. Neurol. Neurosurg. Psychiatry*, 1978a, 41: 193–204.

Kadrie, H.A. and Brown, W.F. Neuromuscular transmission in myasthenic single motor units. *J. Neurol. Neurosurg. Psychiatry*, 1978b, 41: 205–214.

Kadrie, H.A., Yates, S.K., Milner-Brown, H.S. and Brown, W. F. Multiple point electrical stimulation of ulnar and median nerves. *J. Neurol. Neurosurg. Psychiatry*, 1976, 39: 973–985.

Kelkar, P. and Ross, M.A. Variation in compound muscle action potential amplitude and area with muscle contraction and position change. *Muscle Nerve*, 1993, 16: 1084A–1085A.

McComas, A.J. Motor unit estimation: anxieties and achievements. *Muscle Nerve*, 1995, 18: 369–379.

Stålberg, E. and Sanders, D.B. Electrophysiologic tests of neuromuscular transmission. "*Clinical Neurophysiology*" (E. Stalberg and R. Young, Eds.), 1981, pp. 238–264. Butterworth, London.

Stashuk, D.W., Doherty, T.J., Kassam, A. and Brown, W.F. MUNE based on the automated analysis of F-responses. *Muscle Nerve*, 1994, 17: 881–890.

Motor Unit Number Estimation (Supplements to Clinical Neurophysiology Vol. 55)
Editor: M.B. Bromberg

Chapter 27

Correlations between MUNE obtained by the intraneural microstimulation technique and the Appel clinical rating scale

Keisuke Arasaki*

EMG/EEG Laboratory, Department of Neurology, NTT East Kanto Medical Center, 5-9-22 Higashi-Gotanda, Shinagawa-ku, Tokyo 141-0022, Japan

Introduction

The time course of functional spinal alpha motor neuron loss in ALS should provide insight into the natural course of the disease (Dantes and McComas, 1991). Clinical rating scales (Appel et al., 1987; ACTS Group, 1996) are used in current therapeutic trials to document the course of ALS and the effects of drugs, but changes in MUNE values may be a more sensitive outcome measure of this disease (Yuen and Olney, 1997; Olney et al., 1999). Consistent with this idea are the results of our previous study (Arasaki and Tamaki, 1998), in which ALS patients who lost about 70% of their functional SA motor neurons showed only a 15% increase in their Appel ALS scores (Appel et al., 1987). Thus, our present study was aimed at delineating the time course of functional spinal alpha motor neuron loss and changes in a clinical rating scale in ALS patients. Detailed results of the present study are in press (Arasaki et al., 2002).

*Correspondence to: Dr. Keisuke Arasaki, EMG/EEG Laboratory, Department of Neurology, NTT East Kanto Medical Center, 5-9-22 Higashi-Gotanda, Shinagawa-ku, Tokyo 141-0022, Japan. Tel.: 81-3-3448-6455, Fax: 81-3-3448-6458.
e-mail: arasaki@rr.iij4u.or.jp

doi: 10.1016/S1567-424X(03)00027-8

Methods

We obtained a series of MUNE values for each of ten patients, 36–85 years of age, who were diagnosed with definite ALS according to the El Escorial criteria (WFN Research Group, 1994). The time of testing was between 10 and 12, 16 and 18, and 22 and 24 months after the onset of symptoms. At the time of testing, we also examined the patients clinically to obtain their Appel scores (Appel et al., 1987). The Appel score is the sum of five groups of functional scores: medullary functions, respiration, muscle strength, upper extremity functions, and lower extremity functions. The normal score for each functional group is six, making the Appel score for a completely normal person equal to 30. As a patient's condition worsens, the score becomes higher, and the worst score is 164.

The control subjects were 20 patients, 36–80 years of age, with headaches but no other neurological symptoms or signs. In each subject of the control group, MUNEs were obtained twice with an interval of one week in order to document their reproducibility. Before testing, we discussed the procedure with both groups of subjects and obtained their informed consent. Their medical records were reviewed. Our study was approved by the Committee for the Assurance of Clinical Study Quality in our institution.

Our current methods of performing MUNE is different from those described elsewhere (Arasaki and Tamaki, 1998) in that data acquisition and analysis were done using Neuropack MEB-2200 (Nihon Kohden, Tokyo, Japan). We recorded the maximal compound muscle action potentials (CMAPs) and at least ten unitary muscle action potentials (MAPs) from hypothenar and EDB muscles. For the microstimulation of motor axons, fine tungsten-needle electrodes with a tip impedance of 9–13 MΩ at 1000 Hz and 10^{-8} A (Frederick Haer & Co., Brunswick, ME, USA) were inserted into the ulnar and peroneal nerves at the wrist and ankle, respectively. While keeping the same insertion point, we manipulated the needle electrode manually, placing its tip at different points in the nerve trunk to stimulate different single motor axons with an electric square pulse of 0.5–8.0 mA and a duration of 10–50 μs.

Using an MEB-2200 with an integration algorithm installed[6], the area of the negative portion of the maximal CMAP was measured. In order to obtain the mean unitary MAP waveform, at least ten unitary MAP waveforms were recorded and averaged by an off-line computer. An exception to this was that fewer than ten different motor units could be sampled successfully in some patients with advanced ALS and the mean unitary MAP waveform was determined using only those sampled (see below). A MUNE was then calculated by dividing the area of the negative portion of the CMAP by that of the digitally averaged unitary MAP.

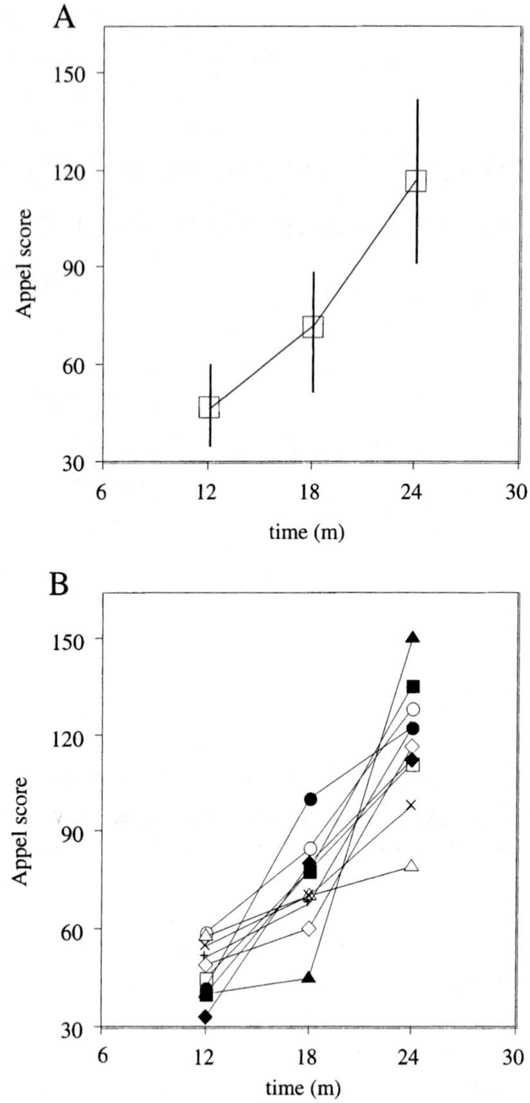

Fig. 1. Changes in Appel's scores. In A, each box and bar indicate the mean and SD of the scores, respectively, at 12, 18, and 24 months after onset of symptoms. In B, the scores of each ALS patient are plotted in the same manner as in A. Individual patients were represented by different symbols.

Results

The Appel score in the group of patients with headaches was 32 ± 2 (mean ± SD, $n = 20$), whereas that in the ALS patient group ($n = 10$) was 47 ± 9 at 12 months after onset, 72 ± 15 at 18 months, and 117 ± 20 at 24 months (Fig. 1A). The rate of progression of the disease in each of the ALS patient group was highly variable. As shown in Fig. 1B, the rate of progression was slow in two cases, whereas it was relatively fast in five. The score included lateral pinch power (see above), which represented the motor strength of intrinsic hand muscles. As we measured the hypothenar MUNE, we paid particular attention to pinch power, which was 5.9 ± 1.6 kg at 12 months after onset ($n = 10$), 4.3 ± 2.5 kg at 18 months ($n = 10$), and 1.4 ± 0.8 kg at 24 months ($n = 8$).

MUNE values from the hypothenar muscle in the control group of patients was 247 ± 94, whereas that of the EDB muscle was 107 ± 56 (n = 20). In the ALS patient group, MUNE values of the hypothenar and EDB muscles decreased to 62 ± 30 (a range of 22–100) and 22 ± 14 (5–48) at 12 months after onset (n = 10), 30 ± 14 (15–58) and 12 ± 18 (3–32) at 18 months (n = 10), and 11 ± 12 (2–40) and 4 ± 5 (0–16) at 24 months (n = 8), respectively (Fig. 2A). As shown in Fig. 2B and C, MUNE values were also variable according to each patient, but what was remarkable was the similarity between changes in the Appel scores and those in the MUNEs. Two ALS patients with slow clinical progression showed a slow decrease in their MUNE values, whereas four ALS patients with a rapid clinical progression showed a similar rapid decrease in their MUNE values.

The relationship between Appel scores and MUNE values is shown in Fig. 3. MUNE values of the hypothenar and EDB muscles of each patient with ALS plotted against Appel scores were variable but seemed to have a negative correlation. In fact, the means of these MUNE values showed a negative hyperbolic correlation with Appel scores, and the decrease in the hypothenar MUNE was steeper than that in the EDB MUNE (Fig. 3C).

Discussion

The present study was a longitudinal assessment, in which we followed ten patients with ALS and performed MUNE studies in each patient at 12, 18, and 24 months after the onset of symptoms. As the patients became more disabled, their Appel scores increased. Although the rate of progression in the scores of individual ALS patients was highly variable, as shown in Fig. 1B, the mean values of the rates showed a slower increase 12–18 months after onset than 18–24 months after onset (Fig. 1A).

As the patients became more disabled, their MUNE values decreased. In ALS patients with severe muscular atrophy, however, we were not always able to sample at least ten motor units, but the number of motor units recorded was consistently equal to the number of remaining functional

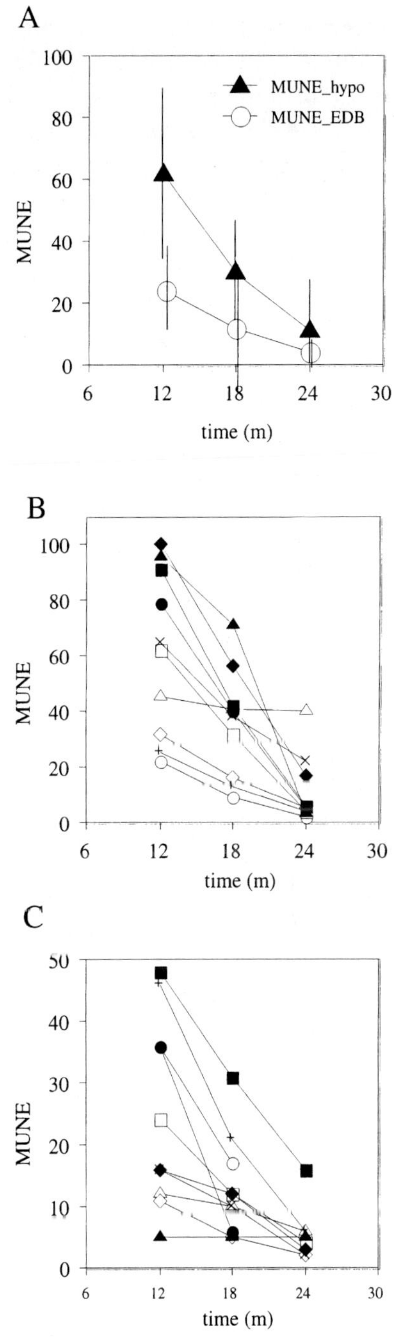

Fig. 2. MUNEs of the hypothenar and EDB muscles in patients with ALS. In A, filled triangles and open circles indicate MUNEs of the hypothenar and EDB muscles, respectively, obtained from ALS patients at 12, 18, and 24 months after onset. B and C show changes in MUNEs of the hypothenar and EDB muscles, respectively, in each ALS patient obtained at 12, 18, and 24 months after onset. Individual patients were represented by different symbols.

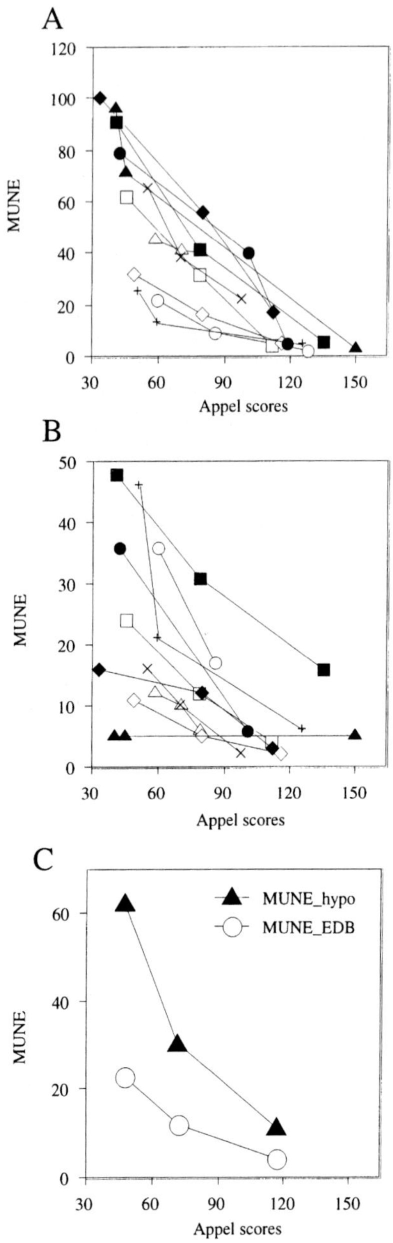

Fig. 3. Relationship between Appel's scores and MUNEs of the hypothenar and EDB muscles in patients with ALS. A and B show the hypothenar and EDB MUNEs, respectively, of each ALS patient plotted against his/her Appel's scores. Three points in each patient's plot represent data obtained at 12, 18, and 24 months after onset. Individual patients were represented by different symbols. In C, filled triangles and open circles indicate the means of the MUNEs of the hypothenar and EDB muscles, respectively, obtained 12, 18, and 24 months after onset. In each figure, the abscissa is Appel's scores, whereas the ordinate is MUNEs.

motor units. It has also been recognized by other authors (Armon et al., 1997; Shefner, 2001) that the fewer the remaining motor units there are, the more consistent are the resulting MUNE values. Therefore, we conclude that MUNE values obtained with our methodology should represent the number of functional motor units in a muscle in a wide range of states, from normal to severe atrophy. Although the rate of decrease in MUNE values in the ALS patient group was highly variable, as shown in Fig. 3B and C, the mean MUNE values showed a steeper decrease at 12–18 months after onset than at 18–24 months after onset.

Although we now use clinical rating scales (ACTS Group, 1996) for the clinical assessment of ALS patients in therapeutic trials, MUNE should have a major impact because such rating scales may not be sensitive enough to detect early changes in ALS (Yuen and Olney, 1997). Rating scales such as Appel scores show composite and average bodily changes in order to define disability. Although a direct comparison between Appel scores and MUNE might seem irrational, changes in the rating scale result from a loss of motor neurons supplying the bulbar, truncal, and limb muscles in ALS patients. Accordingly, a MUNE of a single muscle may well be compared to the part of a scale that is functionally related to that particular muscle, and such a relationship between the MUNE values of a proximal muscle and their isometric strength has already been studied (Bromberg and Larson, 1996).

As clinical rating scales in ALS patients reflect a loss of upper and lower motor neurons, such scales may theoretically be substituted for MUNE of all muscles in the regions being studied. This is technically impractical, but it is interesting to speculate on how many muscles should be tested to obtain a composite MUNE score that may be comparable to the rating scale. In the present study; we suggest that MUNE of the hypothenar and EDB muscles might be sufficient for this purpose. Furthermore, the MUNE values were distributed hyperbolically against Appel scores in Fig. 3C, which means that the former seems more sensitive than the latter in detecting early changes in ALS. Thus, considering the importance of initiating therapeutic intervention as early as possible in the course of ALS, the use of MUNE in the early assessment of a patient's condition may be a better parameter than clinical rating scales.

Despite technical variability, MUNE values obtained using different methods show a close agreement in studies of normal subjects and patients with neurological disorders (Shefner, 2001). The occurrence of significant changes in MUNE in the early stage of ALS has already been reported by previous authors (Brown and Jaatool, 1974; Dantes and McComas, 1991). In these reports, however, MUNE was performed by a manual incremental technique that is subject to technical pitfalls (McComas, 1998), whereas in the present study we used the microstimulation method, the validity of which has been proven by an animal study (Arasaki et al., 1997). Our present data, therefore, strengthen the reliability of the finding that changes in MUNE are more significant than changes in rating scale in patients with early ALS.

Referenccs

Appel, V., Stewart, S.S., Smith, G. and Appel, S.H. A rating scale for amyotrophic lateral sclerosis: description and preliminary experience. *Ann. Neurol.*, 1987, 22: 328–333.

Arasaki, K. and Tamaki, M. A loss of functional spinal alpha motor neurons in amyotrophic lateral sclerosis. *Neurology*, 1998, 51: 603–605.

Arasaki, K., Tamaki, M., Hosoya, Y. and Kudo, N. Validity of electromyograms and tension as a means of motor unit number estimation. *Muscle Nerve*, 1997, 20: 552–560.

Arasaki, K, Kato, Y, Hyodo, A, Ushijima, R and Tamaki, M. Longitudinal study of functional spinal alpha motor neuron loss in amyotrophic lateral sclerosis. *Muscle Nerve*, 2002, 25: 520–526.

Armon, C., Brandstater, M.E. and Peterson, G.W. Motor unit number estimates and quantitative muscle strength measurements of distal muscles in patients with amyotrophic lateral sclerosis. *Muscle Nerve*, 1997, 20: 499–501.

Bromberg, M. and Larson, W.L. Relationship between motor-unit number estimates and isometric strength in distal muscles in ALS/MND. *J. Neurol. Sci.*, 1996, 139(Suppl.): 38–42.

Brown, W.F. and Jaatool, N. Amyotrophic lateral sclerosis. Electrophysiological study. *Arch. Neurol.*, 1974, 31: 242–248.

Dantes, M. and McComas, A. The extent and time course of motoneuron involvement in amyotrophic lateral sclerosis. *Muscle Nerve*, 1991, 14: 416–421.

McComas, A.J. Motor units: how many, how large, what kind? *J. Electromyogr. Kinesiol.*, 1998, 8: 391–402.

Olney, R.K., Yen, E.C. and Engstrom, J.W. The rate of changes in motor unit number estimates predicts survival in patients with amyotrophic lateral sclerosis. *Neurology*, 1999, 52 (Suppl. 2): A3.

Shefner, J.M. Motor unit number estimation in human neurological diseases and animal models. *Clin. Neurophysiol.*, 2001, 112: 955–964.

The ALS CNTF treatment study (ACTS) phase I-II Study Group. The amyotrophic lateral sclerosis functional rating scale. *Arch. Neurol.*, 1996, 53: 141–147.

World Federation of Neurology Research Group on Neuromuscular Diseases. El Escorial World Federation of Neurology criteria for the diagnosis of amyotrophic lateral sclerosis. *J. Neurol. Sci.*, 1994, 124: 96–107.

Yuen, E.C. and Olney, R.K. Longitudinal study of fiber density and motor unit number estimate in patients with amyotrophic lateral sclerosis. *Neurology*, 1997, 49: 573–578.

Motor Unit Number Estimation (Supplements to Clinical Neurophysiology Vol. 55)
Editor: M.B. Bromberg

Chapter 28

Relationships between MUNE and muscle strength

A. Gordon Smith[a,b,*] and Victoria Lawson[a]

[a]*Department of Neurology, University of Utah, Salt Lake City, UT 84132, USA*
[b]*Department of Pathology, University of Utah, Salt Lake City, UT 84132, USA*

Introduction

Muscle weakness is the primary cause of disability among patients with motor neuron disorders and motor predominant peripheral neuropathies. It is therefore appropriate that measures of muscle strength have traditionally provided the primary means of following disease progression and response to therapeutic agents. During the progressive middle phase of amyotrophic lateral sclerosis (ALS), the decline in muscle strength is linear. However, this finding is misleading in that it does not accurately reflect the primary pathology, motor unit loss. There is now great interest in preventing motor unit loss early in the disease course, ideally before the development of symptomatic weakness. Motor unit number estimation (MUNE) provides a means of assessing the primary pathology of motor neuron disorders.

MUNE may also be useful in following clinically relevant processes secondary to a primary pathology. Charcot–Marie–Tooth disease type I (CMT1) is an autosomal dominant disorder involving duplication of the gene for peripheral myelin protein 22 and resultant demyelination. All patients with CMT1, regardless of the degree of weakness, have slowed nerve conduction velocity. Nerve conduction velocity does not correlate well with strength. It has been well demonstrated that strength in CMT1 patients shows higher correlations with measures of axon loss (Krajewski et al., 2000). MUNE is therefore a useful technique in the study of subjects with a primary demyelinating pathology that results in secondary axonal loss, leading to muscle weakness.

This chapter will review the relationship between MUNE and strength and highlight the role of MUNE in assessing the primary process of motor neuron disease, or the secondary axonal loss of CMT1.

Motor neuron disease

There is a growing body of data regarding the use of MUNE in subjects with ALS. In principle, MUNE holds great promise as a means of following motor unit loss, even prior to the development of clinically evident muscle weakness. Several groups have investigated the relationship between strength and MUNE in subjects with ALS. Bromberg et al., (1993). correlated biceps-brachialis MUNE using spike triggered averaging with elbow flexion strength among 31 subjects with ALS. There was not a significant relationship between MUNE and strength ($r = 0.37$). The poor correlation was thought to be secondary to the effects of collateral reinnervation. Armon et al. (1997) found a better

**Correspondence to*: A. Gordon Smith, Department of Neurology, University of Utah, 50 North Medical Drive, Room 3R152, Salt Lake City, UT 84132, USA. Tel.: 801-585-5884, Fax: 801-585-2054.
e-mail: Gordon.smith@hsc.utah.edu

doi: 10.1016/S1567-424X(03)00028-X

correlation between thenar, hypothenar, and toe extensor MUNE and grip or dorsiflexor strength using the manual incremental stimulation technique (correlation coefficients 0.55–067). Their subjects had lower MUNE values and were likely in a phase of the disease where reinnervation was failing.

Longitudinal studies provide further support for the concept that MUNE declines prior the development of muscle weakness because of the effects of collateral sprouting and reinnervation. Felice performed MUNE using multiple point stimulation and measured strength serially in 21 ALS subjects. MUNE declined prior muscle strength and was a more sensitive measure of disease progression (Felice, 1997). Yuen and Olney performed serial MUNE (statistical technique), strength measurements and fiber density in 10 subjects with ALS. As expected, MUNE declined at a greater rate than grip strength although there was a significant correlation between the two ($r = 0.55$, $P < 0.0015$). While fiber density was not correlated with strength ($r = 0.084$), it increased during the study. Furthermore, subjects with a more robust increase in fiber density had slower clinical progression (Yuen and Olney, 1997). While MUNE provides a good measure of the primary pathology of ALS, fiber density measures collateral reinnervation, the compensatory response to motor unit loss. This response explains the relatively poor correlation between MUNE and strength.

The relationship between MUNE and strength is dependent on the muscle group tested. Many investigators have used grip dynamometry to follow upper extremity muscle strength quantitatively. Multi-channel electromyography recordings during grip indicate both forearm and upper arm muscles contribute to grip strength (Bromberg and Larson, 1996). Most MUNE techniques utilize distal muscle groups (thenar or hypothenar). Future studies correlating strength and MUNE should measure strength and MUNE in the same group.

Charcot–Marie–Tooth disease

In contrast to motor neuron disorders, the primary process in CMT1 is considered to be peripheral nerve demyelination. This process, in and of itself, does not result in muscle weakness. In large CMT-1A pedigrees there can be marked variability of phenotypic expression of weakness, but all individuals have markedly slow conduction velocities (Kaku et al., 1993; Birouk et al., 1997). This observation supports the notion that muscle weakness is caused by axonal loss and denervation, not slow conduction velocity, and that the abnormalities of PMP-22 not only affect myelin structure and function but also affect the underlying axon.

There is little specific information on the distribution and degree of denervation because most reports on CMT phenotype focus on the electrodiagnostic measurement of conduction velocity (Birouk et al., 1997). More recently, Krajewski et al. performed MUNE of the thenar muscle group using the statistical method. MUNE was difficult to obtain in patients with severe weakness due to high nerve stimulation thresholds. Despite this technical difficulty, MUNE correlated with thumb abduction strength ($r = 0.51$, $P < 0.01$) but not with median nerve conduction velocity ($r = 0.08$) (Krajewski et al., 2000).

Because of the high stimulation threshold in patients with demyelinating CMT, our group has focused on the use of non-stimulation based techniques to perform MUNE in this patient population. In order to measure strength and MUNE in the same muscle group we have developed a manipulandum that measures strength of fifth finger abduction. The fifth digit is isolated and hand and forearm secured in order to minimize contribution from more proximal muscles. We have performed hypothenar and biceps bachii MUNE using spike triggered averaging in eight subjects with genetically confirmed CMT1A. Results were correlated with motor conduction velocity, hypothenar strength measured with the manipulandum, and grip dynamometry (Jamar).

As anticipated, there was a poor correlation between hypothenar MUNE and ulnar motor conduction velocity (correlation coefficient 0.2). There was a much stronger correlation between hypothenar strength and MUNE (correlation coefficient 0.65). The correlation between hypothenar MUNE and grip strength was less robust

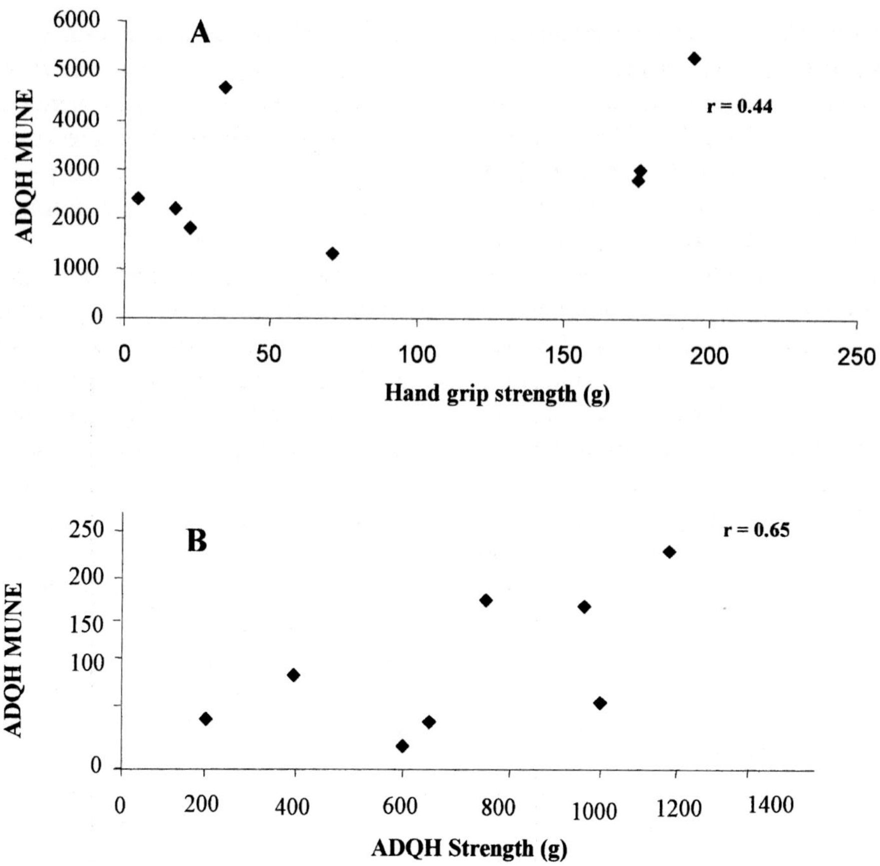

Fig. 1. Grip strength was poorly correlated with ADQH MUNE ($r = 0.44$) (A), while there was a stronger correlation with ADQH strength ($r = 0.65$) (B).

(correlation coefficient 0.45) (Fig. 1). There was a poor correlation between CMAP amplitude and strength, probably because of the effects of collateral reinnervation. The spike triggered averaging technique was well tolerated by all subjects. Our experience suggests stimulation based techniques are both technically challenging and more uncomfortable for CMT1 subjects.

During the collection of surface motor unit action potentials for calculation of MUNE, the waveform characteristics of the averaged intramuscular motor unit action potential were collected. Mean motor unit amplitude in the abductor digiti mini was significantly higher in subjects with CMT1A when compared to 10 control subjects of similar age and gender (1340 vs. 863 μV). This finding is consistent with the presence of ongoing collateral sprouting and reinnervation that compensates for axonal loss.

These results indicate that weakness in CMT1A is due to secondary axonal loss, not primary demyelination. As with motor neuron disease, however, the correlation between MUNE and strength is lessened by the effects of collateral sprouting and reinnervation. MUNE is therefore an appropriate means to follow progression of axonal loss and holds promise as an endpoint measure for treatment trials in hereditary peripheral neuropathy.

Conclusions

While muscle weakness is the primary cause of disability in motor neuron disease and CMT, muscle strength has many determinants that are independent of the disease process. Disuse, premorbid conditioning, nutrition and many other issues influence strength. MUNE is clearly related to strength in patients with progressive denervating conditions. However, MUNE actually provides a more representative measure of the pathophysiologic cause of weakness than strength measurements can provide. MUNE therefore provides a unique and valuable progression measure for use in therapeutic trials in denervating illness. Other progression measures are necessary to follow compensatory reinnervation however. Motor unit action potential amplitude and fiber density are appropriate measures of reinnervation. Compound muscle action potential amplitude and strength measures provide a composite measure of the severity motor unit or axon loss and the success of collateral sprouting and reinnervation.

References

Armon, C., Brandstater, M. and Peterson, G. Motor unit number estimates and quantitative muscle strength measurements of distal muscles in patients with amyotrophic lateral sclerosis. *Muscle and Nerve*, 1997, 20: 449–501.

Birouk, N., Gouider, R., Le Guren, E., Gugenheim, M., Tardieu, S. and Maisonobe, T. Charcot–Marie–Tooth disease type 1A with 17p11.2 duplication: clinical and electrophysiological phenotype study and factors influencing disease severity in 119 cases. *Brain*, 1997, 120: 813–823.

Bromberg, M., Forshew, D., Nau, K., Bromberg, J., Simmons, Z. and Fries, T. Motor unit number estimation isometric strength and electromyographic measures in amyotrophic lateral sclerosis. *Muscle and Nerve*, 1993, 16: 1213–1219.

Bromberg, M. and Larson, W. Relationships between motor unit number estimates and isometric strength in distal muscles in ALS/MND. *J. Neurolog. Sci.*, 1996, 139 (Suppl.): 38–42.

Felice, K. A longitudinal study comparing thenar motor unit number estimates to other quantitative tests in patients with amyotrophic lateral sclerosis. *Muscle and Nerve*, 1997, 20: 179–185.

Kaku, D., Parry, G., Malamut, R., Lupski, J. and Garcia, C. Nerve conduction studies in Charcot-Marie Tooth polyneuropathy associated with a segmental duplication of chromosome 17. *Neurology*, 1993, 43: 1806–1808.

Krajewski, K., Lewis, R., Fuerst, D., Turansky, C., Hinderer, S., Garbern, J., Kamholz, J. and Shy, M. Neurological dysfunction and axonal degeneration in Charcot-Marie-Tooth disease type 1A. *Brain*, 2000, 123: 1516–1527.

Yuen, E. and Olney, R. Longitudinal study of fiber density and motor unit number estimate in patients with amyotrophic lateral sclerosis. *Neurology*, 1997, 49: 573–578.

Discussion after Section VII

Mark Bromberg, Salt Lake City, Utah

Let me ask a question of Ming about the motor unit that later in its lifetime could not keep up with the discharge rate, do you think that was due to central or peripheral failure?

Ming Chan, Edmonton, Alberta

I can only speculate. It is possible that it could be due to a reduction of central descending motor drive to the motor unit. On the other hand, it is also possible that the membrane physiological characteristics in the anterior horn cell could have changed, leading to reduced excitability of the alpha motor neuron itself. In support of the latter, the persistence of the alpha motor neuron response declined markedly over the 2-year period.

Richard Olney, San Francisco, California

We have tracked two or three final surviving motor units in people with the statistical technique. We were still able to electrically stimulate the nerve to activate them every three months for 6–9 months, but often the patients could not recruit the motor units voluntarily. This supports a central failure.

Timothy Doherty, London, Ontario

I have a question for François. In your experience with the AMPS technique, as you follow patients with depleting motor unit pools, did you find it progressively more difficult to isolate individual motor unit potentials, suggesting that there may be problems with either distal branching or decrement in individual potentials?

François Wang, Liége, Belgium

No, it was not more difficult when the motor unit numbers were very low.

Richard Olney, San Francisco, California

I have a question for Robin or Mike. I think that Robin's data showed non-linearity in that units got bigger when more units were activate, and I think that Mike's data from yesterday showed just the opposite effect. I wonder if you or anyone who understands non-linearity well enough can comment on what is going on or how do we explain this difference?

Michael Slawnych, Calgary, Alberta

I can comment on the work I presented yesterday. I presented a simple model system made up as a series of parallel motor units, in which the contribution of a motor unit decreases as the number of active motor units increases. There is not a wealth of data to support this model, and I presented the only data I was able to find by two different groups. One set of data was by Parry and colleagues (*J. Neurol. Sci.* 1977, 33: 283–296), and they looked at motor units under conditions when very few motor units were active and under conditions when many motor units were active. They showed how the contribution of a motor unit decreases by approximately 20–25%. The other group showed a decrease as well, but much smaller, on the order of about 6%.

Robin Conwit, Baltimore, Maryland

We were looking at the average size of motor unit potentials and not the relative contribution of each one. The larger-size units may have affected the average to a greater extent, and that may explain the discrepancy.

Jack Petajan, Salt Lake City, Utah

How did you identify which active units to study at various levels of contraction?

Robin Conwit, Baltimore, Maryland

At first we had hoped to track the same units and follow them at different levels of contraction, but we found it exceedingly difficult, even when we tried using wire electrodes that were left in place. We just looked at representative samples and chose 15–20 surface motor unit potentials at each force level that had the correct size, shape, and seemed to have a firing rate histogram that was physiologic.

Jack Petajan, Salt Lake City, Utah

I have a question for Ming Chan related to the type of exercise when you were "training" the motor units. In a small muscle might the training actually be damaging?

Ming Chan, Edmonton, Alberta

I think it is a mis-advertisement to use the word "training" because high-frequency repetitive stimulation is a highly artificial way of activating those motor units. Those units probably do not fire in that kind of vigorous pattern. We actually counted the number of impulses, 24,000 a day. All of them recovered to their baseline value within 5 weeks after the training program ended, so the changes I showed during training were reversible. We characterized the tetanic tension of these motor units and picked a stimulation frequency that produced a 50% maximum tetanic tension, and that worked out to be between 30 and 40 Hz.

Jasper Daube, Rochester, Minnesota

Two questions. The first based on the question to François regarding decrement with unstable motor units. In the multiple point stimulation technique applied to ALS patients who have unstable motor units, there may be difficulty in identifying single motor unit potentials because they may decrement immediately. Do you find that a difficulty?

Timothy Doherty, London, Ontario

I have found it difficult at times. However, with the multiple point stimulation technique, it can be recognized easily and lessened by reducing the stimulation frequency.

Clifton Gooch, New York, New York

A few comments. I think that decrement occurs in a subpopulation of motor units in ALS, and it may or may not correlate with decrement observed in the CMAP. In my experience, I tend to reject those motor units for analysis or for tracking because it can sometimes be difficult to be certain that they are a single motor unit or whether they represent alternation or recruitment of a second smaller unit.

Jasper Daube, Rochester, Minnesota

The other question is whether there are differences between the spike triggered averaging and the decomposition techniques. Would you expect the same results from the two techniques?

Timothy Doherty, London, Ontario

No direct comparisons have been made between single motor unit spike triggered averaging and multiple unit spike triggered averaging by decomposition. In the decomposition technique, higher threshold motor units and larger amplitude motor units are collected, and this may have an effect.

Section VIII

MUNE in Clinical Practice

Motor Unit Number Estimation (Supplements to Clinical Neurophysiology Vol. 55)
Editor: M.B. Bromberg

Chapter 29

MUNE in the electrodiagnostic clinic

Adrian R.M. Upton and Alan J. McComas*

Department of Medicine (Neurology), McMaster University, Hamilton, ON L8N 3Z5, Canada

Introduction

After motor unit number estimation (MUNE) had been devised (McComas et al., 1971), it was applied as a research tool to different groups of patients with neuromuscular disorders and to control subjects of varying ages. At the same time it was a natural step to see whether the new methodology might have a place in the electrodiagnostic laboratory. Accordingly, we began to apply MUNE routinely to patients with a variety of neurological problems, the only exclusion being those patients with cranial nerve symptoms. By a conservative estimate we, and our trained EMG technologists, have performed more than 20,000 MUNEs on our patients in the electrodiagnostic laboratory since 1971. Only a small fraction of these data has been published, and then mostly that concerning some of the more obvious neuropathic conditions – amyotrophic lateral sclerosis (ALS), spinal muscular atrophy (SMA), and old poliomyelitis – all of which are represented in these Proceedings. For logistic reasons it is not possible to provide a statistical summary of our combined experience with all the other disorders, but the ensuing commentary gives a qualitative account of our findings, together with the protocols which we have followed consistently over the past 30 years.

Methods

All the MUNEs were performed by gradually increasing the stimulus intensity to the motor nerve and analysing the resulting incremental muscle responses. The mean size of the incremental responses were then divided into the maximal response of the same muscle or muscle group, so as to yield the estimated number of units. The great majority of MUNEs were performed manually (McComas et al., 1971) but there was a 2-year period when extensive and successful use was made of the automated incremental method, also developed in our laboratory (Galea et al., 1991). The advantages of the automated method are that it eliminates observer bias, both in the application of stimuli of different intensities and in the recognition of "alternation". Because of the latter capability, the MUNEs obtained automatically tend to be about one-third lower than those derived manually. Unfortunately, and despite its success, the automated system is no longer available on a commercial EMG machine, but there is no reason why individual EMG laboratories, with the necessary resources, should not create their own versions. The manual method, in contrast, can be performed on any EMG machine, even one with a single trace and no storage, and, in experienced hands, is

**Correspondence to*: Dr. Alan J. McComas, Division of Neurology (4U1), McMaster University Medical Centre, 1200 Main Street West, Hamilton, ON L8N 3Z5, Canada. Tel.: (905) 525-9140x22519, Fax: (905) 521-2656. e-mail: mccomas@fhs.mcmaster.ca

doi: 10.1016/S1567-424X(03)00029-1

considerably faster. One important requirement of the manual method is that, because of the subjective component (see above), each electromyographer should compile his or her own set of control data.

It is natural to apply MUNE immediately before or after a motor nerve conduction study, since the same stimulating and recording electrodes can be used. If MUNE is performed first, there is the advantage that the amplitude of the maximal response need not be known until the response increments have been measured. In this way any subconscious bias in the recognition of increments can be avoided. For example, if it was already known that the maximum M-wave was small, there could be an expectation that the MUNE would be reduced, indicating the presence of denervation. However, the putative motor unit potential increments would also be diminished if the subcutaneous tissue overlying a perfectly normal muscle was thickened. If the increments are determined first, such subjective biases are avoided. Once started, a manual MUNE should take no more than 3–5 min to complete.

In relation to the recording electrodes, we now use self-adhesive EKG ones; these are cut in half, with the active electrode being placed over the innervation zone of the muscle whenever possible. The bandwidth of the amplifier system should be set to 0.1 Hz–1 kHz to ensure an optimal signal-to-noise ratio. The muscles that can be used for MUNE, and the electrode placements employed in each case, are shown in Fig. 1. In a patient presenting with neck or arm symptoms, the thenar and hypothenar muscles would be investigated routinely, with the option of including the biceps as well. Similarly, in patients with low back or leg symptoms, the extensor digitorum brevis (EDB) and plantar muscles would always be examined, and sometimes the medial vastus and soleus also. In a patient in whom a generalized process is suspected, the examination would include MUNEs in an arm and a leg, the thenar and EDB muscles usually being those selected.

Table 1 gives the lower limits of the respective normal ranges for MUNEs performed manually in our laboratory. Since the distributions of MUNEs are highly skewed in populations of control subjects, the lower limits are derived from the scatter of values rather than the standard deviations. In view of the motor unit attrition which takes place as part of the normal aging process, particularly in the thenar and EDB muscles, the lower limit is

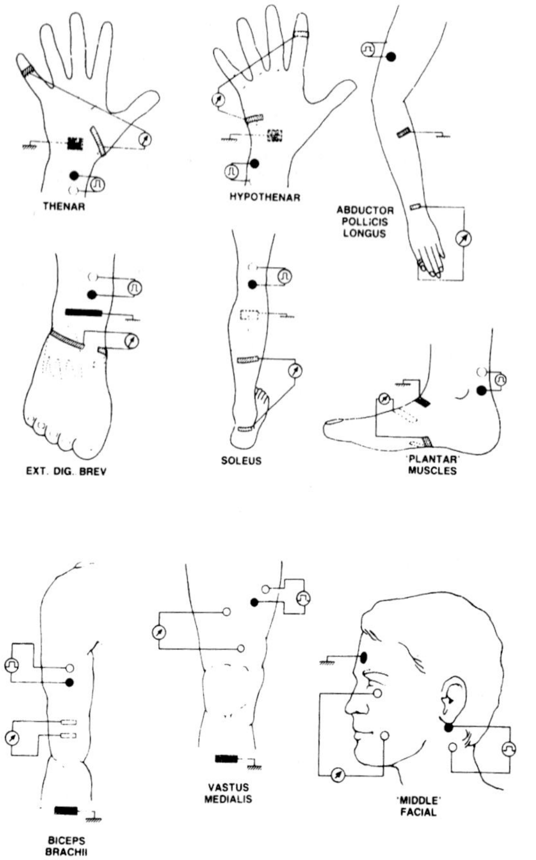

Fig. 1. Different muscles used for incremental MUNE, showing placement of stimulating and recording electrodes. Reproduced with permission from McComas (1991).

TABLE 1

LOWER LIMITS OF MUNE FOR UPPER AND LOWER LIMB MUSCLES, EMPLOYED IN OUR LABORATORY FOR MANUAL INCREMENTAL METHOD

Muscle group	Lower limit of MUNE
Thenar group (median n.)	220
Hypothenar group	250
Biceps brachii	55
EDB	120
Plantar group	250
Vastus medialis	80

relaxed above the age of 60 years. As a rough guide, the lower limits are halved by 70 years and halved again by 80 years.

Results

Generalized neuropathies

The first published reports of MUNEs in generalized peripheral neuropathies were those of Ballantyne and Hansen, who investigated patients with uremic, alcoholic and diabetic types (Hansen and Ballantyne, 1977, 1978; Ballantyne et al., 1980). Our experience is that the sensory nerve fibers are usually affected sooner and more severely than the motor fibers, and this is certainly true for diabetic neuropathy, as Fig. 2 clearly shows. In this figure, the thenar and hypothenar MUNEs have been compared with the aggregate amplitudes of the sensory nerve responses in the same hands. When motor fibers are affected in a generalized neuropathy, the EDB is the first muscle to show a reduced MUNE, followed by the thenar group. In hereditary and vincristine-induced peripheral neuropathies, it is our impression that the vulnerabilities of the sensory and motor fibers are usually rather similar. Even if it is already clear from the sensory

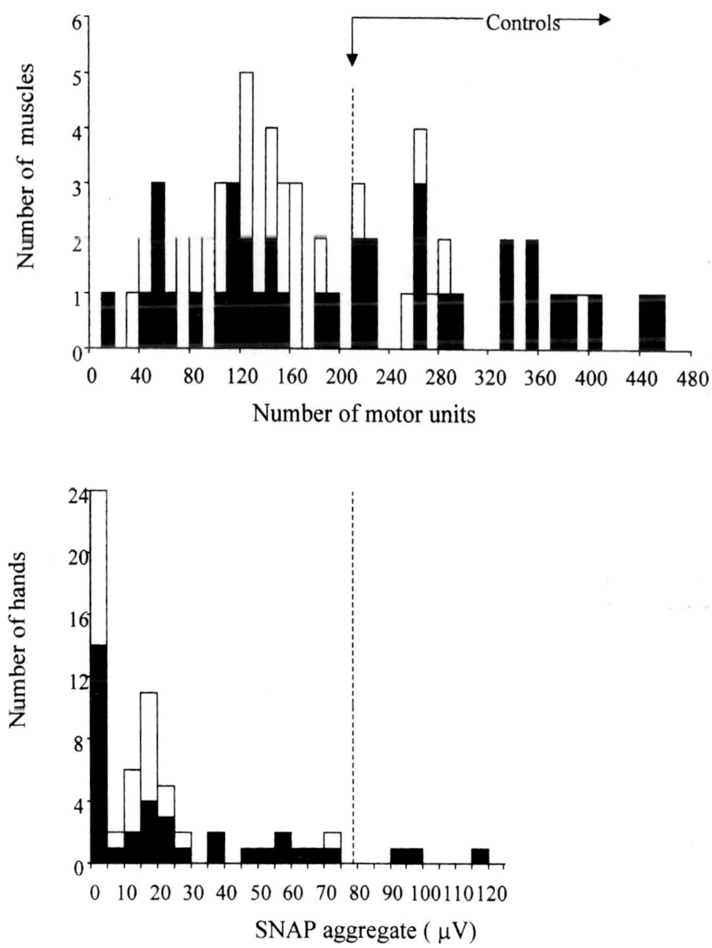

Fig. 2. *Top.* Thenar and hypothenar MUNEs in 67 patients with diabetes mellitus. *Bottom.* The aggregates of the sensory response amplitudes recorded orthodromically from the same hands. The interrupted vertical lines show the lower limits of the control ranges. The filled and open columns represent values in patients below and above the age of 60 years, respectively. Comparison of the two histograms shows that neuropathic involvement is much greater in sensory fibers than in motor ones. Reproduced with permission from McComas (1998).

examination that a generalized peripheral neuropathy is present, MUNE is still of value in documenting the degree of involvement of the motor fibers. In the demyelinating form of Guillain–Barré syndrome, the evoked motor unit responses are dispersed and do not summate linearly in the maximal M-wave, so that MUNE is more difficult to perform. Although the estimate will be less accurate than in other conditions, it is still worthwhile attempting MUNE, in order to gain some idea of the extent of motor fiber involvement.

Regardless of the etiology of the neuropathy, serial MUNEs can be used to follow the progress of the condition. Figure 3 shows the marked loss of functioning motor units in a patient receiving vincristine for a seminoma, and the slow recovery of innervation which occurred after this treatment had been discontinued. In the case of the thenar muscles, the recovery was complete, but this was not true of the EDB.

Localized neuropathies

In most cases of *carpal tunnel syndrome*, MUNE is the last EMG parameter to be affected. In our experience, the earliest abnormality is slowing of sensory nerve conduction, followed by diminution of the sensory nerve responses, and then prolongation of the median nerve terminal motor latency. It is likely that the differential susceptibility of the motor and sensory axons is related to the positions of the respective fascicles in the median nerve trunk under the flexor retinaculum. We always perform a hypothenar MUNE in the same hand, in case an *ulnar neuropathy* is also present. Conversely, when an ulnar neuropathy is the primary diagnosis, a thenar MUNE is carried out as part of the assessment of median nerve function. In the leg, the EDB estimate is usually reduced in a *peroneal neuropathy* at the neck of the fibula. Sometimes, however, the lesion causing weakness of ankle dorsiflexion is situated proximally in the sciatic nerve, and this possibility, or multiple root lesions (see below), should always be considered if the plantar MUNE is also reduced.

Although we do not often carry out MUNE on radial-innervated muscles, it is a useful examination in cases of *radial nerve injury*. A MUNE, performed in exactly the same way but on the non-affected limb, is probably a better reference than reliance on published radial MUNE values. We have not employed MUNE for *facial nerve*

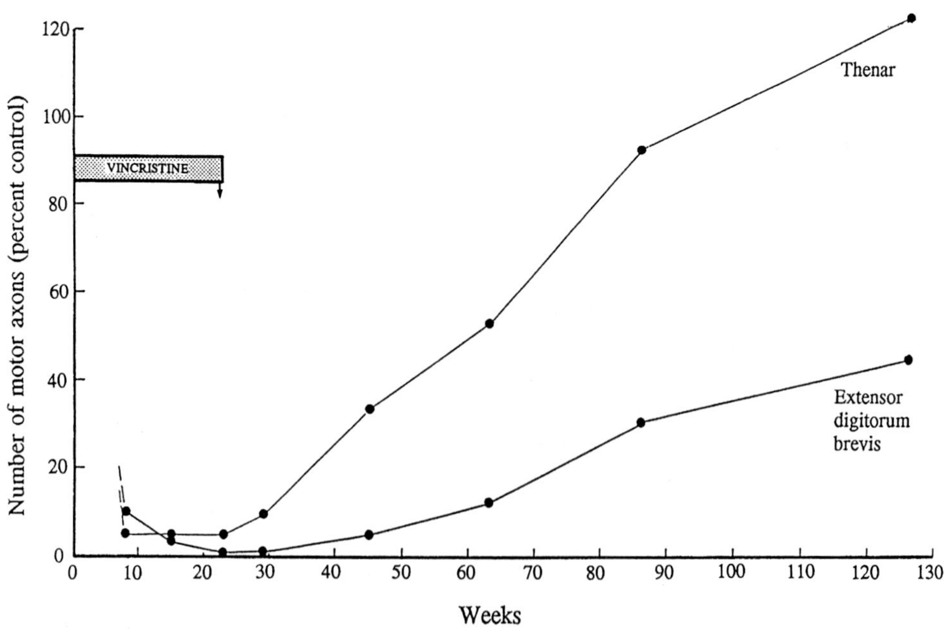

Fig. 3. Serial MUNEs of thenar and EDB muscles in a patient treated with vincristine for a malignancy. Recovery was complete in the thenar muscles but not in EDB.

lesions. However, the method has been used to good effect by Delbeke (1982) in an evaluation of surgical cross-innervation.

Plexopathies and radiculopathies

In brachial plexopathies, we add the biceps to the thenar and hypothenar muscles for MUNE. In *obstetric brachial plexopathies*, MUNE enables an objective assessment of the obstetric damage to be made early on, and the examination is especially useful since needle studies are limited by the inability of the infant to perform voluntary contractions at the electromyographer's request. In late cases MUNE will sometimes show that adequate reinnervation has occurred in a limb which is poorly used. The persisting disability is presumably due to an apraxia, incurred when the infant was unable to develop motor programs at a critical stage in development (see Galea et al., this volume).

In our laboratory *thoracic outlet syndrome* is infrequently diagnosed, since we insist on the presence of reduced MUNEs for both the thenar and hypothenar muscle groups, as well as the demonstration of diminished sensory nerve responses in the ring and little fingers. Most commonly in such referrals, the thenar MUNE is reduced, while the hypothenar MUNE is normal. This discrepancy would be inconsistent with a lesion affecting the lower cord of the brachial plexus, but it would be compatible with a C8 radiculopathy and this is the diagnosis usually favored. In *lumbar plexopathies* from any cause, it is desirable to include the medial vastus as one of the tests, and to compare the result with that on the supposedly normal side.

In *chronic cervical radiculopathies*, which are notoriously difficult to diagnose by conventional EMG, MUNE may be especially valuable. This is because, in a controlled examination of distal muscles in patients with clinical evidence of neuropathic conditions, MUNE was much superior to the needle examination, even with automatic analysis, in detecting denervation (McComas and Sica, 1978; Fig. 4, *left*). The sensory nerve responses are also of great value, in that they can help to distinguish between pre- and post-ganglionic lesions. Because nerve root lesions tend to have unequal effects on the thenar and hypothenar muscles, we have come to regard the median-innervated thenar muscles as being supplied mainly by the C8 root and the hypothenar muscles by T1 (Fig. 5). An example of this differentiation is shown in Fig. 4 (*right*), which shows the first few of the considerably enlarged increments in a thenar MUNE. The patient, a young woman, had slipped on ice, falling on her back, with her legs "going up in the air". Subsequently, she developed persisting pain in her neck, which radiated down her right arm and was associated with numbness and tingling in the ring and little fingers. Although the thenar MUNE was severely reduced, the hypothenar MUNE was normal, presumably because the root innervations

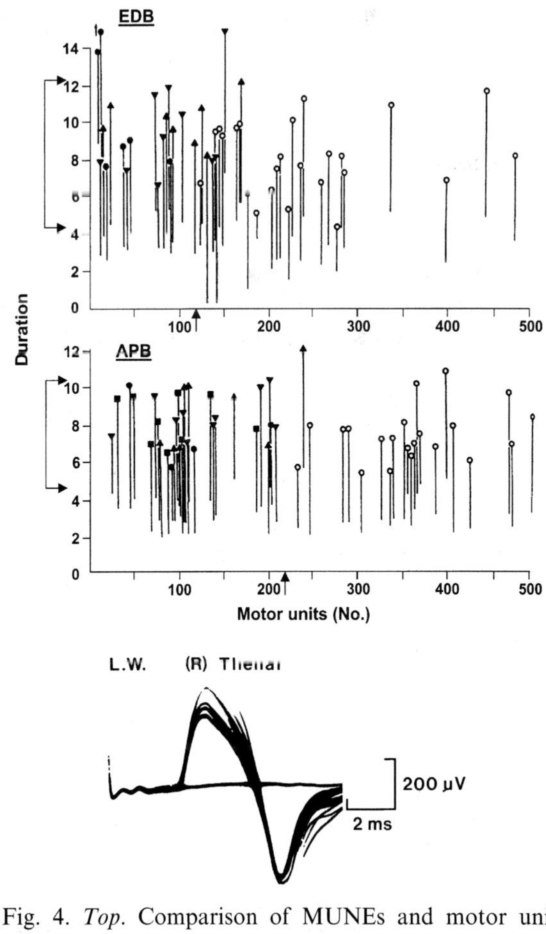

Fig. 4. *Top*. Comparison of MUNEs and motor unit potential durations, recorded with a needle electrode and analyzed automatically by the ANOPS system. Reproduced with permission from McComas and Sica (1978). *Bottom*. The first few thenar MUNE increments in a patient with a recent C8 root lesion; see text.

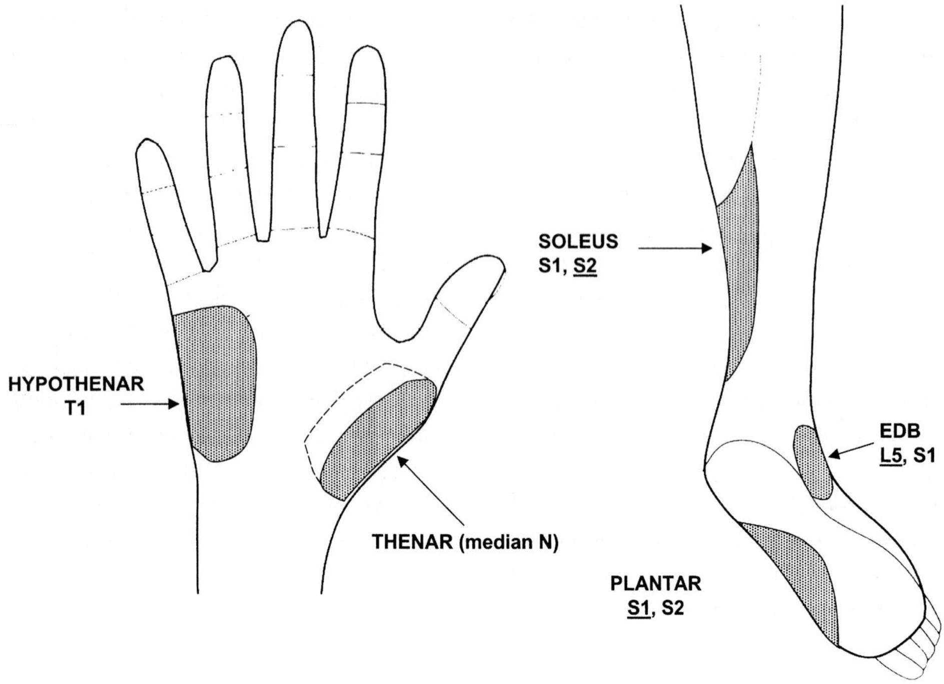

Fig. 5. Probable nerve root innervations, as determined by MUNE, in thenar and hypothenar muscles (*left*) and in EDB and plantar muscles (*right*).

were mainly C8 and T1, respectively. The EMG findings in *monomelic muscle atrophy* may also be consistent with this interpretation of the root innervation of the hand. Thus, we have seen a 16-year-old boy with obvious wasting and weakness of the thenar muscles of one hand, for which no peripheral cause could be found. Whereas the thenar MUNE was severely reduced, the hypothenar value, like all the sensory nerve responses, was well within the normal range (Miller et al., 1999).

A third case is typical of many who are referred because of neck or arm symptoms. The patient, a 51-year-old man, complained bitterly of pain in his neck radiating into his arm, present for several months, and associated with numbness of his thumb. Both the thenar and biceps MUNEs were considerably reduced (93 and 29, respectively, lower limits 220 and 55), while the hypothenar value was borderline (251). These reductions indicated damage at the C6 (biceps) and C8 (thenar) levels and, since the sensory nerve responses were diminished in the thumb and all the fingers, the lesions must have been situated at, or distal to, the respective intervertebral foramina. In this patient the monopolar needle examination happened to be abnormal as well, confirming the presence of denervation in the C6 and C8 myotomes, and in C7 also.

We have found the C8 root to be especially susceptible to *whiplash injuries* and we attribute this to stretch as the C7 vertebra is flexed backwards on T1. In contrast, the T1 root is protected since the T1 and T2 vertebrae, between which it emerges, are braced by the rib cage. In *chronic lumbosacral radiculopathies* it is similarly possible to use MUNE to determine the level of nerve root involvement. Since the EDB and the plantar muscle MUNEs are often affected unequally, it is highly likely that their root innervations differ. Thus the L5 root appears to predominate in the innervation of the EDB muscle while the plantar muscles receive most of their nerve supply from S1 (Fig. 5). The situation is not always clear, however, possibly because of overlap and perhaps also because of pre- and post-fixation of the spinal cord. To complicate matters further, there is sometimes differential involvement of soleus and the plantar muscles, as reflected in their respective MUNEs; this situation would not be expected to occur if both muscles were supplied mainly by S1, as the text books state. There is an obvious need for systematic observations on the distribution of muscle twitches, when nerve roots are stimulated in the operating theatre, to resolve these and other uncertainties.

Motoneuronopathies

The muscles to be examined by MUNE depend on the etiology of the disorder and on the anatomical distribution of the clinical abnormalities. At the very least, we will study both an upper limb muscle, usually the thenar group, and a lower limb muscle, most commonly EDB, for patients suspected of having ALS or SMA. If a limb is clearly affected, as revealed by the initial MUNE, we will often add a second muscle or group for MUNE (e.g. hypothenar muscles or biceps for the arm, and plantar muscles for the leg). Our findings in different types of motoneuronopathy are described elsewhere in these Proceedings (see Turnbull et al., this volume; Fehlings et al., this volume).

Survey of MUNEs in the EMG clinic

Differences in the types of patient referred for EMG, from one clinic to another, are to be expected. Table 2 has been included to show the referring or final diagnoses, and the incidences of normal and abnormal MUNEs, using the automated incremental system (Galea et al., 1991) in 225 consecutive patients during a 2-year period at one of the McMaster University clinics. As might have been expected, the highest incidence of abnormal MUNEs, 68%, was found in patients with ALS and SMA, while approximately half of the estimates were abnormal in patients with generalized peripheral neuropathies. A high incidence of abnormality was also found in patients with low back pain and/or sciatica, but the value for those patients with neck pain or a history of motor vehicle accidents is surprisingly low. However, this is rather misleading for, in a typical case, the thenar MUNE might be reduced on the side of symptoms, while both the ipsilateral hypothenar MUNE and the contralateral thenar MUNE might be normal. Thus, even with two of the three MUNEs being normal, a diagnosis of a unilateral C8 lesion could still be reached.

TABLE 2

INCIDENCE OF NORMAL AND ABNORMAL MUNES IN 225 CONSECUTIVE PATIENTS EXAMINED WITH THE AUTOMATED INCREMENTAL METHOD OVER A 2-YEAR PERIOD[a]

Disorder[b]	Abnormal MUNEs	Normal MUNEs	% Abnormal MUNEs
'None' (fatigability, cramps, affected relatives, etc.)	0	85	0
Neck symptoms	6	48	11
Low back pain, sciatica	21	30	41
Carpal tunnel syndrome	15	48	24
Other focal neuropathies	10	14	42
Generalized neuropathy	19	17	53
Brachial plexopathy	20	23	47
Motor vehicle accidents	2	26	7
Previous polio	7	8	47
ALS, SMA	23	11	68
Muscular dystrophy, myasthenia, collagen disease	2	15	12
CNS, other	2	15	12
Overall	127	340	27

[a] Reproduced with permission from McComas (1998).
[b] ALS, amyotrophic lateral sclerosis; SMA, spinal muscular atrophy; CNS, central nervous system.

Similarly, a patient found to have a carpal tunnel entrapment on one side, would also have a hypothenar MUNE carried out on the same side, in case of an associated ulnar neuropathy. Many patients, of course, are normal altogether, and this conclusion is as important as one of a neuromuscular disorder.

Conclusions

More than 20,000 MUNEs have been performed in the diagnostic EMG clinic over a 30-year period. Most of the estimates were on the intrinsic muscles of the hand and foot. The test has proved of value, not only in detecting muscle denervation and helping in the formation of a neuromuscular diagnosis, but also in the exclusion of abnormality. The highest incidences of abnormal MUNEs were found in patients with motoneuronopathies, generalized peripheral neuropathies, and lumbosacral root lesions.

Acknowledgements

We are grateful for Jane Butler's help in preparing this manuscript, and to Hillary Libbrecht, Heidi Scarfone and Henny Spoelstra for performing many of the MUNEs. Rebecca Newberry kindly prepared the figures.

References

Ballantyne, J.P., Hansen, S., Weir, A., Whitehead, J.R. and Mullin, P.J. Quantitative electrophysiological study of alcoholic neuropathy. *J. Neurol. Neurosurg. Psychiatry*, 1980, 43: 427–432.

Delbeke, J. Electrophysiological evaluation of cross-face nerve graft in a treatment of facial palsy. *Acta Neurochirur.*, 1982, 65: 111–127.

Galea, V., DeBruin, H., Cavasin, R. and McComas, A.J. The numbers and relative sizes of motor units estimated by computer. *Muscle Nerve*, 1991, 14: 1123–1130.

Hansen, S. and Ballantyne, J.P. Axonal dysfunction in the neuropathy of diabetes mellitus: a quantitative electrophysiological study. *J. Neurol. Neurosurg. Psychiatry*, 1977, 40: 555–564.

Hansen, S. and Ballantyne, J.P. A quantitative electrophysiological study of uraemic neuropathy. Diabetic and renal neuropathies compared. *J. Neurol. Neurosurg. Psychiatry*, 1978, 41: 128–134.

McComas, A.J. Invited review: motor unit estimation: methods, results, and present status. *Muscle Nerve*, 1991, 14: 585–597.

McComas, A.J. Motor units: how many, how large, what kind? *J. Electromyogr. Kinesiol.*, 1998, 8: 391–402.

McComas, A.J. and Sica, R.E.P. Automatic quantitative analysis of the electromyogram in partially denervated distal muscles: comparison with motor unit counting. *Canad. J. Neurol. Sci.*, 1978, 5: 377–383.

McComas, A.J., Fawcett, P.R.W., Campbell, M.J. and Sica, R.E.P. Electrophysiological estimation of the number of motor units within a human muscle. *J. Neurol. Neurosurg. Psychiatry*, 1971, 34: 121–131.

Miller, T., Roth, J. and McComas, A.J. Monomelic amyotrophy presenting as isolated thenar wasting after a fall. Abstract: 34th Meeting of the Canadian Congress of Neurological Sciences, 1999.

Motor Unit Number Estimation (Supplements to Clinical Neurophysiology Vol. 55)
Editor: M.B. Bromberg

Chapter 30

MUNE in clinical EMG practice

Benn E. Smith*

Department of Neurology, Mayo Clinic, Scottsdale, AZ 85259, USA

Introduction

While motor unit number estimation (MUNE) has been an important research tool in the study of anterior horn cell physiology, less information is available regarding the use of these techniques in day to day clinical EMG practice. What might be the applications for using MUNE on a non-research clinical basis? The two main groups of patients where MUNE have proven useful are: (1) disorders involving lower motor neurons (including amyotrophic lateral sclerosis, spinal muscular atrophy, monomelic amyotrophy, and others); and (2) benign conditions in which the patient or the referring provider mistakenly suspects a lower motor neuron disorder (isolated fasciculations, fatigue, cramps, age-related muscle atrophy, and others).

In a busy clinical neurophysiology laboratory, excluding subjects studied as part of research trials or those examined for normal control data, 87 MUNE studies were performed over 5 years for clinical reasons alone (Smith, unpublished observations). In patients with spinal muscular atrophy MUNE studies were abnormal in 28/32 (88%) of muscles examined, whereas in definite or probable ALS cases the rate of abnormality was 14/23 (61%). In individuals mistakenly suspected by the patient or the referring physician of having a neurogenic disorder, 0/18 (0%) had abnormal MUNE results.

MUNE in anterior horn cell disorders

In the case of disorders involving the anterior horn cell, MUNE can help to identify involved (and sometimes asymptomatic) spinal segments, thereby allowing a diagnosis of laboratory supported probable ALS (Brooks et al., 2000) for the purpose of inclusion in clinical trials or for diagnosis for justification of prescription of durable medical equipment (Corr et al., 1998). Although concentric needle electromyography is an extraordinarily sensitive method for detecting active denervation, in muscles where reinnervation has kept pace with denervation, there may be little or no active fibrillation potentials despite a significant loss of anterior horn cell numbers.

As to practical considerations in using MUNE for patients suspected of having involvement of anterior horn cells, a number of lessons have been gleaned over the years. (1) It is best to select muscles with normal compound muscle action potential (CMAP) amplitudes. From a previous longitudinal MUNE study of a large number of patients with ALS (Smith et al., 1995) it is apparent that all patients with a low CMAP amplitude will likewise have an abnormally low MUNE value for that muscle. (2) The same study (Smith et al., 1995)

**Correspondence to*: Dr. Benn E. Smith, Mayo Clinic Scottsdale, 13400 East Shea Blvd, Scottsdale, AZ 85259, USA. Tel.: 602-301-7989, Fax: 602-301-8451.
e-mail: Gordon.Smith@hsc.utah.edu

doi: 10.1016/S1567-424X(03)00030-8

demonstrated that the posterior tibial/abductor hallucis muscle remains normal from the MUNE standpoint until relatively late in the course of disease, making it somewhat insensitive as a muscle to establish the presence of lower motor neuron involvement in the lumbosacral segment. The fibular/extensor digitorum brevis muscle is involved at a much earlier time in the disease course of ALS and therefore would be a better choice for detecting early denervation in the lumbosacral territory. (3) Because of the technical demands of performing MUNE, it is best to avoid limbs with marked spasticity, fasciculations, and/or tremor. Any of these alone or in combination can render MUNE data difficult to obtain or of insufficient quality to be useful in making clinical judgements. (4) If MUNE is being used to follow motor unit counts in a particular muscle over time it is important to pay close attention to recording electrode placement so as to maximize reproducibility and reliability of serial measurements. (5) Once the number of motor units falls below 10–20, it is best to transition to manual MUNE, as the statistical method offers the advantage of estimating large numbers while the manual method allows direct assessment of amplitude increments with small numbers of motor unlts (Daube, 1995).

TABLE 1

MUNE STUDIES IN CLINICAL EMG PRACTICE 1997–2001

Diagnosis	MUNE abnormal	MUNE normal
SMA	28/32	4/32
ALS definite or probable	14/23	9/23
ALS possible	2/4	2/4
Normal	0/18	18/18
Focal neurogenic	2/2	0/2
Myopathy	0/1	1/1
Uncertain	2/7	5/7
Total	48/87 (55%)	39/87 (45%)

MUNE in benign conditions

It is a relatively common occurrence for individuals with professional or personal acquaintance with motor neuron disease to suspect that common benign symptoms, such as exercise-induced fasciculation or cramps, in themselves or others might be due to motor neuron disease. These people are often physicians, other healthcare providers, former competitive athletes, or relatives of patients with proven anterior horn cell disease. One reasonable approach to this clinical situation is to perform a thorough history, neurological examination, nerve conduction studies, and concentric needle examination, and when these are all found to be normal, to consider MUNE so as to "leave no stone unturned". Our experience mirrors that of Windebank in studying patients with isolated fasciculations in that to date none have gone on to have anterior horn cell disease (Blexrud et al., 1993). Once detailed clinical and electrodiagnostic studies (including MUNE) have been found to be normal, the worried individual can be reassured that there is no evidence that a life-threatening neuromuscular disorder is present. When an isolated MUNE abnormality is found in such individuals, it is advised to seek an alternative explanation for this finding, such as an old neurogenic process as previous trauma. If no such explanation can be uncovered, longitudinal assessment should be recommended, perhaps every 4–6 months. In the current series (see Table 1) of 20 patients referred for possible neurogenic disease because of fasciculations, fatigue, or muscle cramps in the face of a normal neurologic examination, 18 were normal and two were found to have an old mononeuropathy or radiculopathy. No patient in this group had an unexplained low MUNE.

References

Blexrud, M.D., Windebank, A.J. and Daube, J.R. Long-term follow-up of 121 patients with benign fasciculations. *Ann. Neurol.*, 1993, 34(4): 622–625.

Brooks B.R., Miller R.G., Swash M and Munsat T.L. World Federation of Neurology Research Group on Motor Neuron Diseases. El Escorial revisited: revised criteria for the diagnosis of amyotrophic lateral sclerosis. *Amyotrophic Lateral Sclerosis & Other Motor Neuron Disorders*, 2000, 1(5): 293–299.

Corr, B., Frost, E., Traynor, B.J. and Hardiman, O. Service provision for patients with ALS/MND: a cost-effective multidisciplinary approach. *J. Neurol. Sci.*, 1998, 160 (Suppl. 1): S141–S145.

Daube, J.R. Estimating the number of motor units in a muscle. *Journal of Clinical Neurophysiology*, 1995, 12: 585–594.

Smith, B.E. Unpublished observations.

Smith B.E., Stevens, J.C., Litchy W.J., Daube J.R., Olney R.K., Bromberg M.B. and Yuen E.C. Longitudinal electrodiagnostic strategies in amyotrophic lateral sclerosis patients treated with recombinant human ciliary neurotrophic factor. American Academy of Neurology, 1995.

Section IX

MUNE in Clinical Trials

Motor Unit Number Estimation (Supplements to Clinical Neurophysiology Vol. 55)
Editor: M.B. Bromberg

Chapter 31

The use of statistical MUNE in ALS to predict prognosis

Richard K. Olney*

Department of Neurology, University of California, San Francisco, CA 94143-0114, USA

Introduction

Experience with the statistical motor unit number estimation (MUNE) technique in amyotrophic lateral sclerosis (ALS) has increased since 1993 though its usage as a secondary endpoint measure at a number of participating centers in multicenter randomized controlled treatment trials of ciliary neurotrophic factor (CNTF) and brain-derived neurotrophic factor (BDNF). Neither CNTF nor BDNF showed a significant effect on the course of ALS by the primary endpoints nor showed a detectable effect on rates of decline of MUNE values (ALS CNTF Treatment Study Group, 1996; BDNF Study Group, 1999). However, the lack of detectable effect on MUNE rates of decline may have been influenced by the relatively small number of patients studied and the fact that many patients had initial low MUNE values preventing the detection of a meaningful change. Furthermore, patients frequently experience an initial rapid loss of motor units followed by stability of the remaining units, and thus MUNE studies performed during the stable stage of the disease may not show a change in values during the trial. In support of this, three of the four patients in the CNTF trial at UCSF who had an initial MUNE below 10 had a similar MUNE at the end of the 9-month trial (Olney and Lomen-Hoerth, 2000).

Our group has continued to explore the use of MUNE in clinical trials. Our initial intent was to use MUNE in ALS as a secondary end-point that would provide insight into mechanisms of therapeutic benefit. We considered two physiological mechanisms; a decreased rate of motor unit loss, or an increased rate of collateral sprouting from surviving motor units. If a therapeutic benefit was due to a neuroprotective effect on the anterior horn cells, we expected to see a slower rate of loss in MUNE values in the active treatment group compared with the placebo-treated group. If a therapeutic benefit was due to enhanced collateral sprouting, we expected to see a less steep rate of decline in strength and compound muscle action potential (CMAP) amplitude and an associated increase in the average single motor unit potential amplitude.

With no effective trials to date, we have shifted our attention to validating the clinical utility of the statistical MUNE technique and refine technical aspects as they might influence MUNE results.

Methods

We are currently studying muscles innervated by the ulnar (hypothenar group) or peroneal (tibiolis anterior) nerves for longitudinal assessment of MUNE. Nerve-muscle selection criteria are based on the following. First, the limb selected needs to be

**Correspondence to*: Dr. Richard K. Olney, Neurology, Box 0114, UCSF, San Francisco, CA 94143-0114, USA. Tel.: 415-353-1986, Fax: 415-353-8578.
e-mail: olney@itsa.ucsf.edu

doi: 10.1016/S1567-424X(03)00031-X

one that has lower motor neuron loss, or is expected to involved in the near future. Second, the initial MUNE needs to be greater than 10, although we prefer an initial MUNE that is close to normal. If both upper limbs are weak and atrophic, the stronger limb is chosen as long as the MUNE is well above 10. If the stronger upper limb has a MUNE less than 10, then a lower limb is chosen. If neither upper limb has obvious atrophic weakness, the hypothenar group on the side with the more severely affected lower limb or with the more prominent upper motor neuron signs is selected. In our experience, a hypothenar group with a normal MUNE value may not be useful to measure the rate of progression, unless these muscles develop weakness during the course of longitudinal observation.

Results

We asked whether MUNE provides different or additional information compared to muscle strength measurements or CMAP amplitude. In a study of 10 patients, we compared the changes in grip strength, CMAP amplitude and MUNE values (Yuen and Olney, 1997). Because collateral sprouting is able to compensate partially for the effects of motor unit loss on strength and CMAP amplitude, we predicted that MUNE would show greater changes than the other two measures. This was the case for these 10 patients, with hypothenar MUNE values decreasing significantly over three months, whereas grip strength and CMAP amplitude did not. Furthermore, MUNE values decreased significantly greater over six months than did grip strength and CMAP amplitude. Other investigators have reported that MUNE, determined by the multiple point stimulation MUNE technique, is a more sensitive measure of progression in ALS than are strength and CMAP amplitude as well as forced vital capacity and the Appel scale (Felice, 1997).

We have performed post hoc analysis on these 10 patients based on length of their survival (Yuen and Olney, 1997). Five patients with the shortest total survival, measured from symptomatic onset to death, were grouped as "rapid", and the other five were grouped as "slow". MUNE values decreased significantly faster at 3 and 6 months in the rapid than in the slow group. In contrast, neither strength nor CMAP amplitude was significantly different between groups at 3 or 6 months. We conclude that statistical MUNE is able to detect differences in the rate of progression between two small groups that have non-overlapping duration for total disease course.

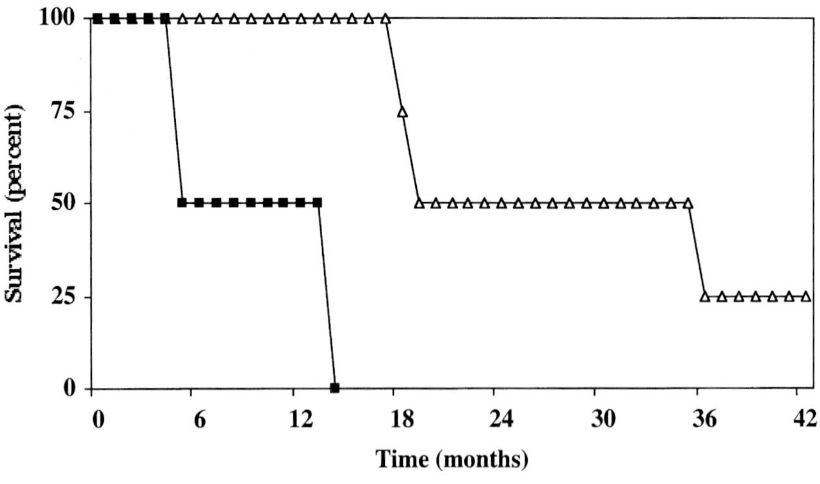

Fig. 1. Survival analysis of six patients with ALS based on statistical MUNE determination from the hypothenar muscle group. Two patients represented by the black squares had a greater than 40% decrease in MUNE values over the first 3 months of the trial. Four patients represented by the open triangles had less than a 40% decrease in MUNE values over three months.

We have also studied whether MUNE determinations of the rate of change can be used to predict prognosis. We found that patients who have the most rapid rates of clinical progression usually have a rapid loss of MUNE values over the first three months of observation (Olney et al., 1999). The degree of change that is required to predict a poor prognosis is in part dependent on the technical reproducibility of the MUNE technique as well as on the selection of an informative nerve-muscle. The reproducibility of statistical MUNE was less in our hands during the CNTF trial than in subsequent studies. This can be a limiting factor as the following example illustrates: two patients who had a decrease in MUNE values of greater than 40% over the first three months of observation had a much worse prognosis than the four who had a decrease in MUNE less than 40% (Olney and Lomen-Hoerth, 2000). This is showed in Fig. 1. We have focused efforts to identify technical factors that affect reproducibility and to develop modifications to the statistical technique that reduce technical variations (Olney et al., 2000; Lomen-Hoerth and Olney, 2001). Reproducibility of statistical MUNE is well below the 30% change that preliminary analysis of our BDNF era data suggests is a biologically meaningful threshold for identifying patients who have significant progression.

Conclusions

We have explored uses of MUNE in clinical trials, and have focused on identifying factors affecting MUNE reproducibility and its use to predict rates of progression. Several technical issues have been identified to improve reproducibility of the statistical technique, and a consensus on methods for performing statistical MUNE was reached during this meeting and is included in a separate section.

References

ALS CNTF Treatment Study Group. A double-blind placebo-controlled clinical trial of subcutaneous recombinant human ciliary neurotrophic factor (rHCNTF) in amyotrophic lateral sclerosis. *Neurology*, 1996, 46: 1244–1249.

BDNF Study Group. A controlled trial of recombinant methionyl human BDNF in ALS. *Neurology*, 1999, 52: 1427–1433.

Felice, K. A longitudinal study comparing thenar motor unit number estimates to other quantitative tests in patients with amyotrophic lateral sclerosis. *Muscle Nerve*, 1997, 20: 179–185.

Lomen-Hoerth, C. and Olney, R. Effect of recording window and stimulation variables on the statistical technique of motor unit number estimation. *Muscle Nerve*, 2001, 24: 1659–1664.

Olney, R. and Lomen-Hoerth, C. Motor unit number estimation (MUNE): how may it contribute to the diagnosis of ALS? *Amyotroph. Lateral Scler. Other Motor Neuron. Disord*, 2000, 1(Suppl. 2): S41–S44.

Olney, R., Yuen, E. and Engstrom, J. Statistical motor unit number estimation: reproducibility and sources of error in patients with amyotrophic lateral sclerosis. *Muscle Nerve*, 2000, 23: 193–197.

Olney, R.K., Yuen, E.C. and Engstrom, J.E. The rate of change in motor unit number estimates predicts survival in patients with amyotrophic lateral sclerosis (ALS). *Neurology*, 1999, 52(Suppl 2): A3.

Yuen, E. and Olney, R. Longitudinal study of fiber density and motor unit number estimate in patients with amyotrophic lateral sclerosis. *Neurology*, 1997, 49: 573–578.

Motor Unit Number Estimation (Supplements to Clinical Neurophysiology Vol. 55)
Editor: M.B. Bromberg

Chapter 32

Multiple point stimulation MUNE with single motor unit tracking in a therapeutic ALS trial

Clifton L. Gooch[a,*], Petra Kaufmann[a] and Yadollah Harati[b]

[a]*Columbia Presbyterian Medical Center, Columbia University College of Physicians and Surgeons, 710 West 168th Street, New York, NY 10032, USA*
[b]*Baylor College of Medicine, One Baylor Plaza, TX 77030, USA*

Introduction

Motor unit number estimation (MUNE) techniques can provide unique insights into the pathophysiology of motor unit survival and loss in human subjects. MUNE can also be used as outcome measures in therapeutic trials, particularly those involving amyotrophic lateral sclerosis (ALS) (McComas et al., 1971; Daube, 1988; Dantes and McComas, 1991; Bromberg et al., 1993; Doherty and Brown, 1993; Stashuk et al., 1994; Felice, 1995; Gooch and Harati, 1997; Yuen and Olney, 1997; Armon and Brandstader, 1999; Shefner et al., 1999). The multiple point stimulation (MPS) MUNE technique uses percutaneous nerve stimulation to elicit a number of individual single motor unit action potential waveforms (S-MUAPs) (Doherty and Brown, 1993). The principles of the MPS can be used to identify and track S-MUAPs over time (Doherty and Brown, 1994; Gooch and Harati, 1997; Chan et al., 1998). This led to a modification of the MPS MUNE method that integrates S-MUAP tracking. The accuracy and reproducibility of this modification has been discussed in Chapter 8. We have used MPS MUNE with tracking to follow a group of ALS patients enrolled in a multicenter controlled trial of xaliproden with and without riluzole. Data analysis is ongoing and will be the subject of a future publication, but summary results of an interim analysis are described below.

Methods

The methodology of the modified MPS MUNE technique with tracking are described in an earlier chapter. All electromyographers and technicians performing MUNE were blinded to patient randomization.

MUNE studies were performed in the same hand in each patient at 1- to 4-month intervals for 18 months or until death or tracheostomy. Patients were randomized to one of six study arms: Placebo alone or riluzole (50 mg BID) plus placebo; xaliproden (1 mg/day) alone or xaliproden (1 mg/day) plus riluzole; xaliproden (2 mg/day) alone or xaliproden (2 mg/day) plus riluzole.

Interim analysis

The interim analysis is limited because data are from 10 months of the study and randomization is

**Correspondence to*: Dr. Clifton Gooch, Columbia Presbyterian Medical Center, Columbia University College of Physicians and Surgeons, 710 West 168th Street, New York, NY 10032, USA.
e-mail: CLG33@columbia.edu

doi: 10.1016/S1567-424X(03)00032-1

known only with respect to which patients are taking riluzole but not who were receiving xaliproden or placebo. MUNE values remained static in five patients (four on riluzole), increased in seven (six on riluzole), and declined in 38 (11 on riluzole). Average S-MUAP amplitude values remained static in three patients (two on riluzole), increased in 20 (13 on riluzole), and declined in the remaining 16 (eight on riluzole). Average rates of MUNE decline for all patients during this interval approached 50% at 6 months, similar to rates previously reported. Plots of S-MUAP amplitude against MUNE values demonstrated no significant changes until MUNE values fell below 50–100, at which point significant increases in S-MUAP amplitude were noted. This suggests more aggressive collateral reinnervation at low MUNE levels. Similar relationships were noted between thenar strength and MUNE values, with strength in the normal to near normal range until MUNE values dropped below 50–100, at which point more substantial weakness was noted. S-MUAP tracking was also assessed, and 106 S-MUAPs were identified for tracking at the start of the trial. By 10 months, 29 S-MUAPs could still be followed, while 77 could no longer be elicited.

Summary

MUNE combining routine MPS and S-MUAP tracking is possible in a clinical trial, and can provide important information not obtained by either technique alone. Interim analysis of our data suggests a possible effect of riluzole on motor unit preservation in patients with ALS. In addition, there appears to be a threshold for more aggressive compensatory reinnervation when MUNE values fall below 50–100 motor units. Despite the increase in S-MUAP size there is a progression of weakness. These observations remain preliminary, and will be more rigorously tested when the full and unblinded data are analyzed. Longitudinal MPS MUNE-T provides an important tool for the sensitive and early quantitative measure of denervation and compensatory reinnervation in patients with ALS, enabling early recognition of the effects of experimental therapy.

References

Armon, C. and Brandstader, M.E. Motor unit number estimate-based rates of progression of ALS predict patient survival. *Muscle Nerve*, 1999, 11: 1571–1575.

Bromberg, M.B., Forshew, D.A., Nan, K.L., Bromberg, J., Simmons, Z. and Fries, T.J. Motor unit number estimation, isometric strength and electromyographic measures in amyotrophic lateral sclerosis. *Muscle Nerve*, 1993, 12: 1218–1219.

Chan, K.M., Stashuk, D. and Brown, W.F. A longitudinal study of the pathophysiological changes in single human thenar motor units in ALS. *Muscle Nerve*, 1998, 21: 1714–1723.

Dantes, A. and McComas, A. The extent and time course of motor neuron involvement in ALS. *Muscle Nerve*, 1991, 14: 416–421.

Daube, J.R. Statistical estimates of number of motor units in thenar and foot muscles in patients with amyotrophic lateral sclerosis or the residue of poliomyelitis. *Muscle Nerve*, 1988, 11: 957-A.

Doherty, T.J. and Brown, W.F. The estimated numbers and relative sizes of thenar motor units as selected by multiple point stimulation in young and older adults. *Muscle Nerve*, 1993, 16: 355–366.

Doherty, T.J. and Brown, W.F. A method for the longitudinal study of human thenar motor units. *Muscle Nerve*, 1994, 17: 1029–1036.

Felice, K.J. Thenar motor unit number estimates using the multiple point stimulation technique: reproducibility studies in ALS patient and normal subjects. *Muscle Nerve*, 1995, 18: 1412–1416.

Gooch, C.L. and Harati, Y. Longitudinal tracking of the same single motor unit in amyotrophic lateral sclerosis. *Muscle Nerve*, 1997, 20: 511–513.

McComas, A.J., Fawcett, P.R.W., Campbell, M.J. and Sica, R. E.P. Electrophysiological estimation of the number of motor units within a human muscle. *J. Neurol. Neurosurg. Psychiatry*., 1971, 34: 121–131.

Shefner, J.M., Reaume, A.G., Flood, D.G., Scott, R.W., Kowall, N.W., Ferrante, R.J., Siwek, D.F., Upton-Rice, M. and Brown, R.H. Mice lacking cytosolic Cu/ZN SOD display a distinctive motor axonopathy. *Neurology*, 1999, 53: 1239–1246.

Stashuk, D.W., Doherty, T.J., Kassam, A. and Brown, W.F. Motor unit number estimates based on the automated analysis of F-responses. *Muscle Nerve*, 1994, 17: 881–890.

Yuen, E.C. and Olney, R.K. Longitudinal study of fiber density and motor unit number estimate in patients with amyotrophic lateral sclerosis. *Neurology*, 1997, 49: 573–578.

Motor Unit Number Estimation (Supplements to Clinical Neurophysiology Vol. 55)
Editor: M.B. Bromberg

Chapter 33

MUNE in an ALS treatment trial

Jeremy M. Shefner*

Department of Neurology, Upstate Medical University, Syracuse, NY 13210, USA

Introduction

The goal of any clinical trial is to evaluate the effect of a potential therapeutic agent using the minimum number of patients and the shortest possible time period. The choice of the primary outcome measure has a dramatic impact on both duration and size of the study. The ideal measure will have high test–retest reliability, and will change in a meaningful fashion as a function of disease progression. The most commonly used primary outcome measures in amyotrophic lateral sclerosis (ALS) clinical trials have been patient survival, quantitative strength measures, and pulmonary function. Each has strengths and weaknesses. The advantage of survival as an endpoint is that it is clinically meaningful, and has little variability of measurement. However, its use obligates a long trial duration. Quantitative strength measurements are not as directly related to clinical status, but are attractive in a disease such as ALS where weakness is a primary symptom. Variability of measurement can be a problem, in part because the measure requires active patient participation. Pulmonary function tests also require patient participation, and reflect activity in a combination of muscle groups that may vary from patient to patient and with disease duration. Other measures have been used, including functional rating scales. Such measures often have low variability of measurement, but their relationship to disease state may be indirect.

Clearly, none of the above are perfect outcome measures for ALS trials. Motor unit number estimation (MUNE) offers several potential advantages as an outcome measure. An important attraction is the intuitive relationship between MUNE and disease progression in ALS. Patients progress clinically in large part because of progressive loss of functional motor units; this loss is exactly what MUNE techniques are designed to assess. The time course of motor unit loss in patients with ALS was first studied with the incremental stimulation technique by Dantes and McComas (1991). Their data suggested that motor unit loss occurred more rapidly early in the disease, with the slope of motor unit decline leveling off after the first year. Using a variation of the multiple point stimulation (MPS) technique, Arasaki et al. (1997) also found that MUNE dropped by 70% in the first year after diagnosis. This rapid decline in MUNE early in the disease raises the potential utility of MUNE as an outcome measure, as most clinical studies aim to attract mildly affected patients for which other potential outcome measures are changing quite slowly. Evidence that MUNE is in fact more sensitive in detecting patient progression in a clinical

**Correspondence to*: Dr. Jeremy M. Shefner, Department of Neurology, 750 E. Adams St., HSC Syracuse, Syracuse, NY 13210, USA.
Tel.: 315-464-4627, Fax: 315-464-5006
e-mail: shefnerj@upstate.edu

doi: 10.1016/S1567-424X(03)00033-3

trial comes from a study in which MPS MUNE, compound motor action potential (CMAP) amplitude, hand grip, strength testing, and vital capacity were all measured at regular intervals (Felice, 1997). MUNE showed a higher percent change than any other measure, and had a higher likelihood of detecting a criterion change in response than any of the others. Similarly, a study comparing the statistical MUNE technique to grip strength and CMAP amplitude showed a significant decrease in MUNE at within 3 months, but no significant change in other measures (Yuen and Olney, 1997).

As MUNE techniques have been refined, test–retest reliability has improved, further increasing its potential utility as an outcome measure. Across a number of MUNE techniques, correlation coefficients range between 0.85 and 0.98 for normal subjects, and tend to be higher in patients with neurogenic lesions (Felice, 1995). One important attribute that contributes to reducing test–retest variability is that the measure is independent of patient effort. Especially late in the course of the disease, effort can be quite variable and can affect results of both pulmonary function and quantitative strength measures.

As part of a clinical trial to test the efficacy of creatine in patients with ALS, MUNE is used as a secondary outcome measure. The statistical MUNE techniques was chosen for use because of its high test–retest reliability, and because it was felt that it could be well standardized across multiple centers with appropriate training.

Methods

Subjects

Subjects with probable or definite ALS are recruited to take part in a clinical trial evaluating the efficacy and safety of creatine, taken orally at a dose of 5 g per day. Inclusion and exclusion criteria for the study include age between 18 and 80 years, without other concurrent diseases that would interfere with their ability to participate in a clinical trial, and without any history of superimposed neuromuscular disease. As the primary outcome measure is quantitative strength measurements in the upper extremity, all subjects have at least two evaluable muscle groups out of a total of eight. Subjects will be studied monthly over a 6-month trial period, for a total of eight evaluations.

Prior to evaluating patients, all 17 participating trial sites were required to study four control subjects without neuromuscular disease. These subjects were studied to establish test–retest reliability; each subject was studied twice, with a time interval between study of at least 3 h.

MUNE technique

A modification of the statistical technique originally proposed by Daube was employed (Daube, 1988; Shefner et al., 1999). The muscle for study is either the median innervated abductor pollicis brevis (APB), or the ulnar innervated abductor digiti minimi (ADM), on either side. Choice of muscle is made using a combination of clinical and electrophysiological criteria. If all potential muscles are above MRC grade 4 strength, the weakest muscle is chosen for study. If all muscles are less than MRC grade 4, the strongest muscle is selected. If multiple muscles are graded at grade 4 strength, CMAPs are obtained, with stimulation at wrist and recording over the muscle of interest, and the muscle with the greatest amplitude CMAP is chosen for study. Once selected, that muscle will be studied repeatedly over the course of the trial period.

All studies are performed with the subject laying supine on an examining table, with self-adhesive recording electrodes placed on the muscle in standard fashion. Stimulating electrodes are also self adhesive circular patch electrodes, placed over the nerve after the location of minimum threshold had been determined. A scan of the response range is then obtained, starting from a stimulus strength that is just subthreshold for evoking a response and progressing to a stimulus producing a just supramaximal response over 30 equal stimulus strength increments. The scan is visually inspected, and the presence or absence of large breaks in the response range is determined; the presence of such breaks are taken as suggesting the presence of a large amplitude motor unit at that level. The criterion for further investigation of such a break is that it encompassed 15% or more of the entire response range. If such a break is present, it is further evaluated by obtaining responses to 30 successive stimuli of an intensity set to produce responses in the range from just below to just above the break. This closer investigation often revealed responses within the range that were skipped in the original scan. Under this circumstance, the gap is not felt to indicate the presence of a large unit in this region. However, if a gap in the response of greater than 10% of the total response range remains, it is felt to represent a single large motor unit of amplitude determined by the size of the gap. Such units are independently counted, and are removed from the statistical analysis. All large breaks in the stimulus response curve are treated in this fashion.

Assuming the absence of large breaks in the stimulus response curve, four areas are chosen for statistical study. Units are evaluated in the ranges of 10–20%, 25–35%, 40–50%, and 55–65% of the maximum response. For each range, or window, a stimulus is chosen that evoked a response within it. A total of 120–300 responses to the stimulus are recorded, with stimuli presented at a frequency of 1–2 Hz, and evaluated in blocks of 30 responses. The variability of the responses to the repeated constant intensity stimuli are used to estimate the amplitude and area of the single motor unit potentials (SMUPs) present in that area of the response range. The estimates of SMUP size from each of the four response ranges are combined to form a single estimate of SMUP size using the weighted average method reported previously (Shefner et al., 1999; Lomen-Hoerth and Olney, 2000).

If no large units are from the scan as described above, the estimate of the SMUP size is divided into the maximum CMAP to yield the MUNE. The presence of large units, however, requires modification in two ways. First, if a large unit is present in the part of the range mandated to be studied (i.e. 10–65%), the windows are altered so that ranges are studied above and below that area of the response range. Secondly, if a large unit is detected, it is counted manually, and therefore its amplitude is subtracted from the CMAP used to calculate the MUNE. For example, if the maximum CMAP is 8 mV, but a large unit of 1.5 mV is detected, the MUNE would be calculated by dividing the estimate of SMUP size into the residual CMAP of 6.5 mV. The total MUNE would be the result of that calculation, plus 1 for the large unit that was excluded.

In order to maximize reliability of measurement, MUNE determinations were performed twice in succession for each patient and control evaluation, with electrodes staying in place between measurements. The average of the two MUNE determinations was taken as the final estimate. For test–retest evaluations, pairs of MUNE measurements were repeated at an interval of at least 3 h, with electrodes removed and reapplied.

Results

Patients

Patients are currently being recruited for participation in the clinical trial; at this writing, 96 patients are currently enrolled. No data are available at present for this group.

Control subjects

Four subjects were studied on two separate sessions at each of the 17 sites. In most subjects, the APB was studied. Mean MUNE for 66 subjects was 101, with SD of 20.3. MUNE as a function of age is shown in Fig. 1. From site to site, average MUNE values were quite similar (Fig. 2). Test–retest reliability was expressed as percent variability; the criterion for participation in the clinical trial was that percent variability for normal subjects be less than 20%.Variability across sites is shown in Fig. 3.

Discussion

An absolute requirement for an outcome measure to be useful in a multicenter clinical trial is that it is reproducible and that measurement can be standardized across treatment sites. Just as

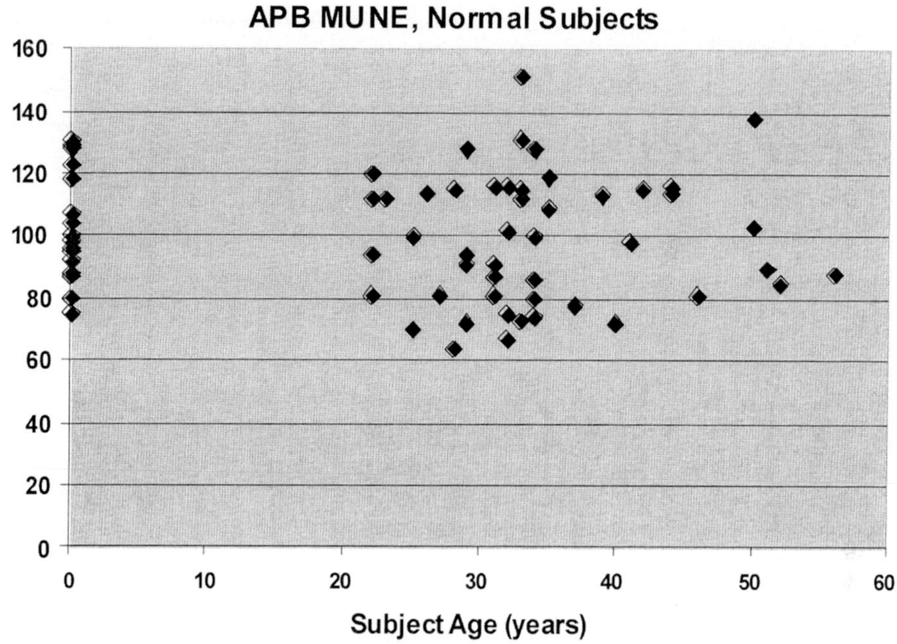

Fig. 1. MUNE for control subjects from APB muscle. Each MUNE is average of two evaluations performed in succession with electrodes in place. Subjects for whom age is unkown are plotted at 0.

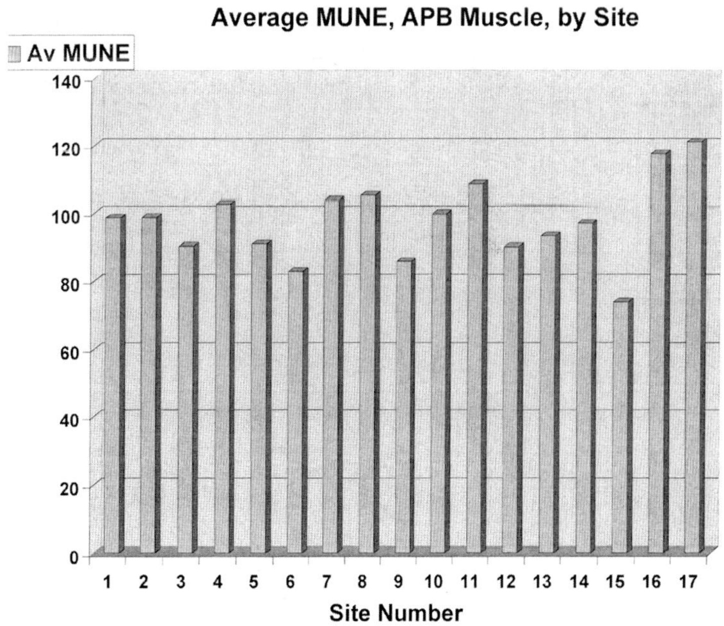

Fig. 2. MUNE for normal subjects by participating site.

important, the measure must be shown to change reliably with disease progression. Data to address this second concern are currently being acquired. However, we have shown that statistical MUNE can produced estimates in normal subjects that are satisfactory with respect to test–retest variability, and that MUNE values are quite similar from site to site. Of 17 sites involved in the creatine/ALS

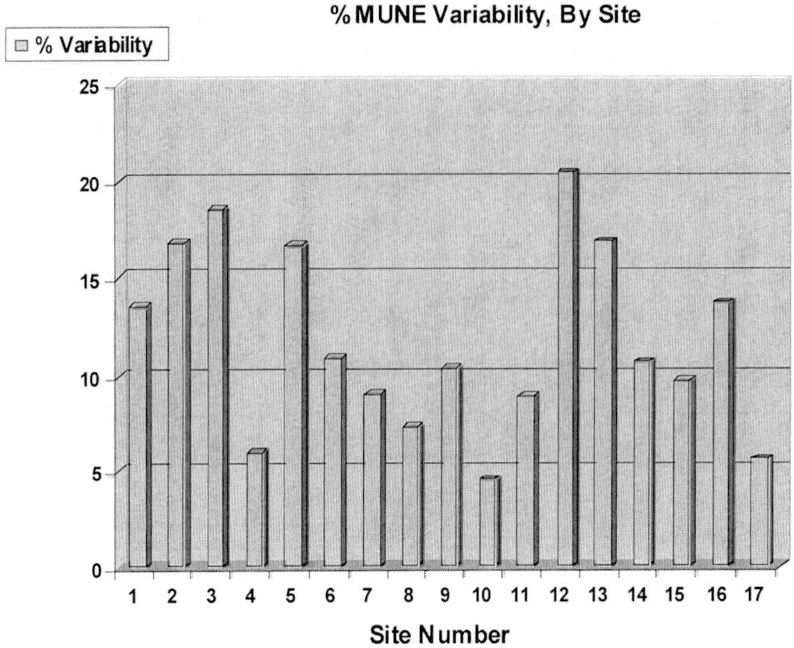

Fig. 3. Percent variability by participating site.

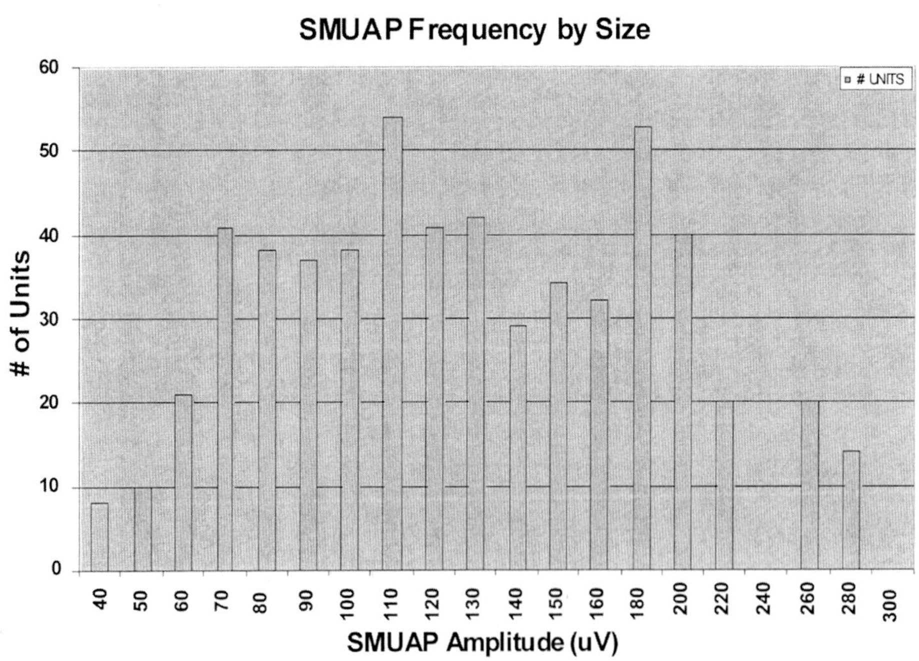

Fig. 4. SMUP sizes for 66 normal subjects from ABP muscle.

treatment study, average MUNE values were between 80 and 120 in all but one site. Test–retest variability was mandated to be less than 20%; this was achieved with training in all sites. At 12 sites, variability was less than 15%, and it was less than 10% in eight sites.

Comparison of MUNE in normal subjects using the statistical technique modified as described here shows that MUNE values are somewhat smaller. Average MUNE values in normal subjects using the spike triggered average, incremental, MPS, and F wave techniques show values that range from 151 to 270 (Shefner, 2001). The smaller MUNE values derived with the statistical technique occur because of a larger estimate of mean SMUP amplitude. Figure 4 shows the distribution of SMUP sizes in normal subjects across sites. Out of more than 500 units estimated across all subjects, only 18 were less than 60 μV in size. This is in clear contrast with units recorded with the MPS technique, in which the average SMUP size in normal subjects is less than 100 μV. It is not clear which method produces an estimate that is most closely related to anatomic fiber counts; in the context of a clinical trial, standardization and reliability of measurement may be more important than anatomic correlation.

Acknowledgements

Electrophysiologists participating in the Northeast ALS Clinical Trials Group ALS/Creatine treatment study: Dr. L. Krivickas, Boston; Drs. R. Olney, K. Lomen-Hoerth, San Francisco; Dr. C. Gooch, New York; Drs. D. Jillapalli, J. Shefner, Syracuse; Dr. M. Al-Lozi, St. Louis; Dr. G. Sachs, Providence; Dr. H. Horak, Indianapolis; Dr. E. Pioro, Cleveland; Dr. M. Ross, Louisville; Drs. E. Sorensen, J. Daube, Rochester; Dr. K. Sharma, Miami; Dr. R. Conwit, Baltimore; Dr. J. Caress, Winston-Salem; Dr. T. Fries, Burlington.

References

Arasaki, K. et al. Validity of electromyograms and tension as a means of motor unit number estimation. *Muscle Nerve*, 1997, 20(5): 552–560.

Dantes, M. and McComas, A. The extent and time course of motoneuron involvement in amyotrophic lateral sclerosis. *Muscle Nerve*, 1991, 7: 416–421.

Daube, J. Statistical estimates of number of motor units in the thenar and foot muscles in patients with amyotrophic lateral sclerosis. *Muscle Nerve*, 1988, 11: 957–958.

Felice, K.J. Thenar motor unit number estimates using the multiple point stimulation technique: reproducibility studies in ALS patients and normal subjects. *Muscle Nerve*, 1995, 18(12): 1412–1416.

Felice, K.J. A longitudinal study comparing thenar motor unit number estimates to other quantitative tests in patients with amyotrophic lateral sclerosis. *Muscle Nerve*, 1997, 20(2): 179–185.

Lomen-Hoerth, C. and Olney, R.K. Comparison of multiple point and statistical motor unit number estimation. *Muscle Nerve*, 2000, 23(10): 1525–1533.

Shefner, J.M. Motor unit number estimation in human neurological diseases and animal models. *Clin. Neurophysiol.*, 2001, 112: 955–964.

Shefner, J.M., Jillapalli, D. and Bradshaw, D.Y. Reducing intersubject variability in motor unit number estimation [In Process Citation]. *Muscle Nerve*, 1999, 22(10): 1457–1460.

Yuen, E.C. and Olney, R.K. Longitudinal study of fiber density and motor unit number estimate in patients with amyotrophic lateral sclerosis. *Neurology*, 1997, 49: 573–578.

Motor Unit Number Estimation (Supplements to Clinical Neurophysiology Vol. 55)
Editor: M.B. Bromberg

Chapter 34

Increasing muscle sampling to improve MUNE power in the clinical trial setting

E.J. Sorenson*, J.R. Daube and A.J. Windebank

Department of Neurology, Mayo Clinic, Rochester, MN 55905, USA

Introduction

A number of techniques have been developed to estimate the number of motor units innervating a muscle or muscle group. These have collectively been termed motor unit number estimation (MUNE). For obvious reasons the ability to quantitate the number of surviving motor neurons is attractive as an outcome measure in clinical trials of the motor neuron diseases. MUNE has already been used in amyotrophic lateral sclerosis (ALS) therapeutic trials and in natural history studies of post-polio (Daube et al., 1995; Windebank et al., 1996; McComas et al., 1997). However, for MUNE to become more widely acceptable as an outcome measure in a clinical trial a number of issues remain to be addressed. Among these is how to obtain the most power from the techniques.

Clinical trial power is driven by four variables: type 1 error rate, type 2 error rate, the magnitude of change one is interested in detecting, and the variability of the outcome measure within the study population. Types 1 and 2 error rates are independent of the outcome measure and may, for the purposes of comparing outcome measures, be considered constants. The magnitude of change is largely driven by the intervention being tested including the expected magnitude of benefit and the likelihood and severity of adverse effects.

Therefore, when assessing power of outcome measures comparing population variability is sufficient. Population variability can be improved upon by increasing the number of muscles sampled per subject. By increasing the sample size the effect of outlying values and the effect of test–retest variability is minimized resulting in a more uniform population. In the case of MUNE, increasing the number of muscles studied per subject from 1 to 4 should have the effect of improving population variability and improving power when used as an outcome measure. To test this hypothesis, we have assessed the effects of muscle sampling on power using the statistical method of MUNE in patients with prior paralytic poliomyelitis.

Methods

Fifty subjects were randomly chosen from a population-based cohort of 298 patients with a remote history of paralytic poliomyelitis. The demographics of the study population have previously been described in detail (Windebank et al., 1991). All 50 subjects underwent MUNE analysis using the statistical technique as described by Daube (1995). Four muscle groups were sampled

*Correspondence to: Dr. Eric J. Sorenson, Department of Neurology, Mayo Clinic, Rochester, MN 55905, USA. e-mail: Sorenson.Eric@mayo.edu

doi: 10.1016/S1567-424X(03)00034-5

in all subjects: bilateral thenar muscles and peroneal motor (extensor digitorum brevis). For each subject, MUNE was calculated and averaged for four sample sizes: one muscle sampled (left thenar), two muscles sampled (left thenar and peroneal motor), three muscles sampled (bilateral thenar and left peroneal motor), and four muscles sampled (bilateral thenar and bilateral peroneal motor).

For each muscle sample size a population mean and standard deviation were calculated. A coefficient of variation was generated by dividing the standard deviation by the population mean. From the coefficients of variation a subject sample size was calculated for a theoretical clinical trial. The theoretical clinical trial was based on the following assumptions: powered to detect a 20% change in the MUNE, type 1 error rate of 0.05, and type 2 error rate of 0.20.

Results

MUNE mean values were as follows: for the left median 107 (SD 68), for the left peroneal 60 (SD 58), right median mean 106 (SD 67), and right peroneal mean 73 (SD 53). Mean MUNE values for the muscle sample size groups were 126 (SD 73), 99 (SD 49), 109 (SD 49) and 102 (SD 43) for the one, two, three, and four muscle sample sizes, respectively (Fig. 1). This resulted in coefficients of variation (expressed as a percent) of 58, 49, 45 and 42% for muscle sample sizes of one, two, three, and four, respectively (Fig. 2). Given that the mean and

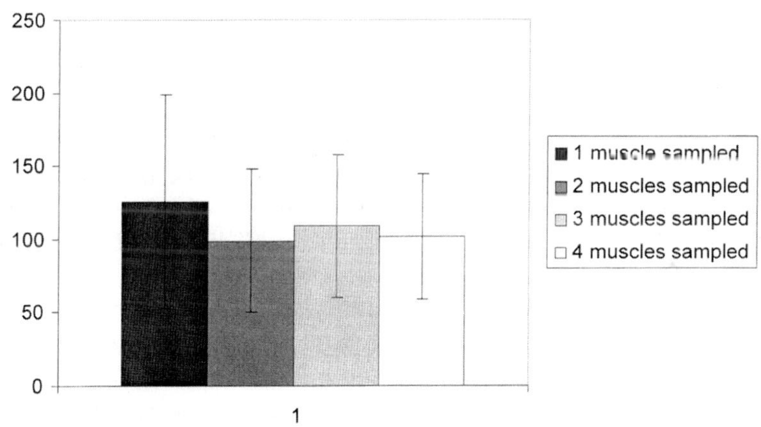

Fig. 1. Mean motor unit number estimates plotted by sample size with standard deviations indicated by the error bars.

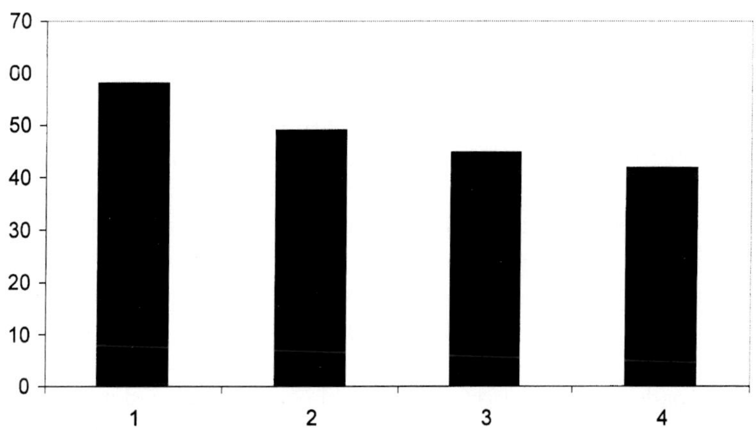

Fig. 2. Coefficients of variation (expressed as a percent) for sample sizes from 1 to 4 muscles sampled.

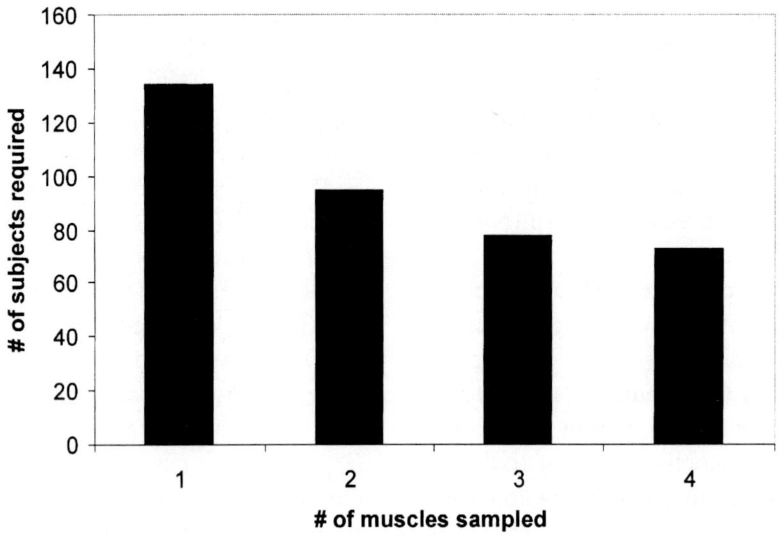

Fig. 3. Number of subjects required for a clinical trial with varying the muscle sample size (assumes a type I error rate of 0.05, type II error rate of 0.20, and a power to detect a change in the mean by 20%).

standard deviations of the individual four muscles is not uniform, the order in which one places the muscles does alter the curve slightly. However, in all combinations the trend and the final coefficient of variation remain unchanged. Based upon these coefficients of variation, subject sample size calculations for a theoretical clinical trial powered to detect a 20% change in the mean (type 1 error of 0.05 and type 2 error rate of 0.20) would require 134, 95, 78, and 73 subjects per treatment arm for muscle sample sizes one, two, three, and four, respectively (Fig. 3).

Discussion

In planning a clinical trial, careful thought must be given to the objectives and to the outcome measures used to assess these objectives. Power calculations remain a central feature to trial design. Clinical trial power is largely driven by population variability. When comparing population variability between outcome measures one can compare the coefficients of variation between techniques. There are two elements to population variability: test–retest reproducibility (i.e. test noise) and the inherent or true variability among individuals within the population. Some of the current MUNE techniques have achieved test–retest variation of under 20% (Olney et al., 2000; Simmons et al., 2001). Because of this, most of the population variability seen with these measures will be that of the inherent population variability, with a minority from test noise. While test–retest reproducibility remains important to MUNE as an outcome measure, as test–retest variation drops to 10% or below, further improvements will have relatively little impact upon study power. Potentially much larger impacts upon study power could be achieved by addressing the inherent variability within the individuals of a population.

There are two potential strategies to improve population variability: to enrich the subject population by selecting subjects based upon uniformity, or to increase the intra-subject sampling. Enriching the subject population by selecting a smaller, more uniform, subgroup is attractive. However, while power will be improved, the number of subjects diminishes. Commonly, this reduction in subjects negates any advantage offered by subject uniformity.

If we elect to assess how the number of muscles sampled per subject affected population variability, Increasing the sample size offers two advantages: it allows for any test–retest variability to be averaged out over an increased number of muscles, and minimizes the effect of outlying values. Both of these factors will trend toward improving population variability. Both factors, however, would be expected to have their greatest impact within the first few muscles sampled, and diminishing returns as sample size increases further. Based upon this, one would expect the greatest improvement in population variability within the first few muscles averaged and lesser improvement by the addition of subsequent muscles.

Our findings are consistent with these predictions. We have shown that increasing the sample size from one to four muscles does reduce the population variability. This will in turn improve clinical trial power for a given subject sample size. It appears from this data that sampling an individual muscle per subject is insufficient when used as a trial outcome measure. While the ideal number to sample is unknown, given the diminishing improvement with successive sample sizes, it appears that four muscles sampled per subject is sufficient and allows for a technically feasible muscle to be sampled from each limb. Additionally, sampling beyond four muscles likely offers little further gain in power while requiring a prohibitive time commitment.

References

Daube, J.R. Estimating the number of motor units in a muscle. *J. Clin. Neurophysiol.*, 1995, 12(6): 585–594.

Daube, J.R., Windebank, A.J. and Litchy, W.J. Electrophysiologic changes in neuromuscular function over five years in polio survivors. *Ann. N.Y. Acad. Sci.*, 1995, 753: 120–128.

McComas, A.J., Quartly, C. and Griggs, R.C. Early and late losses of motor units after poliomyelitis. *Brain*, 1997, 120 (Pt 8): 1415–1421.

Olney, R.K., Yuen, E.C. and Engstrom, J.W. Statistical motor unit number estimation: reproducibility and sources of error in patients with amyotrophic lateral sclerosis. *Muscle Nerve*, 2000, 23(2): 193–197.

Simmons, Z., Epstein, D.K., Borg, B., Mauger, D.T., Kothari, M.J. and Shefner, J.M. Reproducibility of motor unit number estimation in individual subjects. *Muscle Nerve*, 2001, 24(4): 467–473.

Windebank, A.J., Litchy, W.J., Daube, J.R., Kurland, L.T., Codd, M.B. and Iverson, R. Late effects of paralytic poliomyelitis in Olmsted County, Minnesota. *Neurology*, 1991, 41(4): 501–507.

Windebank, A.J., Litchy, W.J., Daube, J.R. and Iverson, R.A. Lack of progression of neurologic deficit in survivors of paralytic polio: a 5-year prospective population-based study. [see comments]. *Neurology*, 1996, 46(1): 80–84.

Discussion after Session IX

Jasper Daube, Rochester, Minnesota

In returning to the question of what is the smallest motor unit to include, we should not make decisions based on "what it feels like", but based on data. Our investigation that I described yesterday shows that the greatest single motor unit potential variation is 25 μV ms or 10 μV. Motor unit potential variation is not sufficient to account for what you presented to us. Smaller motor unit potentials are not seen in the normal population because the technique that has been selected, a 10% window, biases against them. That is in contrast to what we have seen with each of the other MUNE techniques, incremental or multiple point stimulation, where you see many more small motor unit potentials. So, I think that motor unit potential variation will not cause what you have seen and you do not see it in normal subjects because you are biasing against it by how you are setting the window.

Richard Olney, San Francisco, California

I am not as convinced that this cannot reflect motor unit variation, and I have some data that might speak to that. These certainly might be small units. The question is how to deal with them when you have a method that selectively reduces your ability to see them under one set of circumstance (normal muscles), and in other circumstances (denervated muscle) selectively accentuates your ability to see them. We do not see reduced numbers of smaller motor units in circumstances of normality because there is presumably a reduced number of them.

Jasper Daube, Rochester, Minnesota

You have shown the answer on your slide when Kathy widened the window. You can modify the window on the basis of what is appropriate for what you see. The original technique arbitrarily selected 10% window widths, and said we are going to stick with 10% all the time.

Jeremy Shefner, Syracuse, New York

I would like to say that it is not just widening the window, because if you adjust the stimulus intensity in a certain way, no matter how wide the window and how many stimuli you provide, you will only get a normal distribution of the data. The way to get a skewed distribution is not just by widening the window but by changing the stimulus intensity so that you are somewhere in the middle of the window. Therefore, it is a combination of widening the window and changing the stimulus intensity. Is there an alternate suggestion? Given that there may be small units, is there a way with the statistical technique to go back and include the small units in the original estimate in normal subjects so that we can be more physiologic and not ignore this population that may be important?

Mark Bromberg, Salt Lake City, Utah

I would like to ask questions about the riluzole data. I do not understand how, over a couple of months on riluzole, there can be an increase in MUNE values. What is the physiologic mechanism? The response seems to be fairly robust, yet clinically I do not hear patients telling me they can function better after started riluzole.

Clifton Gooch, New York, New York

Our speculation is that there may be a pool of sick motor neurons, motor neurons that are functioning at a bare threshold of survivability, that are not well enough to respond to extrinsic stimulation or perhaps even volitional stimulation. But that with a little help, in this particular case from riluzole, they can be pushed beyond that threshold, and that process may be relatively rapid, over a period of 2–3 months.

The clinical effect is modest in our population as well. The clinical effects in the trials that gained approval for riluzole were modest. I would say that the slight but statistically positive effect we saw on MUNE values was probably not dramatic enough to make a clinical impact. The importance of the data would be not so much that riluzole causes a very dramatic change, but that it is causing a measurable electrophysiologic change, and may be doing something important at the level of the anterior horn cell. This might promote or encourage further investigation along those lines to produce a more potent drug.

Jasper Daube, Rochester, Minnesota

I would like to ask a practical question of Eric Sorenson with regard to the conclusions that he came to of sampling multiple muscles for motor unit number estimates. Right now, I am part of the multicenter creatine trial in which we study one muscle and sample it twice. Eric, would we be better off sampling two muscles once or one muscle twice?

Eric Sorenson, Rochester, Minnesota

I can give you my thoughts without looking at data. My feeling is you would probably reduce your population variability by sampling two muscles rather than one muscle twice. Test–retest reproducibility of the MUNE technique is actually quite reasonable doing it just one time. I am not sure that you are adding that much by testing the same muscle twice.

Catherine Lomen-Hoerth, San Francisco, California

We showed that the coefficient of variation is 7% with a single test in an ALS patient with intermediate motor unit loss, a patient group with the greatest variability.

Richard Olney, San Francisco, California

In ALS, weakness starts regionally and spreads. Eric, how much would we benefit from making sure that if we performed an MUNE study in one upper limb and one lower limb muscle?

Eric Sorensen, Rochester, Minnesota

We can consider our experience with muscle strength testing. If you test limbs that are affected, we found a fairly low ability of predicting which limb would subsequently show the most change. Therefore, one or two muscles is not enough. If you are going to use a technique, I would sample one muscle in each limb.

Mark Bromberg, Salt Lake City, Utah

It would be valuable to have consensus on a number of issues related to MUNE. We may not be able to reach them at this moment, but should discuss these issues and they can be incorporated into a section in the proceedings.

One is whether we can eliminate some MUNE techniques that are not particularly viable, hard to use, not reliable, etc. There is a lot of discussion about the statistical technique, and it is probably the one that is used the most. On the other hand, there are a lot of issues surrounding it. We have had discussions about the multiple point and the adapted multiple stimulation techniques, and they seem to have advantages and at least do not have the issues that are surrounding the statistical technique. The spike triggered averaging technique in some sense is being revived with the decomposition program, with more people interested in it and its use in different applications such as proximal muscles and questions of recruitment order.

Another is how to express test–retest data. One runs the risk of being too dogmatic in telling people how to collect test–retest data and express the variability. I think it is reasonable to leave it open, but state explicitly what was done – whether the electrodes were kept on or were taken off and reapplied, whether another person came in to repeat the test, and so on. People may have different questions they are asking. Variability can be expressed in a number of ways, but agreeing on one common way would be valuable. Carmel expressed that it is preferable to take the difference between tests 1 and 2 in absolute terms and then divided that by the mean of both of them. You can express that as a number or multiply it by 100 and express it as a percentage.

Eric Sorenson, Rochester, Minnesota

That will give the variation of a single test, but not for a population. In fact, if you want to do test–retest assessment of a population of multiple individuals being tested twice, what you really need to do is an interclass correlation co-efficient. You get a unitless R value that can be compare directly across all the techniques. That is a much more standard way of assessing variance than it is going to be by doing what he suggested.

Mark Bromberg, Salt Lake City, Utah

A third issue is where we apply our recording electrodes. Alan suggests we place the stigmatic electrode over the endplate zone; then most motor unit potentials will be initially negative and there will be much less dispersion in time.

A fourth issue relates to the preferred metric for single motor units size. This group seems to agree that if it is possible, we use negative peak area. Then the second metric is between negative peak amplitude and peak-to-peak amplitude.

Each of us has our own reasons for doing things in a particular way. There will not be any requirements that people do it a particular way. These are just suggestions and their reasons, to try to get us to do things in a similar way. I think the extent to which a group does things more similarly makes it more likely that it will be acceptable to others outside this group.

Kathryn Swoboda, Salt Lake City, Utah

In our work, we have published three numbers: peak-to-peak amplitude, negative peak amplitude, and negative peak area. It becomes very confusing for people who are not MUNE aficionados, and I think we should publish one number, based on the negative peak area.

Jasper Daube, Rochester, Minnesota

I get a lot of MUNE papers to review, and I think we as reviewers can help guide some consensus that we reached in this group.

Mark Bromberg, Salt Lake City, Utah

Another issue is terminology and abbreviations for the various potentials, especially with the spike triggered averaging techniques where surface and intramuscular potentials are recorded.

Daniel Stashuk, Waterloo, Ontario

I do not think we need the word "single" because "motor unit" implies that it is an individual motor unit, and I do not think we need the words "action potential". I suggest in place of single motor unit action potential the term "surface motor unit potential". If it were intramuscular potentials they would be referred to as "intramuscular motor unit potential".

Section X

MUNE in Animal Studies

Motor Unit Number Estimation (Supplements to Clinical Neurophysiology Vol. 55)
Editor: M.B. Bromberg

Chapter 35

MUNE studies in mouse models of motor neuron disease

Jeremy M. Shefner*

Department of Neurology, Upstate Medical University, 750 E. Adams St., HSC Syracuse, Syracuse, NY 13210, USA

Introduction

Some patients with familial ALS have missense mutations in the gene encoding cytosolic copper–zinc superoxide dismutase (SOD1) (Rosen et al., 1993). Similarly to patients with familial ALS, mice bearing a transgene encoding an FALS-associated mutation in the SOD1 gene (mFALS mice) are born and develop normally but then experience an adult-onset motor neuron disease and die within 4–7 months (Gurney et al., 1994). These mice express normal amounts of murine SOD1 in addition to the mutated human enzyme, suggesting the hypothesis that in this model motor neuron disease can arise from a toxic gain of function. Studies on mFALS mice have provided important insights into the pathophysiology of ALS. Histological studies have shown abnormalities in motor neuron morphology, but no loss of axons prior to any behavioral evidence of weakness. Dal Canto and Gurney (1994) noted abnormal inclusions in mice at 73 days, but no axon dropout. Similarly, Kong and Xu (1998) found degeneration of mitochondria within motor neurons prior to symptomatic weakness, but no loss of axons in ventral roots until animals began to rapidly decline in strength.

Correspondence to: Dr. Jeremy Shefner, Department of Neurology, 750 E. Adams St., HSC Syracuse, Syracuse, NY 13210, USA. Tel.: 315-464-4627, Fax: 315-464-5006. e-mail: shefnerj@upstate.edu

doi: 10.1016/S1567-424X(03)00035-7

Motor unit number estimation (MUNE) provides a unique tool to correlate physiological and histological changes in this model. With MUNE, both total number of motor neurons innervating a muscle group and changes that might occur within a motor unit may be repeatedly assessed prior to and during the course of disease. This is potentially useful not only in identifying events that eventually lead to behavioral consequences, but also in determining the effects of experimental therapeutic agents. In this paper, two methods of MUNE in the mouse model will be described. Results in wild-type mice will be presented, followed by a summary of data on mice with mFALS as well as a related form of motor nerve degeneration.

Methods

The studies to be described were performed on normal mice, mice hemizygous for the FALS mutation, mice homozygous for the FALS mutation, and mice with targeted inactivation of the SOD1 gene (SOD1 knockout mice or SOD1-KO). The hemizygous mFALS mice carried a human transgene with a missense mutation substituting alanine for glycine at codon 93 (G93A). Animals homozygous for the transgene were bred at the Massachusetts General Hospital from the hemizygous animals described above. These animals have more rapidly progressive disease, with earlier mean onset and death. SOD1-KO mice were bred at Cephalon Inc. (Reaume et al., 1996).

mFALS mice were studied four times, starting at day 60 and approximately every 20 days thereafter. As SOD1-KO mice have a much longer lifespan, their studies were more dispersed, as discussed below. Animals were also observed behaviorally to determine onset of disease. This assessment was somewhat subjective, but included speed of movement, posture while being held inverted, and grip strength. Mice were anesthetized with sodium pentobarbital (5 mg/ml) injected intraperitoneally at a dose of 50 mg/kg body weight. The abdomen and distal hindlimbs were shaved, and animals were taped prone to a Styrofoam board. The stimulating electrodes were 0.7 mm needles insulated with Teflon. The cathode was placed close to the sciatic nerve at the proximal thigh, and the anode was placed subcutaneously 1 cm proximally. Motor responses were recorded from a pregelled, self-adhesive surface recording strip cut to a length of 1.5 cm and a width of about 0.5 cm. This electrode was placed circumferentially around the animal's distal hindlimb and thus recorded activity in both flexor and extensor compartments. The reference electrode was a monopolar needle placed subcutaneously in the foot, 1.5–2 cm distal to the recording electrode. Distance between stimulating and recording electrodes was 1.2–1.6 cm. Both the right and left hindlimbs were studied.

Stimuli were 0.1 ms monophasic pulses of constant current delivered through a constant current stimulator with fine intensity control. Recordings were made through motor amplifiers for off-line analysis. Filter settings were 500 Hz and 5 kHz.

Incremental stimulation MUNE technique was performed at a standard amplifier gain using a modification of the technique described by McComas (McComas et al., 1971; Dantes and McComas, 1991). Using a repetition rate of 1/s, stimulus intensity was slowly increased from subthreshold levels until a small, all-or-none response was evoked. The stability of this response was established by observing the identical response three to four times. The response was then accepted and recorded digitally. The intensity was slowly increased until the response increased in a quantal fashion. The increased response was again observed for stability before a tracing was accepted for analysis. This process was repeated for a total of 10 increments. After 10 increments, a supramaximal compound muscle action potential (CMAP) response was obtained. This response was used to calculate distal motor latency, as well as the maximum CMAP amplitude (measured peak-to-peak). Individual motor unit amplitudes were obtained by subtracting amplitudes of each response from that of the prior response. The individual values were averaged to yield an estimate of average single motor unit action potential (SMUP) amplitude. This value was divided into the peak-to-peak amplitude of the maximum CMAP to yield the MUNE value.

To perform multiple point stimulation (MPS) MUNE (Brown and Milner-Brown, 1976), the supramaximal response was obtained in a manner identical to that described above. Individual motor unit responses were obtained by moving the stimulating electrode and isolating threshold responses with distinct morphologies. Given the small size of the animals, the length of nerve available for stimulation was restricted, but 5–6 individual motor unit responses could usually be elicited. Peak-to-peak amplitude was determined, and averaged to yield the average SMUP amplitude.

Results

MUNE in normal mice

Twenty-nine limbs from 15 normal mice were studied (Shefner et al., 1999). The mean distal motor latency was 1.42 ± 0.17 ms; the distance between the stimulus and recording electrodes varied between 1.2 and 1.6 cm. The mean supramaximal CMAP amplitude was 10.32 ± 2.14 mV. Despite the fact that recordings were made from multiple muscle groups simultaneously, an initial negative phase response was almost always observed, implying proximity to the motor points.

An example of a normal supramaximal CMAP is shown in Fig. 1, with incremental responses from which motor unit estimation was performed. In this

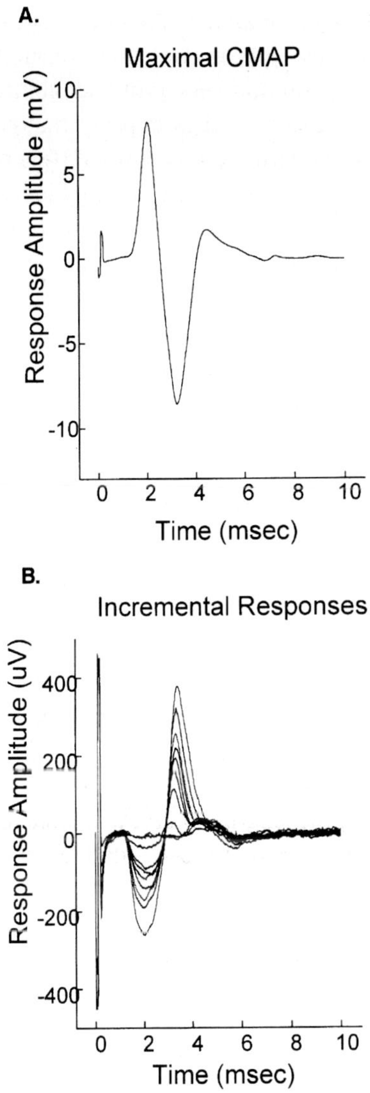

Fig. 1. Incremental MUNE for wildtype mouse. (A) Maximum compound motor action potential (CMAP). (B) Incremental responses starting from threshold levels. From: Shefner et al. (1999), with permission.

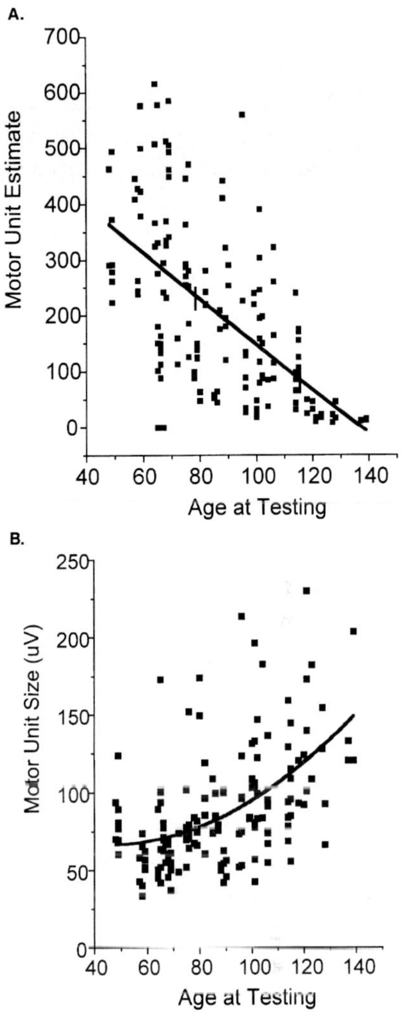

Fig. 2. Changes in MUNE (A) and SMUP amplitude (B) as a function of age in mFALS mice. Data are presented from 24 mice. Values are calculated for both hindlimbs, then averaged for each animal. The solid vertical lines denote average onset of behavioral abnormalities and average age at death. The data are fit to a second order polynomial regression model. From Shefner et al. (2001a), with permission.

mouse, stimulus increments produced additive responses without a significant latency shift. For 15 normal animals, the mean MUNE was 310 ± 100 with an average SMUP of 69 ± 19 μV.

MUNE in mFALS mice

Fig. 2 shows changes in MUNE and SMUP size as a function of age, using the incremental stimulation technique (Shefner et al., 2001a). From a normal value, MUNE fell rapidly, and by clinical onset, had dropped by 31%. The concomitant rise in SMUP amplitude was delayed; by the time of clinical onset, amplitude was increased by only 15% over baseline. CMAP fell nearly linearly throughout the entire period of study (Fig. 3), dropping by 25% by the time of clinical onset.

These data show striking similarities in the physiological properties of motor neurons and the

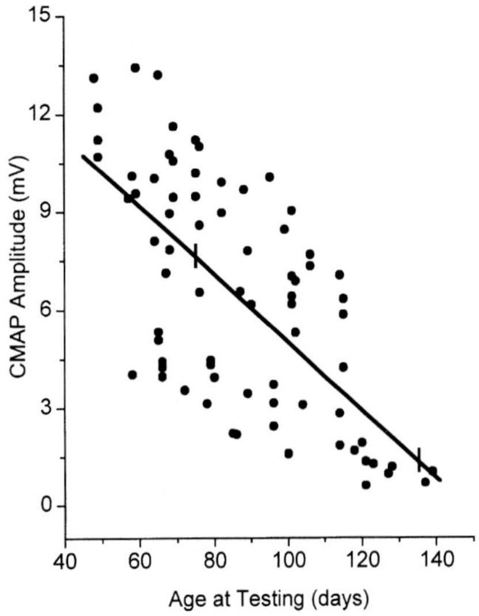

Fig. 3. Compound motor action potential changes with age in mFALS mice. Data are presented from 24 mice. CMAPs are calculated for both hindlimbs, then averaged for each animal. Vertical lines are as in Fig. 1. Data are fit to a second-order polynomial regression model. From Shefner et al. (2001a), with permission.

motor units in mFALS mice and humans with ALS. In humans, it is difficult to obtain clear description of the physiological changes in the motor neuron before the disease is clinically apparent; however, MUNE progressively declines as the disease progresses, while MUS increases in response to axon loss. In the mouse model, CMAP, MUNE, and SMUP amplitude are normal prior to disease onset. Mice begin to show behavioral abnormalities at approximately 11 weeks of age; by that time, MUNE has already decreased from normal values by approximately 30%. While CMAP amplitude is preserved in ALS patients until well into the course of the disease (Dantes and McComas, 1991; Felice, 1997; Yuen and Olney, 1997), amplitude drops in the mFALS mice by the time any behavioral abnormality is seen. This difference between human and mouse studies almost certainly reflects the rapidity of the murine disease process. In both diseases, MUNE drops rapidly after symptom onset, while MUS increases, often with a delay.

In contrast to histological studies, a drop-out in numbers of motor neurons is seen beginning at or prior to 60 days of age, significantly before the onset of any signs of weakness. As noted above, histological studies appear to show normal motor neuron and axon numbers until after clinical weakness has appeared. It thus appears that there is a physiological disruption of axonal function that precedes motor neuron cell death and loss of motor neuron cell bodies and axons. This discontinuity likely reflects a disparity between the physiological properties of a degenerating axon and its histological status and serves as a caveat that a full understanding of the pathophysiology of motor neuron degeneration requires both electrophysiological and histological analysis.

Comparison of incremental and multiple point stimulation MUNE

In a small number of animals, both incremental and MPS MUNE were performed concurrently as disease progressed (Shefner et al., 2001b). This was done partially to serve as an internal validation of method, as well as to provide insight into differences that might exist between the two methods. MUNE from both incremental and MPS techniques declined monotonically from day 60 (Fig. 4). The incremental technique yielded estimates approximately 10% lower than the MPS technique early in the course of the disease, with the difference becoming less as the number of motor units declined. Similarly, SMUP amplitude was lower as calculated using the MPS technique compared with the incremental method.

Correlation coefficients relating MUNE and SMUP values from the two methods were 0.71 for SMUP amplitude and 0.95 for MUNE ($P<0.001$ for both comparisons). Thus, both incremental and MPS MUNE methods yield similar absolute results and change in a similar fashion in mFALS mice. A tendency was noted throughout the disease course for the MPS technique to estimate smaller SMUP amplitudes than the incremental technique, although this trend was less apparent at very low MUNEs. This suggests that, in general, the first motor unit recruited with electrical stimulation is smaller than other units with higher electrical thresholds. However, the differences are quite small, and do not speak to the relative merit of the two methods.

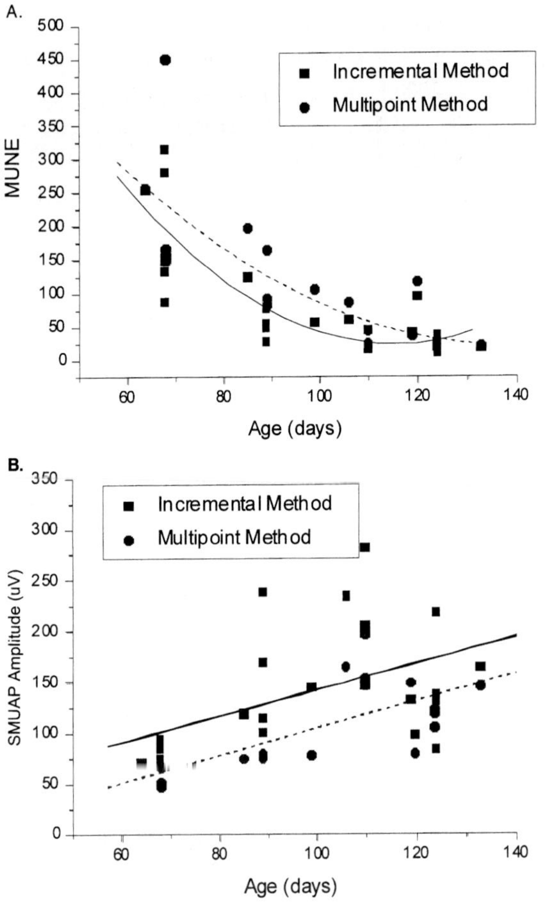

Fig. 4. Change in MUNE (A) and SMUP amplitude (B) over time using both multiple point and incremental techniques. Curves are second order polynomial functions fit to the data; dashed line is fit to the multiple point data, solid line to the incremental data. From Shefner et al. (2001b), with permission.

Assessing efficacy of experimental therapeutic agents with MUNE

Neurophilin ligands are small molecule compounds that promote neurite outgrowth in vitro and improve outcomes in vivo in animal models of traumatic nerve injury, diabetic neuropathy, toxin-induced neuropathy, spinal cord injury, and Parkinson disease (Costantini et al., 1998; Madsen et al., 1998; Costantini and Isacson, 2000a,b). Two similar neurophilin ligands were administered to mFALS mice to determine whether they had any effect of survival or disease progression (Shefner et al., 2001a). Mice were treated with either V-13,670 or V-10,367 by oral gavage, five times weekly starting at day 30 of life. Untreated littermates served as controls. Studies were performed at two different dose levels (26.5 and 53 mg/kg/day for V-10,367, and 39.5 and 79 mg/kg/day for V-13,670), each of which had separate control groups.

Incremental MUNE technique was performed on all animals between 50 and 120 days of age. MUNE in animals treated with V-13,670 declined at the same rate as the control animals (Fig. 5), with no dose effect noted. However, a dose related effect of V-13,670 was seen on motor unit size. SMUAPs increased more rapidly in treated animals, and reached a greater ultimate size ($P < 0.001$). For animals treated with V-10,367, neither the decline in MUNE or the increase in SMUPs showed significant changes.

The observation that a neurophilin ligand increased motor unit size is consistent with previous reports from in vitro studies documenting that these compounds augment the outgrowth of neurites (Gold et al., 1997). SMUP amplitude should be a direct reflection of the ability of the terminal axon to sprout. In this model, however, such a change did not prove beneficial. One might anticipate that a treatment that enhances the capacity of the ALS motor neuron to sprout might slow the overall process of motor neuron degeneration and death. On the other hand, one could also speculate that forced sprouting of the dying motor neuron might have an overall adverse effect on rate of death of the cell. In this study, the dose-dependent increase in motor unit size produced by one of the agents was neither beneficial nor detrimental clinically. The absence of clear survival benefit suggests that the rapid, aggressive course of motor neuron disease in these mice overwhelms any potential benefit of terminal sprouting.

MUNE in SOD1-KO mice

Given that mutations in the human gene for SOD1 are responsible for some forms of familial ALS, the effect of complete removal of SOD1 on the motor system is of some interest. Mice with targeted inactivation of the SOD1 gene (SOD1 knockout mice or SOD1-KO) live at least

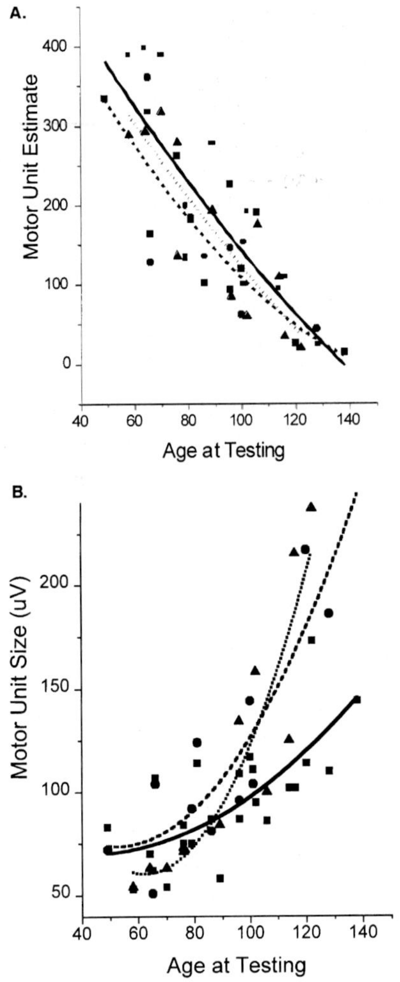

Fig. 5. Changes in MUNE (A) and SMUP amplitude (B) with time for control animals and animals treated with two dose levels of a neurophilin ligand. MUNE is calculated for both hindlimbs, then averaged for each animal. Data were obtained from 24 control animals and 12 animals from each dose level. Squares are from control animals, circles are from the low dose, and triangles are from the high dose. From Shefner et al. (2001a), with permission.

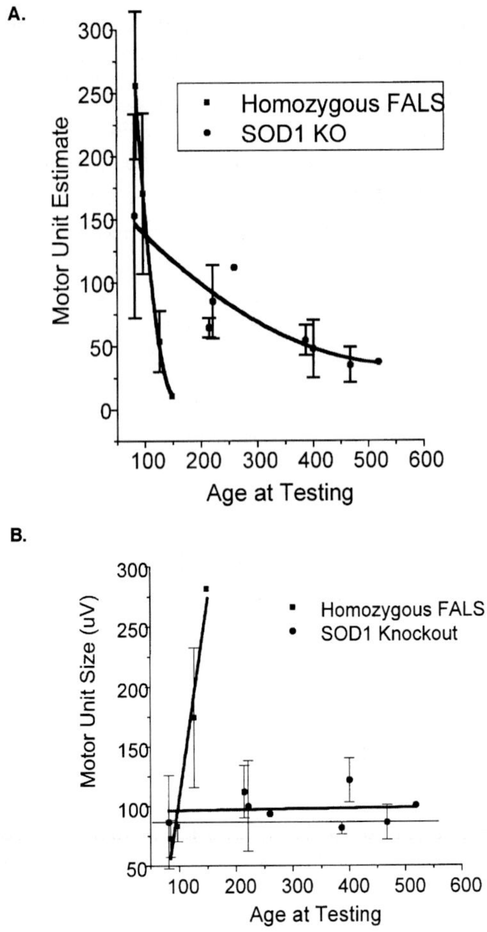

Fig. 6. MUNE (A) and SMUP amplitude (B) changes with age for mFALS mice and SOD1-KO mice. From Shefner et al. (1999), with permission.

18 months (Reaume et al., 1996). They display normal motor behavior in the first 3–4 months but show evidence of subtle motor impairment by six months of age. Thus, although SOD1-KO mouse is not a good model of human ALS, their motor deficits suggest that a loss of SOD1 function may also be relevant to motor neuron degeneration.

Incremental stimulation MUNE was performed in 19 SOD1-KO mice aged 82–518 days (Shefner et al., 1999). MUNE and SMUP amplitude changes were quite distinct from both wildtype and mFALS mice. At the earliest time point (Fig. 6), MUNE was significantly reduced from normal. With time, further reductions were seen, but at a rate significantly slower than that observed in the mFALS animals. SMUP amplitude was mildly increased as compared to wild type; however, no changes were seen with age to indicated continued terminal reinnervation; that is, there was no tendency for increased SMUP amplitude with continued decline in MUNE.

Thus, MUNE studies suggest a slowly progressive loss of motor unit function, without significant distal reinnervation. Interestingly, morphometric counts of motor neurons in the ventral horns or

SOD1-KO mice show an increase in the number of small neurons, but normal total neuron counts, suggesting a distal locus of pathology. Consistent with this hypothesis, muscle biopsies show mild denervation as early as two months of age. This is more evident at 4–6 months (Reaume et al., 1996; Flood et al., 1999). Axons approaching the neuromuscular junction are abnormally tortuous, suggesting involvement of the distal axon. Proximal axons in the ventral root are normal in number at 6 and 17 months, although some shrunken axons are present.

Summary

MUNE studies in mice with motor system degeneration has proven useful in characterizing the pathophysiology of disease processes, and can provide important information about how potential therapeutic agents affect the motor system. Potential new applications include the study of MUNE changes with stem cell transplantation, as well as study of other pharmacological agents. MUNE is also adaptable to other animal models of motor neuron disease, widening its application in the study of new therapies for ALS.

References

Brown, W.F. and Milner-Brown, H.S. Some electrical properties of motor units and their effects on the methods of estimating motor unit numbers. *J. Neurol. Neurosurg. Psychiatry*, 1976, 39: 249–257.

Costantini, L.C. and Isacson, O. Immunophilin ligands and GDNF enhance neurite branching or elongation from developing dopamine neurons in culture. *Exp. Neurol.*, 2000a, 161: 60–70.

Costantini, L.C. and Isacson, O. Neuroimmunophilin ligand enhances neurite outgrowth and effect of fetal dopamine transplants. *Neuroscience.*, 2000b, 100: 515–520.

Costantini, L.C., Chaturvedi, P., Armistead, D.M., McCaffrey, P.G., Deacon, T.W. and Isacson, O. A novel immunophilin ligand: distinct branching effects on dopaminergic neurons in culture and neurotrophic actions after oral administration in an animal model of Parkinson's disease. *Neurobiol. Dis.*, 1998, 5: 97–106.

Dal Canto, M.C. and Gurney, M.E. Development of central nervous system pathology in a murine transgenic model of human amyotrophic lateral sclerosis. *Am. J. Pathol.*, 1994, 145: 1271–1279.

Dantes, M. and McComas, A. The extent and time course of motoneuron involvement in amyotrophic lateral sclerosis. *Muscle Nerve*, 1991, 7: 416–421.

Felice, K.J. A longitudinal study comparing thenar motor unit number estimates to other quantitative tests in patients with amyotrophic lateral sclerosis. *Muscle Nerve*, 1997, 20: 179–185.

Flood, D.G., Reaume, A.G., Gruner, J.A., Hoffman, E.K., Hirsch, J.D., Lin, Y.G., Dorfman, K.S. and Scott, R.W. Hindlimb motor neurons require Cu/Zn superoxide dismutase for maintenance of neuromuscular junctions. *Am. J. Pathol.*, 1999, 155: 663–672.

Gold, B., Zeleny-Pooley, M., Wang, M., Chaturvedi, P. and Armistead, D. A nonimmunosuppressant FKBP-12 ligand increases nerve regeneration. *Exp. Neurol.*, 1997, 147: 269–278.

Gurney M.E., Pu H., Chiu A.Y., Dal Canto M.C., Polchow C.Y., Alexander D.D., Caliendo J., Hentati A., Kwon Y.W., Deng H.X. et al. Motor neuron degeneration in mice that express a human Cu,Zn superoxide dismutase mutation [see comments] [published erratum appears in Science 1995 Jul 14; 269(5221): 149]. *Science*, 1994, 264: 1772–1775.

Kong, J. and Xu, Z. Massive mitochondrial degeneration in motor neurons triggers the onset of amyotrophic lateral sclerosis in mice expressing a mutant SOD1. *J. Neurosci.*, 1998, 18: 3241–3250.

Madsen, J.R., MacDonald, P., Irwin, N., Goldberg, D.E., Yao, G.L., Meiri, K.F., Rimm, I.J., Stieg, P.E. and Benowitz, L.I. Tacrolimus (FK506) increases neuronal expression of GAP-43 and improves functional recovery after spinal cord injury in rats. *Exp. Neurol.*, 1998, 154: 673–683.

McComas, A., Fawcett, P., Campbell, M. and Sica, R. Electrophysiological estimation of the number of motor units within a human muscle. *J. Neurol. Neurosurg. Psychiatry.*, 1971, 34: 121–131.

Reaume, A., Elliott, J., Hoffman, E., Kowall, N., Ferrante, R., Siwek, D., Wilcox, H., Flood, D., Beal, F., Brown, R., Scott, R. and Snider, W. Motor neurons in Cu/Zn superoxide dismutase deficient mice develop normally but exhibit enhanced cell death after axonal injury. *Nat. Genet.*, 1996, 13: 43–47.

Rosen D.R., Siddique T., Patterson D., Figlewicz D.A., Sapp P., Hentati A., Donaldson D., Goto J., O'Regan J.P., Deng H. X. et al. Mutations in Cu/Zn superoxide dismutase gene are associated with familial amyotrophic lateral sclerosis [published erratum appears in Nature 1993 Jul 22; 364(6435): 362] [see comments]. *Nature*, 1993, 362: 59–62.

Shefner, J.M., Reaume, A.G., Flood, D.G., Scott, R.W., Kowall, N.W., Ferrante, R.J., Siwek, D.F., Upton-Rice, M. and Brown, R.H. Jr. Mice lacking cytosolic copper/zinc superoxide dismutase display a distinctive motor axonopathy. *Neurology*, 1999, 53: 1239–1246.

Shefner J., Brown R.J., Cole D., Chaturvedi P., Schoenfeld D., Pastuszak K., R.M., Upton-Rice M., Cudkowicz M. Effect of neurophilin ligands on motor units in mice with SOD1 ALS mutations. *Neurology* 2001, 57: 1857–1861.

Shefner J., Cudkowicz M., Brown R., Jr. A comparison of incremental with multipoint MUNE methods in transgenic ALS mice. *Muscle Nerve*, 2002, 25: 39–42.

Yuen, E.C. and Olney, R.K. Longitudinal study of fiber density and motor unit number estimate in patients with amyotrophic lateral sclerosis. *Neurology*, 1997, 49: 573–578.

Motor Unit Number Estimation (Supplements to Clinical Neurophysiology Vol. 55)
Editor: M.B. Bromberg

Chapter 36

MUNE by intraneural microstimulation: animal studies

Keisuke Arasaki*

EMG/EEG Laboratory, Department of Neurology, NTT Kanto Medical Center, 5-9-22 Higashi-Gotanda, Shinagawa-ku, Tokyo 141-0022, Japan

Introduction

Motor unit number estimation (MUNE) is based on obtaining a value representing the activity of all motor units in a muscle and then a value representing the average activity of a unitary motor unit, and dividing the former by the latter. There are at least nine techniques of obtaining unitary motor units from which to derive an average. There are several methods to calculate the average unitary motor unit. These techniques are based upon recording the electrical activity of motor units, but the mechanical activity or tension of motor units can also be used to calculate MUNE values.

Animal experiments are useful for evaluating the validity of different techniques for obtaining unitary motor units and comparing MUNE values to actual alpha motor neuron counts. Several studies have counted alpha motor neurons, but none have compared anatomical counts to MUNE values (Eisen et al., 1974; Peyronnard and Lamarre, 1977). The goals of our animal study were to derive MUNE values by electrophysiological and mechanical techniques and to compare values to anatomical counts of alpha motor neurons. In addition, we assessed two methods of calculating the average unitary motor unit.

Methods

Physiologic MUNE in the rat medial gastrocnemius muscle

Details of the experimental methods have been published elsewhere (Arasaki et al., 1997). Sixteen Sprague–Dawley (S–D) female rats (8–9 weeks of age) were anesthetized by intraperitoneal administration of urethane (700 mg/kg). The fifth lumbar ventral root was exposed and teased fiber techniques were used to isolate filaments containing single functionally intact alpha motor axons innervating the medial gastrocnemius (MG) muscle. The criterion for isolating a single motor axon was an all-or-none response to antidromic nerve action potentials evoked by electrical shocks to the MG motor nerve. Isolated single axons were stimulated orthodromically to obtain unitary or single muscle action potentials (SMAPs) and twitch tensions. The maximal compound muscle action potential (CMAP) and twitch tension of the muscle was also obtained (Fig. 1).

Surface EMG recordings were made with two chloride-coated silver ball-point electrodes attached to the belly of the muscle and connected to a differential amplifier. Mechanical tension was recorded simultaneously by a strain gauge connected to a

**Correspondence to*: Dr. Keisuke Arasaki, EMG/EEG Laboratory, Department of Neurology, NTT Kanto Medical Center, 5-9-22 Higashi-Gotanda, Shinagawa-ku, Tokyo 141-0022, Japan. Tel.: 81-3-3448-6455; Fax: 81-3-3448-6458.
e-mail: arasaki@rr.iij4u.or.jp

doi: 10.1016/S1567-424X(03)00036-9

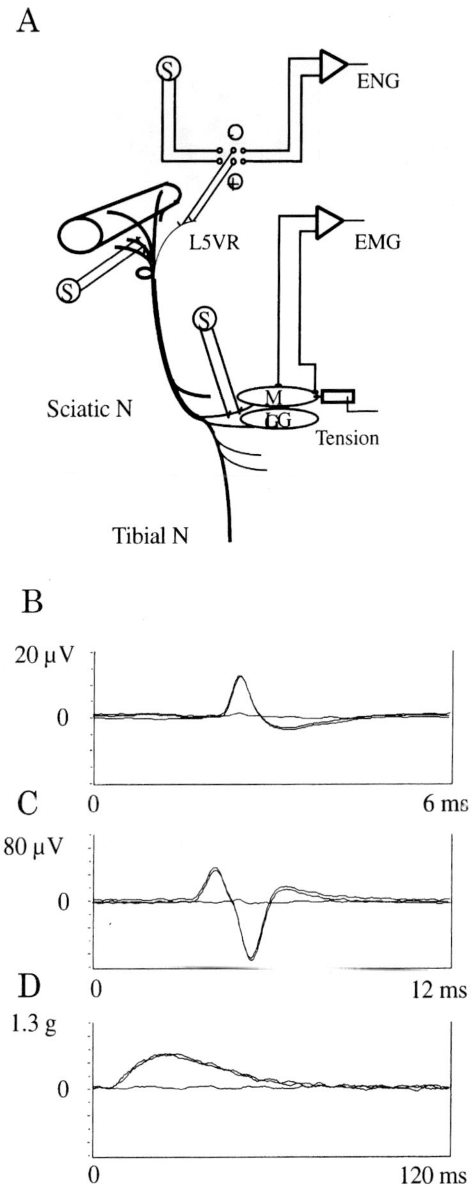

Fig. 1. Diagram of experimental setups used to record the unitary MAP and muscular tension, as well as the maximal CMAP and tension of the rat MG muscle. As shown in (A), L5 and L6 ventral roots were mutually stimulated to obtain the maximal CMAP of the MG muscle. The MG muscle nerve was then stimulated. A bipolar electrode placed on a dissected ventral root filament was used to record the unitary antidromic action potential occurring in the all-or-none manner, as shown in (B). (C) shows the unitary MAP evoked by stimulation of the dissected single axon and recorded by a bipolar electrode placed on the muscle belly. (D) is a sample recording of the unitary muscle twitch tension produced by stimulation of the same single MG axon.

DC amplifier. Negative peak areas of the unitary MAP and the maximal CMAP were determined. Electrophysiologic MUNE values were obtained by dividing the area of the maximal CMAP by the mean unitary MAP. Similarly, the maximal tension curve was divided by the mean unitary tension in order to acquire a mechanical MUNE value.

Morphological determination of the number of spinal alpha motoneurons innervating the MG muscle

Ten S–D female rats of the same age were anesthetized with the intraperitoneal injection of pentobarbital (50 mg/kg). Under the aseptic condition, the fascia of the MG muscle was impaled with a glass micropipette filled with a fresh solution of 0.5% cholera toxin subunit B (CTB), and 2 µl of the CTB solution was injected into the muscle by air pressure. The muscle fascia was then covered with glue. One week later, the rats were sacrificed and perfused transcardially with physiologic saline, followed by 300 ml of 10% formaldehyde and 0.2% glutaraldehyde in 0.1 M phosphate buffer. The spinal cord of the first to the sixth lumbar segments was removed and 40 µm-thick serial sections were stained by Vectastain ABC kit (Vector Labs Inc., USA). MG motoneurons were identified by the presence of retrograde transport of CTB in their cell bodies when the entire nuclei were visible. Alpha motoneurons were differentiated from gamma ones by the larger area of their somas, and only alpha motoneurons were counted.

Results

Electrophysiologic and mechanical MUNEs

The average areas of unprocessed unitary MAPs was 2.6 ± 0.6 (mean ± SD) mV ms, and the average areas of the digitally averaged unitary MAPs was 1.6 ± 0.4 mV ms. The average area of the maximal CMAPs was 148.0 ± 29.4 mV ms, leading to an average electrophysiologic MUNE value from unprocessed unitary MAPs of 57 ± 11, and an average value from digitally averaged MAPs of 93 ± 22

TABLE 1

MUNE VALUES OBTAINED BY THREE DIFFERENT METHODS: UNPROCESSED EMG, DIGITALLY AVERAGED EMG, AND MECHANICAL TENSION

Methods	N	MUNE
MUNE by the unprocessed unitary MAP	7	57 ± 11^a
MUNE by the averaged unitary MAP	7	93 ± 22^b
MUNE by tension	7	117 ± 21^b
Number of SA motor neurons	4	103 ± 16

The number of spinal alpha motoneurons innervating the MG muscle is shown at the bottom of the table. Note that the MUNE values by the digitally averaged EMG and mechanical tension methods are not significantly different from the actual number of spinal alpha (SA) motorneurons (Mann–Whitney test, $P > 0.2$)
[a] $P < 0.01$ (Mann–Whitney test).
[b] $P > 0.2$ (Mann–Whitney test).

(Table 1). The average areas of the unitary tension recordings was 19.8 ± 5.0 gms, while the average maximal tension was 1822.7 ± 392.9 gms, leading to an average mechanical MUNE of 117 ± 22. The tension MUNE values were significantly larger than the MUNE values from unprocessed MAPs (paired t-test, $P < 0.01$), but not statistically different from MUNE values from digitally averaged MAPs (paired t-test, $P > 0.05$) (Table 1).

Morphological alpha motoneuron counts

The cross sectional soma areas of MG spinal motoneurons showed a bimodal distribution, and somas greater than 600 μm^2 were counted as alpha motoneurons (Fig. 2). The average alpha motoneuron number was 103 ± 16 ($n = 4$, Table 1).

MUNE comparisons

Electrophysiologic MUNE values by unprocessed MAPs was statistically smaller than by anatomical counting (Mann–Whitney test, $P < 0.01$). MUNE values by tension and digitally averaged MAPs were not statistically different from the anatomical number (Mann–Whitney test, $P > 0.2$) (Table 1).

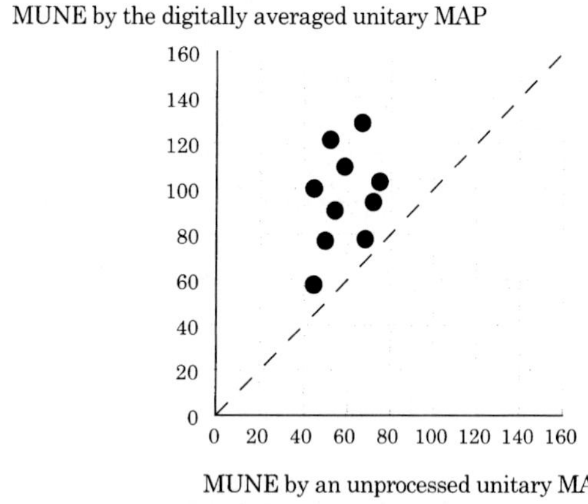

Fig. 2. Scattergram showing the relationship between the MUNE obtained by the digitally averaged unitary MAP and that obtained by unprocessed unitary MAPs. A filled circle represents each rat from which these MUNEs were obtained. The abscissa and the ordinate show the MUNE by unprocessed unitary MAPs and that by the digitally averaged unitary MAP, respectively. Note that all filled circles are located above the dotted line showing the relationship of $y = x$.

Discussion

This study is unique because it compares motor unit estimates based on electrical and mechanical recordings from isolated single units with anatomical motor neuron counts (Arasaki et al., 1997). A previous study compared the incremental stimulation MUNE technique (McComas et al., 1971) with anatomical motor neuron counts and found a statistically different difference between the two methods different ($P < 0.03$, Mann–Whitney test) (Peyronnard and Lamarre, 1977). Another comparison study estimated the number of alpha motor axons by counted the number of motor nerve axons and assumed that alpha motor axons comprised 50% of the larger myelinated fibers (Eisen et al., 1974).

We obtained MUNE values by three different methods. All were immune to the problem of alternation (McComas, 1998) because we stimulated isolated motor axons innervating the MG muscle. However, the electrophysiologic MUNE based on unprocessed MAPs was subject to the problem of phase cancellation (Stein and Yang, 1990) because the waveforms were not monophasic. As shown in Table 1, this electrophysiologic MUNE was

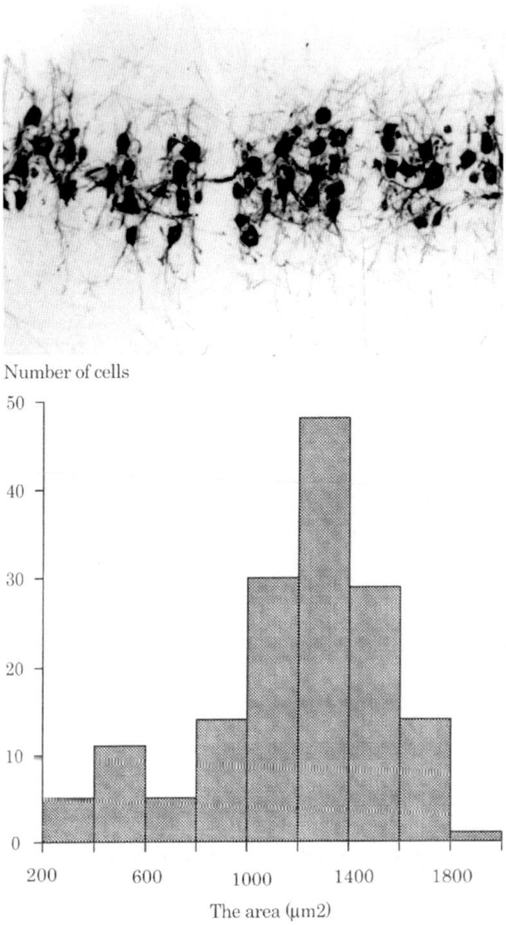

Fig. 3. (A) Photomicrographs of a sagittal spinal cord section. The MG motoneurons containing the cholera toxin were stained by the immunohistochemical method (see text for details). Magnification ×200. (B) A histogram of the area of the somata of the labeled spinal motoneurons shows its bimodal distribution. Larger ones with an area of 800 μm^2 or more most likely represent alpha motoneurons.

significantly smaller than MUNE by tension, probably because of phase cancellation. On the other hand, the MUNE by digitally processed MAPs was statistically not different from that by tension, which suggested that phase cancellation was overcome by computer averaging of the MAP waveforms (Fig. 3).

According to Hashizume (Hashizume et al., 1988), the number of MG alpha motoneurons in 5 month-old Fisher rats is 98 ± 2. There is good agreement, except for a smaller SD, with our results 118 ± 18 MG alpha motoneurons (Table 1). MUNE values by tension and digitally averaged waveforms were not statistically different from the anatomic numbers, and they are probably better estimates of the motor unit number than that by electrophysiological methods. In most clinical neurophysiology laboratories, it is impractical to record tension of a muscle for obtaining MUNEs. Therefore, we recommend that unitary MAPs be obtained by computer averaging when calculating MUNE values.

References

Arasaki, K., Tamaki, M., Hosoya, Y. and Kudo, N. Validity of electromyograms and tension as a means of motor unit number estimation. *Muscle Nerve*, 1997, 20: 552–560.

Eisen, A., Karpati, G., Carpenter, S. and Danon, J. The motor unit profile of the rat soleus in experimental myopathy and reinnervation. *Neurology*, 1974, 24: 878–884.

Hashizume, K., Kanda, K. and Burke, R.E. Medial gastrocnemius motor nucleus in the rat: age-related changes in the number and size of motoneurons. *J. Comp. Neurol.*, 1988, 269: 425–430.

McComas, A.J. Motor units: how many, how large, what kind?. *J. Electromyogr. Kinesiol.*, 1998, 8: 391–402.

McComas, A.J., Fawcett, P.R.W., Campbell, M.J. and Sica, R. E.P. Electrophysiological estimation of the number of motor units within a human muscle. *J. Neurol. Neurosurg. Psychiatry*, 1971, 34: 121–131.

Peyronnard, J.-M. and Lamarre, Y. Electrophysiological and anatomical estimation of the number of motor units in the monkey extensor digitorum brevis muscle. *J. Neurol. Neurosurg. Psychiatry.*, 1977, 40: 756–764.

Stein, R.B. and Yang, J.F. Methods for estimating the number of motor units in human muscles. *Ann. Neurol.*, 1990, 28: 487–495.

Discussion after Section X

Benn Smith, Scottsdale, Arizona

I have a question for Ken. Having performed motor unit counts in the central nervous system in a similar preparation, I understand the technical difficulties associated with serial sections and wanting to avoid counting one motor neuron twice. What methods did you use to ensure that did not happen?

Ken Arasaki, Tokyo, Japan

First, we identified sections that contained the nucleoli. There are formulae from the anatomical literature that take into account the depth of the section and the diameter of the nucleus. We counted only neurons with nucleoli on that particular section and multiplied that by the number of sections.

Benn Smith, Scottsdale, Arizona

So you used the statistical anatomic motor unit number estimation method!

Clifton Gooch, New York, New York

I have several questions for Jeremy. Am I correct that you reported that paralysis in your animals tended to begin when motor unit numbers dropped below a level of approximately 50? I am asking because that correlates with some of the data we have from the human studies regarding the development of clinical weakness. The other question relates to reinnervation. You noticed what appears to be a defect in reinnervation, but it also appears that during the time course of the study many animals did not fall below the 50 motor unit threshold. In our human data, which I will talk about later today, and Alan McComas' data from ALS patients, it seems that reinnervation really begins to take off when motor unit numbers fall to levels of 50–100 units. So, I am wondering if in the SOD mice, because of their slower loss of motor units, is this in part responsible for the lack of reinnervation seen?

Jeremy Shefner, Syracuse, New York

To the first question, you have to remember that these mice are not examined in the same way that people are examined. The first indication of weakness was a sense that they were not moving normally; falling off a rod, posturing when they are held up by their tail, etc. This is a very subjective measure that something is wrong, but you do not know quite what. The second indication that reflected hind-limb paralysis occurred when there were about 50 motor units remaining. I would be comfortable with a rough correlation between that and human studies, but nothing more than that. To the second question, if you compare the SMUP amplitude in the FALS transgenic mouse at the level of motor unit dropout that we saw with the SOD knockout mice, they had bigger motor units. Therefore, I do not think you can explain the lack of motor unit enlargement solely on the basis of the idea that the number of units had not dropped to a critical level. If you compare the two animal lines, at that point in time, the units had already started to reinnervate. In terms of the clinical state of the animals who had 50 units or so, they were not paralyzed, but they were clearly slow-moving. They could not hold onto a bar or hang upside down on the cage the way other mice did, but they were not paralyzed at that level of motor unit loss.

Alan McComas, Hamilton, Ontario

I have a comment on your point about the relationship between the size and the number of surviving motor units. We have looked at this in a number of muscles in ALS and, in every case, we find that the data points tend to form a rectangular hyperbola so that as the denervation becomes greater there is a progressive increase in the sizes of the surviving motor units. This relates to mean sizes because there is always quite a scatter. It seemed that the amount of reinnervation was always proportional to the numbers of denervated muscle fibers available for adoption.

Richard Lewis, Detroit, Michigan

Jeremy, I noticed in your slide that your highest amplitude motor units occurred after your fifth and sixth motor unit. We observed the same pattern with some of our SOD mice. My question is, were you dealing with a greater degree of alternation at that point, leading to a false estimate?

Jeremy Shefner, Syracuse, New York

I do not have an absolute answer to this question. I would be surprised if it were due to alternation because we take care that there is not a response within the jump. Alternatively, is there more of an electrical-size principle acting in animal nerves? There seems to be a tendency to see larger units later on in the incremental process. That was one reason that I compared the incremental with the multiple point stimulation technique, and may account for why the multiple point results are slightly greater in terms of total number of motor units.

Jasper Daube, Rochester, Minnesota

Ken, is your study the first to try to correlate a peripheral electrophysiologic measurement with an anatomic measurement of the number of anterior horn cells?

Ken Arasaki, Tokyo, Japan

Surprisingly, no one else has made the comparison.

Jasper Daube, Rochester, Minnesota

Jeremy, in human subjects, the variation in rate of progression of motor neuron loss makes a big difference in the degree of reinnervation. Are there differences in rates of progression among your animals? If so, does that account for some of the variation in your results?

Jeremy Shefner, Syracuse, New York

The disease in mice is much less variable human ALS. These animals died about 127 days plus-or-minus 7 days. On the other hand, early in the disease there seems to be some variability. I neglected to say that when I study animals, I always study both hind limbs. And so I will occasionally see animals where the units and counts look normal in one leg and are quite deficient in the other leg. But by the second time I examine them, which is usually 20 days later, they are very much equal so there seems to be a slight variability in onset, but they catch up to each other quite quickly. This could add to some of the variability.

Jasper Daube, Rochester, Minnesota

That leads me to another question. In human patients with ALS, Alan and Bill Brown nicely showed that there is an initial rapid loss followed by a much slower loss of motor neurons. Did you find the same thing in the animal model?

Jeremy Shefner, Syracuse, New York

I did not, and the reason might be that I am not recording from a single muscle group. I record from a large number of muscles at the same time, and that might average-out some of these changes.

Alan McComas, Hamilton, Ontario

If I could respond to Jasper Daube's first question. There was one quite important study comparing anatomical and electrophysiological estimates of motor unit numbers, and this was performed on the extensor digitorum muscle in the monkey in the 1970s by Peyronnard and Lamarre (J Neurol Neurosurg Psychiatry 1977, 40: 756–764). They looked at about 10 animals, and my recollection is that there was a very acceptable agreement between the result of the manual incremental estimate and the anatomical study. The one exception was an animal that inadvertently had partial denervation.

Ken Arasaki, Tokyo, Japan

I want to add that Peyronnard and Lamarre and others studied the number of larger myelinated nerve fibers after rhizotomy, but did not look into the number of motor neurons.

Section XI

MUNE Relationship with Industry and Regulatory Agencies

Motor Unit Number Estimation (Supplements to Clinical Neurophysiology Vol. 55)
Editor: M.B. Bromberg

Chapter 37

Software issues in MUNE

Mark B. Bromberg*

Department of Neurology, University of Utah, Salt Lake City, UT 84132, USA

Introduction

Motor unit number estimation (MUNE) is a unique tool that provides information not available by any other electrophysiological methodology, and has the potential to be used widely in clinical and research applications. However, there are impediments to expanding its usage. The original incremental stimulation MUNE technique could be performed on any EMG machine. The subsequent development of other MUNE techniques has led to a dependence upon special computer algorithms for data collection and analysis. Some algorithms are unique to a specific investigator, while others are unique to a specific EMG machine and constitute proprietary software. The impediments to free access to the spectrum of MUNE techniques have been frustrating to those interested in developing and promoting the field. This chapter will review the current status of MUNE software availability and the unique relationship between investigators and the EMG equipment industry. It will conclude with a set of suggested goals and directions for solutions. The opinions expressed represent the author's personal view.

**Correspondence to*: Dr. Mark Bromberg, Department of Neurology, University of Utah, 50 North Medical Drive, Salt Lake City, UT 84132, USA. Tel.: 801-581-6873. e-mail: mark.bromberg@hsc.utah.edu

doi: 10.1016/S1567-424X(03)00037-0

MUNE techniques and software requirements

MUNE techniques can be divided into three categories with respect to software needs (Table 1). Manual techniques require software that is available on most EMG machines as standard programs. Software-assisted techniques can be performed on most EMG machines, but can be facilitated with special software. Software-dependent techniques cannot be performed without special software.

Impediments limiting software availability

The majority of MUNE research is conducted on commercially available EMG machines by clinical neurophysiologists working in academic institutions. Investigators are hampered in their ability to purchase different EMG machines because they are expensive clinical diagnostic tools that are most commonly funded by the academic institution. Funds for EMG equipment oriented to research are limited. This impedes research on comparisons between different MUNE techniques. The ability of investigators to participate in multicenter collaborative projects and clinical trials is restricted if they do not have the EMG machine with the particular MUNE software selected for the study.

TABLE 1

MUNE TECHNIQUES AND THEIR DEPENDENCE UPON SPECIAL SOFTWARE

Software needs	MUNE techniques
Manual techniques	Manual incremental stimulation Multiple point stimulation Adapted multiple point Spike-triggered averaging Single motor unit tracking
Software-assisted techniques	F-wave Multiple point stimulation Adapted multiple point
Software-dependent techniques	Automated incremental stimulation Statistical Decomposition spike-triggered averaging Surface motor unit recording

Access to computer software programming expertise is frequently limited in clinical neurophysiology laboratories. It is challenging to find software specialists to forge ahead with new ideas, and research funds for such endeavors are limited. If specialists are available, MUNE software available on specific EMG machines is usually not documented in the manuals, and can not be readily accessed for modification.

From the perspective of EMG equipment companies, MUNE, at this time, represents an area of limited interest. Allocation of engineers to provide documentation or to make modifications is limited.

Challenges for EMG equipment companies

Given the basic dependence of academic neurophysiologists interested in MUNE research on commercially available EMG machines, the former must appreciate the challenges of equipment companies. EMG machines are designed for clinicians who focus on routine neuromuscular issues. Special quantitative EMG software, including MUNE, may not be a competitive commercial advantage at this time.

Hardware and software development is expensive for equipment manufacturers, and they must focus on the average electromyographer. It would be gratifying to academic clinicians if they felt that their research was contributing to the advancement of clinical neurophysiology. It has been difficult to fill the role of advisor to equipment manufacturers. Many EMG equipment companies represent subsidiaries of larger companies. As such, financial interests commonly take precedence over pursuing research into new methodologies.

Challenges for MUNE research

Given the basic dependence by academic clinical neurophysiologists interested on MUNE research on commercially available EMG machine, by mutatis mutandis, the latter must also appreciate the challenges of the former. Academic neurophysiologists have made numerous requests for additions or changes in MUNE software. The responses from EMG equipment companies have ranged widely, from no interest, to verbal interest, and to active participation.

Proposal for collaboration

A supportive relationship between academic clinical neurophysiologists and industry will be of benefit to everyone, and will advance the field of electromyography in general and MUNE in particular. Several areas for agreement and collaboration are presented.

Investigator agreement

There are issues related to MUNE that need to be discussed and worked out by investigators. EMG equipment companies should be consulted for lesser numbers of well-defined proposals as opposed to larger numbers of individual proposals.

Open MUNE software architecture

It would be advantageous for academic clinical neurophysiologists interested in advancing MUNE development to have access to MUNE software. In return, EMG equipment manufacturers could incorporate advances into their software packages.

Standard input/output formats

For academic EMG laboratories that have programming expertise, it would be advantageous to be able to use EMG machine as input/output devices for subsequent data analysis. Translation of EMG data output into a common format that can be read by commonly available programs would facilitate this (Jabre and Salzsieder, 2002).

Software and hardware availability

It would be ideal to make all MUNE techniques available to every investigator. Given the differences between EMG equipment, MUNE software based on universally available software programs would be desirable. An open architecture based on Microsoft Windows® is suggested for consideration. This would allow MUNE software to run on any PC computer. Standardization of input/output formats would permit the use of commercially available amplifiers and stimulators. A relatively inexpensive package of equipment could thus be assembled in any EMG laboratory.

Summary

The advantages of free access of electrophysiologic software are many; MUNE development will advance, industry can share in making the most usable techniques available to all clinical neurophysiologists, MUNE can be used as endpoint measures in clinical trials. It is hoped that this symposium which included participation from industry will represent a first step in this process.

References

Jabre, J. and Salzsieder, B. Defining extensible markup language standards for electromyography data transmission across the world-wide web. *Muscle and Nerve*, 2002 (Suppl. 11): S72–S76.

Motor Unit Number Estimation (Supplements to Clinical Neurophysiology Vol. 55)
Editor: M.B. Bromberg

Chapter 38

Product program development in industry

John Leedham*

1331 Tinsmith Lane, Oakville, ON LGM 3C8, Canada

Introduction

This article is to provide the EMG researcher and clinician with a more thorough understanding of the processes that industry follows to bring new products and applications to the EMG market. There are specific steps required to bring products to market, and after their initial release there are efforts to continue development of the products. These issues will be presented and discussed to help bring industry and research closer together.

Regulatory compliance

All companies selling medical diagnostic products into the U.S. market must comply with all regulations established by the Food and Drug Administration (FDA). There are similar regulatory agencies in place for Europe (CE Mark), Canada, Japan. Many countries accept the standards of the FDA or CE. These regulations are less stringent for "research" products.

A number of questions must be answered in order to attain regulatory approvals. They include:

- Does the device adhere to patient safety regulations?
- Has the system been appropriately tested and validated?
- Does the company comply with Good Manufacturing Processes (GMP)?
- Is the device substantially equivalent to another device or does it represent a newly emerging technology?

Product development process

Every medical device manufacturer has an established Quality Control program that oversees all aspects of product development, manufacturing and technical support. The quality assurance team develops guidelines and documentation for the product development process. Listed below is a generic product development process used by most medical device manufacturers.

1. Market analysis – This step documents a need for the product. During this stage of the process information about the market segment is collected via surveys, focus groups, feedback from field sales representatives, associations with leading academic centers and through other information channels. This information is analyzed and the following questions are asked:
   - Is there a market for the product?
   - Can a profit be made in this market segment? What is the return on investment?
   - Can the product pass regulatory approvals?

**Correspondence to*: John Leedham, Neuroscan, 18713 Potomac Station Drive, Leesburg, VA 20176, USA. Tel.: (703) 777-3957.
e-mail: JSLeedham@aol.com

doi: 10.1016/S1567-424X(03)00038-2

- Can we establish a meaningful point of difference compared to our competition?
- Does it fit with the philosophy of our company?

2. Planning the process – Once it is determined that the new product is a viable product and is a fit with the company's agenda the next step is to put together a plan to move the development forward. The following considerations are made:
   - What resources will be required verses the budgeted research and development budget?
   - Where in the product development schedule should this product be placed?
   - Planning within the strategic objectives of the company.

3. Designs input file – After the overall plan has been created the primary focus shifts to the creation of a design inputs file. This documentation is imperative in the process and ultimately defines the specifications that the market demands. This information is attained from:
   - Customer feedback
   - Competitive analysis
   - New trends in technology
   - A historical perspective
   - Evolving techniques and methods

4. Software development – Prior to the initiation of the software (and/or hardware) development all of the documentation in the design inputs file is reviewed. At this point in the process the following decisions are made:
   - Which features will be incorporated in the device?
   - What human factors considerations will be made? Examples of these considerations are: Screen layouts, colors, how it will interact with other user interface components, how many steps are needed to complete tasks.
   - Creation of the actual programming and incorporation of algorithms.

   During this stage of product development the engineering teams must be diligent in the documentation of all steps and changes that are made. It is estimated that for every hour of software programming time the software engineer spends 3 hours generating supporting documentation.

   Development continues until a specified "release target" has been attained. This target has previously been established as a logical break point in the development process.

5. Testing – Once a release candidate has been established the software must go through a rigorous testing procedure to ensure that a quality product will be shipped to the customer. Listed below is a typical testing procedure:
   - Initial, in-house, testing – During this stage of testing the product is reviewed and obvious errors are identified and corrected.
   - Validation – During this stage test scenarios are created and the product is put through a thorough test of all imaginable scenarios. Errors are identified and labeled for correction. Of particular importance in the diagnostic device market are: degree of accuracy, efficacy, robustness and stability of the product and ease of use.

   After all of the errors have been identified and corrected a "release candidate" is created which will be distributed to beta test sites.
   - Beta testing – The selection of beta test sites is crucial to the continued development of the product. Beta sites must be selected which are patient enough to tolerate minor inconveniences but objective enough to isolate and report any errors that were not identified in-house. Feedback from beta-test sites not only provides feedback with respect to errors, accuracy and ease of use but will often lead to constructive comments, which when incorporated lead to improvements in the final product.

6. Product release – After the product has been through the testing process it needs to be properly released to the market. There are many issues that must be addressed prior to the product being released to the end-user (electromyographer). These steps include:
   - Documentation – All supporting documentation that was generated during the previous

stages of development must be compiled and filed in such a fashion that a clear "paper trail" of all decisions, algorithms, analyses, feedback etc. can be followed.
- Preparation of User Manuals or updates to the existing manual must be completed. Any software releases must be properly prepared such that the software is burned to a CD and that it can be easily loaded from the CD to the instrument's computer by the end-user. Release notes must be created which accompany the product or upgraded version of the product. These release notes will inform the end-user of the "latest and greatest" features.
- Distribution – An accurate database of all end-users, serial numbers, model numbers and the ship-to addresses must be maintained. In order to distribute the product or upgrade to the installed base in an accurate and timely manner technical support staff must access this database to create mailing lists. The shipping department must then package all product and coordinate shipments such that the correct box goes to the correct end-user.
- Follow-up and technical support – Shortly after a new product or upgrade is released to the end-user it is important for the technical support team to follow-up with correspondence with the end-user to ensure successful installation of the product and to attain any valuable feedback from the market.
- Incorporation of customer feedback into the design inputs file – Any feedback is logged and filed into the design inputs file for future product development or enhancement

The above procedure provides a general overview of the process many medical device manufacturers around the world follow during the design, testing and manufacture of their devices.

Collaboration between the researcher and industry

Given the regulatory issues, rigid procedural parameters, product liability issues and industry's proprietary concerns that the medical device industry must work within, how can the relationship between industry and the research clinician be leveraged to best create and supply products that can assist with and enhance collaboration within areas such as MUNE and DQEMG?

Historical perspective

This has proven to be a very difficult hurdle to overcome. Manufacturer's form alliances whereby they provide the research community with sponsorship funding, test equipment, proprietary software programming and in return they receive exclusive rights to specific applications. Since these applications may not be the prime consideration of the end-user when purchasing new equipment the dispersion of the instruments into the market is limited to those end-users who purchase the proprietary hardware. This need for the manufacturer to have a competitive advantage over their competition becomes an impediment to new applications being widely used in the market.

Example 1: Access to "source" code

Some EMG companies have developed sufficiently secure relations with specific research teams that they have entrusted key components of the source code to the researcher. This, in conjunction with a non-competition and exclusive distribution agreement, allows the researcher to develop the new software applications(s) for research purposes on specific hardware. This type of arrangement allows the manufacturer to bring new applications and products to market quickly while minimizing expenditures. When using this type of arrangement the manufacturer typically assumes control of the distribution of the product and any inherent liabilities that may be associated with the product or it's operation on the manufacturer's hardware platform.

Example 2: Access to "source code" plus resource allocation

Using a strategy similar to Example 1, companies may go further and provide some financial assistance to the researchers to hire programming staff. This staff is overseen by the researcher but receives remuneration directly from the company on a contract basis. This strategy can be made into a win–win situation when the researcher hires graduate students as part of a work–study co-op program as the labor is less expensive, the researcher is familiar with the capabilities of the student and maintains direct control of the project.

Discussion

During the discussion that followed this topic at the MUNE Symposium suggestions were made by the research community that were constructive but were problematic for industry. Problems were typically due to liability concerns on the part of the manufacturer.

Proposed strategies

1. Open (generic) source – Creation of research applications using code that can read data files from many different manufacturer's instruments or that can read the real-time data stream from these instruments. The export of data in a common data format would be preferred by industry as it would not risk the release of proprietary code.
2. Software sharing – Sharing of software amongst the research community would allow for collaboration in areas of common interest and would minimize costs. The drawback to this strategy is the need for industry to maintain and track all devices in the field (regulatory concerns) and also that proprietary hardware would also be needed.

Conclusions

Industry recognizes the important and mutually fruitful relationship with research. There are challenging obstacles between an ideal for a feature on an EMG machine and its implementation that researchers must be aware of. It is hoped that this symposium was informative for industry to see what researchers are focusing on and the constraints that industry faces.

Motor Unit Number Estimation (Supplements to Clinical Neurophysiology Vol. 55)
Editor: M.B. Bromberg

Chapter 39

MUNE as an endpoint in clinical trials

Wilson W. Bryan*

Division of Clinical Trial Design and Analysis, Office of Therapeutics Research and Review, Center for Biologics Evaluation and Research, United States Food and Drug Administration, 1401 Rockville Pike, Room 230N, Rockville, MD 20852, USA

Introduction

Clinical trials in motor neuron disorders have traditionally used either survival or some measure of muscle strength as the primary endpoint. Survival is a clinically meaningful endpoint but generally requires long duration studies and large sample sizes if the treatment has only modest efficacy. Measures of muscle strength may be more sensitive than survival to disease progression but may also be more difficult to interpret clinically. Motor unit number estimation (MUNE) is a relatively new outcome measure with potential to serve as an endpoint in studies of interventions for motor neuron disorders. However, evaluation of MUNE as an endpoint requires consideration of the stages of drug development, the requirements of an endpoint, the special requirements of a surrogate endpoint, and the strengths and weaknesses of MUNE.

Stages of drug development

There are several stages of drug development, although the stages are not always discrete, and in certain situations, the stages may be shortened or collapsed. Initial development of a new agent traditionally begins with in-vitro studies and preclinical animal studies. Agents which appear promising in preclinical studies are administered to humans in phase 1 trials. These initial trials are primarily designed to coarsely assess the safety of the study agent and usually have very small sample size. Phase 1 clinical trials often also look for preliminary evidence of study drug activity. Phase 2 trials are designed to obtain initial evidence of efficacy while exploring dosing regimens, outcome measures, and target populations. Participation in phase 1 and phase 2 trials is often limited to a few, highly experienced research centers. These initial studies include intensive evaluation of subjects and have limited ability to detect less common adverse events. Agents that appear promising in phases 1 and 2 then enter phase 3 trials, which are often large, multi-center studies designed to provide definitive evidence of efficacy and safety.

Endpoint measures

Different endpoints are appropriate for different phases of drug development. Phase 1 and phase 2 trials may explore a variety of endpoints in order to guide the selection of endpoints for the future phase 3 trials. For phase 3 clinical trials, the primary

**Correspondence to*: Division of Clinical Trial Design and Analysis, Office of Therapeutics Research and Review, Center for Biologics Evaluation and Research, United States Food and Drug Administration, 1401 Rockville Pike, Room 230N, Rockville, MD 20852, USA. e-mail: bryanw@cber.fda.gov

doi: 10.1016/S1567-424X(03)00039-4

endpoint should generally be the single best clinically meaningful indicator of the treatment effect. A clinically meaningful efficacy endpoint is one that directly measures how a study subject feels, functions, or survives. Secondary endpoints should support the primary endpoint and are especially important when the primary endpoint is subjective. Demonstration of a positive effect on a single primary and multiple secondary endpoints may improve confidence in the reliability of evidence indicating benefit of the intervention. No single endpoint is ideal for all phases of all clinical trials in all motor neuron diseases.

A surrogate endpoint is a measurement or physical sign used as a substitute for a clinically meaningful endpoint. Changes induced by a therapy on a surrogate endpoint are expected to reflect or predict changes in a clinically meaningful endpoint (Temple, 1995). Although MUNE is not clinically meaningful, MUNE may have the potential to serve as a surrogate endpoint for survival or muscle strength, both traditional clinically meaningful endpoints in motor neuron studies.

Surrogate endpoints may offer many potential advantages over more traditional, clinically meaningful endpoints:

1) Responds to the intervention more rapidly than the true desired clinical outcome (e.g. survival in amyotrophic lateral sclerosis or late-onset spinal muscular atrophy, SMA). More rapid measurements may allow shorter duration trials to demonstrate a clinical effect.
2) More sensitive to effects of an intervention, thereby allowing a smaller sample size.
3) Less variability in measurement, thereby allowing a smaller sample size.
4) More objective than the true desired clinical outcome (e.g. fatigue as an endpoint in post-polio syndrome trials).
5) Easier to measure.
6) Less expensive to measure.

Therefore, surrogate endpoints have a theoretical potential to lead to clinical trials that are faster, smaller, easier, more objective, and less expensive. Surrogate endpoints have several potential roles in drug development:

1) Activity measure in phase 1 and phase 2 trials
   a) To determine dosing regimen for phase 3 trial.
   b) To select population for phase 3 trial.
   c) To estimate treatment effect in order to calculate sample size for phase 3 trial.
2) As secondary endpoint in phase 3 trial.
3) As primary endpoint in phase 3 trials to demonstrate efficacy in support of marketing approval if the surrogate has been validated to predict a clinically meaningful outcome.
4) As a primary endpoint in phase 3 trials under the special circumstances of accelerated approval (Accelerated Approval of New Drugs, 2001). The Food and Drug Administration's Accelerated Approval regulations permit market approval based on demonstration of an effect on a surrogate endpoint. The surrogate endpoint must be reasonably likely to predict clinical benefit, and the study results must support a determination that the study agent provides meaningful therapeutic benefit over existing treatments. Market approval of a new agent under the Accelerated Approval program requires the sponsor to study the drug further to verify and describe the drug's true clinical benefit. If these subsequent studies fail to demonstrate a true clinical benefit, marketing approval may be withdrawn.

The ideal surrogate endpoint is measured easily and reliably, responds quickly to the intervention, and is sensitive to small effects of the intervention on the true clinical endpoint. However, enthusiasm for these potential advantages must be countered by recognition of the potential hazards of the use of surrogate endpoints to assess efficacy in phase 3 studies:

1) To support accelerated approval, the surrogate must be *reasonably likely* to predict the presence or absence of a clinical benefit. This usually requires knowledge of the surrogate's role in the disease, and of the mechanism of the drug's effect on the surrogate.

2) A surrogate deemed reasonably likely to predict benefit may turn out not to predict benefit.
3) Even if a surrogate predicts benefit, it is very difficult to estimate the extent of benefit on a clinically meaningful endpoint based on an effect on a surrogate. Benefits on a surrogate are difficult to weigh against clinically meaningful toxicity in a risk/benefit analysis.
4) Poor reliability, especially if the methodology is not well-defined.
5) Low feasibility if:
   a) Not acceptable to patients.
   b) Require expensive equipment and highly-trained staff.
6) May facilitate clinical trials with small sample sizes sufficient to demonstrate efficacy but not sufficient to demonstrate safety or address other important issues (e.g. differential efficacy in subgroups).
7) Trial conclusions may not be generally acceptable to physicians and/or patients.

Most importantly, the ideal surrogate accurately predicts the effect of the intervention on the true clinical endpoint. Some surrogates are accepted as validated, such as change in blood pressure as a surrogate for morbidity and mortality in studies of hypertension. Unfortunately, no surrogate has ever met the standard of being fully predictive of the true clinical endpoint.

Surrogate endpoints have been shown to not correlate with the endpoint of clinical interest in previous clinical trials (Fleming and DeMets, 1996). Tumor response did not correlate well with survival in clinical trials of leucovorin for colorectal cancer. Suppression of premature ventricular contractions did not accurately predict the effect on mortality in clinical trials of encainide and flecainide in patients with asymptomatic or minimally symptomatic ventricular arrhythmia (Echt et al., 1991). A surrogate can fail in a variety of ways:

1) The surrogate may be independent of the true clinical endpoint. For example, a measure of cognitive dysfunction might not be a good surrogate for survival in ALS clinical trials. Although cognitive dysfunction may occur in ALS, there is little evidence of a predictable relationship between the severity of cognitive dysfunction and survival.
2) The surrogate endpoint may only partially predict the true clinical endpoint. For example, upper and/or lower motor neuron loss can cause motor dysfunction in ALS patients. Therefore, MUNE, which measures only lower motor neuron loss, may only partially predict severity of motor dysfunction in ALS. Patients with severe spasticity may lose the ability to walk without a corresponding change in MUNE.
3) The intervention being studied affects the surrogate endpoint but not the true clinical endpoint. For example, natural history studies have established a correlation between arm strength and survival. On this basis, arm strength has been used as a surrogate for survival in ALS trials. However, an intervention such as exercise training of the upper extremities might improve arm strength without improving survival.
4) The intervention being studied could affect the true clinical endpoint through a mechanism not reflected by the surrogate endpoint. For example, ventilatory support improves survival in ALS patients. However, this improvement in survival is unlikely to be due to any effect of ventilation on the disease process. Surrogate markers for disease progression, such as MUNE and limb strength, would be unlikely to detect the survival benefit provided by ventilatory support.
5) The intervention being studied has separate and independent effects on the surrogate endpoint and the true clinical endpoint. For example, creatine may have direct effects on both muscles and on motor neurons. A surrogate marker for motor dysfunction, such as MUNE, might detect the effect of creatine on motor neurons but miss the effect on muscle. This problem would be most confounding in a clinical trial of an intervention with a positive effect on either the surrogate or the true clinical endpoint and no effect (or a negative effect) on the other.
6) The intervention being studied may have dual effects, and even opposite effects, on the true clinical endpoint – one mediated through the surrogate and the other not. For example, a drug could improve motor neuron survival but also

cause pulmonary fibrosis. Survival surrogates, such as MUNE or limb strength, might detect the "beneficial effect" on motor neurons but not detect the toxicity to the lungs. The drug might cause an overall decrease in survival, while the surrogate would measure only a beneficial effect.

MUNE as an endpoint measure

Is MUNE a viable endpoint for clinical trials in motor neuron disorders? A definition of viable is that an endpoint must be both valid and feasible. A valid endpoint is reliable and clinically meaningful. The process of validation includes determination of reliability (both intra- and inter-rater), comparison of the endpoint with available standard measures or endpoints, and obtaining experience with the endpoint in clinical trials.

For a surrogate endpoint, the process of validation is even more rigorous, requiring not only the steps outlined above for any endpoint, but also the establishment of the relationship between the surrogate and a "gold standard" true clinical endpoint. As noted in the above examples of why surrogates sometimes fail, the value of a surrogate is critically dependent on the inter-relationships of the disease process, the intervention, the surrogate, and the true clinical endpoint. These relationships should be understood, as much as possible, prior to initiating a trial with a surrogate as a primary or secondary endpoint.

How can neuromuscular specialists evaluate the viability of MUNE as a clinical trial endpoint? First, the validity and feasibility of MUNE must be explored. The validity of an endpoint depends on the disease and intervention being studied, as noted in the examples above. The feasibility of an endpoint depends on many factors, including the stage of drug development and the role of the endpoint in the clinical trial. Therefore, the appropriateness of MUNE as an endpoint depends on the specific clinical trial. The validity and feasibility of MUNE are likely different in trials of SMA and post-polio syndrome, which have primarily lower motor neuron dysfunction, than in trials of ALS, where subjects have varying proportions of upper and lower motor neuron dysfunction. MUNE may be useful in phase 1 and phase 2 trials, as a relatively objective and sensitive measure of the activity of an intervention. However, limited patient tolerance and the requirement for special expertise may limit the feasibility of MUNE to serve as a surrogate in phase 3 trials. Unless validity is well established, MUNE may not be acceptable to the community of physicians and patients as a primary endpoint for a phase 3 trial. Also, as noted in the examples provided above, the validity of a surrogate such as MUNE depends on the intervention being studied.

Summary

MUNE appears to have the most immediate potential as an endpoint in exploratory phase 1 and phase 2 clinical trials. In these trials, multiple endpoints are useful to look for activity of the intervention. In this role, MUNE offers the advantages of being relatively objective and of suggesting an effect on the pathophysiology of motor neuron disorders. For pivotal phase 3 trials, MUNE presently has no role as a primary endpoint due to its lack of established clinical meaning or ability to predict a clinical outcome. However, MUNE may be useful as a relatively objective secondary endpoint that supports a primary endpoint by suggesting an effect on the presumed pathophysiology. Research to establish the validity and feasibility of the use of MUNE as a surrogate for clinically meaningful endpoints, such as survival and muscle strength, may facilitate the development of new treatments for motor neuron disorders.

Acknowledgements

I appreciate the assistance of Mary Foulkes, Ph. D., Jay P. Siegel, M.D., Marc K. Walton, M.D., Ph.D., and Karen D. Weiss, M.D., in the preparation of this manuscript.

References

Accelerated Approval of New Drugs for Serious or Life-Threatening Illnesses. *United States Code of Federal Regulations.* 21 CFR 314 (Subpart H). April 1, 2001.

Echt, D.S. and Liebson, P.R., Mitchell, L.B. et al. Mortality and morbidity in patients receiving encainide, flecainide, or placebo: the Cardiac Arrhythmia Suppression Trial. *N. Engl. J. Med.*, 1991, 324: 781–788.

Fleming, T.R. and DeMets, D.L. Surrogate end points in clinical trials: are we being misled? *Ann. Intern. Med.*, 1996, 125: 605–613.

Spilker, B. *Guide to Clinical Trials.* Lippincott Williams & Wilkins, Philadelphia, 1991.

Temple, R.J. A regulatory authority's opinion about surrogate endpoints. "*Clinical Measurement in Drug Evaluation*" (W. S. Nimmo and G.T. Tucker, Eds.), John Wiley & Sons.

Temple, R. Current definitions of phases of investigation and the role of the FDA in the conduct of clinical trials. *Am. Heart J.*, 1995, 139: S133–S135.

Yusuf, S. Challenges in the conduct and interpretation of Phase II (pilot) randomized trials. *Am. Heart J.*, 2000, 139: S136–S142.

Discussion after Section XI

Jack Petajan, Salt Lake City, Utah

The previous talk emphasizes the consequences of standardization. Once you standardize a technique, there can be consequences that other techniques will not be accepted and will not be considered valid. The consequences of standardization may have a dampening effect on research and utilizing other MUNE techniques.

Mark Bromberg, Salt Lake City, Utah

Your comments are good, but my use of the term standardization refers to the availability of software for MUNE. Currently, there are limitations on the availability of proprietary and investigator-based MUNE software. Using standardized formats could allow sharing of software.

Jack Petajan, Salt Lake City, Utah

How do you bill for MUNE studies?

Mark Bromberg, Salt Lake City, Utah

Personally, I bill an MUNE study as a motor nerve CPT code, and I justify the MUNE study in the report.

Jasper Daube, Rochester, Minnesota

I would like to support Mark's suggestion, and I think of standardization the same way. Without standardization we lack the ability to use the spectrum of available techniques. Nicolet Biomedical engineers have put in a lot of time and effort on the statistical platform, and if there was a way that other manufacturers could incorporate the statistical program in their machines, that would be of value to anyone who wanted to make comparisons between techniques. Similarly, if Nicolet Biomedical could incorporate programs like the multiple point or the incremental techniques, that would be an advantage to all of us.

Daniel Stashuk, Waterloo, Ontario

I think the development of open software might have advantages to industry as well. Once software as has been developed in Windows, it could be put on their machines for use by electromyographers.

Sanjeev Nandedkar, Hawthorne, New York

I think what Jasper said is very important. We should be able to perform different tasks on our EMG machines. I have looked at this issue in a different way. I conducted a survey of all the EMG manufactures at the American Academy of Neurology meeting by asking them specific questions about their machines, not necessarily targeted to MUNE specifically. For example, can you do triggered averaging in two channels, or can you record 100 F-waves, or can you get 200 responses? I was delighted to find that if you dig into your EMG machine a little bit, you can perform literally every technique except the automated decomposition technique or the index technique that I recently developed. Most machines will allow you to do spike triggered averaging technique. Most machines will allow you to do multiple point stimulation. And if you dig into your software, most of the machines will allow you to do the statistical method also. The only difference is that it is not automated. So if you are willing to sit down with your instrument manufacturers, tell them what you need to do, most likely they will show you a way to get your result. You may need an extra calculator and things will not happen automatically. I would say every machine, regardless of which brand you have, will allow you to do two or three different methods. Just be patient with it and ask your manufacturer.

I have several comments related to developing software. Although developing software, even a simple formula, appears straight forward, there is a lot of work to incorporate it into the EMG machine. For example, you need to create a display window to show the values and buttons to make entries. In short, you will need to have a programmer and somebody to test the software. If you make one change in a Windows environment, you take one step forward and three steps backwards with the bugs that you create. And that is the reason it takes so long. From my personal viewpoint, I will give you the signals in an ASCII format; hire a graduate student and they will do the job.

Jaap Kap, Nicolet Biomedical, Madison, Wisconsin

I think we have heard a good overview of what industry does. I think what we should do is recognize the existence of the partnership between researchers or methods developers and practitioners. This is the first MUNE meeting and I get the impression that this is somewhat of a special interest group. I think good points were made about the status and the task of industry. I would like to say from the point of industry, that we need three things in order to participate appropriately. One is a consensus. I think we are going along that path right now, but I think you have to realize that it is a requirement for industry to really get involved in an honest way. The second is that we need clinical validation. As soon as we put the method on a system, we bear a responsibility with regard to the customers who are going to use it. We have to be able to support it. The third is to standardize the methods. I do not mean standardization in the sense of determining exactly how it is going to be, but a transfer into a very usable clinical method that can stand by itself. I think recognizing that there is a circle with researches, industry and feedback from practitioners will improve our working together.

Alan McComas, Hamilton, Ontario

Perhaps I could go back and support what Jack Petajan said. We can likely agree on the principles of electrode placement, the size of signal that is acceptable and so forth, and that there are half a dozen techniques that will give reliable results. However, I would hate to feel that if someone did something beyond that, tinkered with the system, came up with a new idea, that that work would not be accepted in a journal because of the rigidity of a reviewer. The field will move on because we currently have techniques which can be applied to ALS and other denervating disorders for diagnosis, management, therapeutic trials, and so on. But we do no more than that, then there is going to be a terrible sterility in the field. That is why there must always be room for accepting ideas that go beyond what we now accept.

Daniel Stashuk, Waterloo, Ontario

I do not think that just because you have standards in place, that they preclude new ideas coming forth if the new ideas are valid and are based on solid assumptions, and so forth. New ideas in time may become the standard. It would be a poor journal reviewer that would reject a valid study just because it was not a standard study. So I think it is unfair to say that because you have got a standard in place, you are going to curtail original thought. Having standards may put a stronger test on nonstandard measures.

John alluded to the possibility that if there are standards that companies would have difficulties differentiating their machine from their competitors. I do not think this is necessarily true. There are human factors, human–computer interaction designs that can separate one machine from another.

As Sanjeev suggested, if there standards for transferring data between manufacturer's equipment, similar to the drivers that Windows software uses to communicate with a printer, then third-party software developers could be hired by a research group. This group effort could combine research funds and could sponsor software that would allow the statistical and multiple point stimulation techniques to run on different machines.

Sanjeev Nandedkar, Hawthorne, New York

I have a comment regarding the development of "drivers" and such. From my personal experience, I would strongly keep away from them because writing drivers can be very expensive, you need to pay $70 to $80 an hour. My suggestion is to look at the files that have been generated on a system, and they can be deciphered very easily. Let me give you as example. An investigator was working with one of the files on our EMG machine, and he had absolutely no idea what to do, so he just plotted the entire file as a graph. Right in the middle, he saw the EMG signal and said I need to throw away the first 200 bites, take the next 1000, and he had the waveform. He was up and running in less than half a day. My recommendation is read the files rather than the driver.

The second point is that once you start writing your own software, I have absolutely no idea whose responsibility it is in terms of the safety of the instrument if your driver fails and if it gives a repetitive stimulus at 100 mA and the patient gets a burn. I cannot be held responsible, and that is why I have strong objection to anyone using my software and hardware to do something on their own.

Jasper Daube, Rochester, Minnesota

I would like to ask ourselves, as the folks who want to form a partnership with industry, to think about what we do in forming that partnership. Many of us have formed a partnership with industry that is beneficial to us. The statistical program was developed originally on a separate computer that looked nothing like what it looks like on a Nicolet EMG machine now. Ten years ago they had the foresight to say maybe this is worth putting on their machine. They came to me to find out what I was doing and how I was doing it. They then built what you see. I suggested the 30 steps and the other features, but they built the program. At that time, as a salaried member of the Mayo Clinic staff, our rules stated that since I did this on clinic time, the EMG laboratory got two free EMG machines, and that was the end of the relationship. There is no longer any royalty. So, that has been my relationship with Nicolet Biomedical regarding the statistical MUNE program. I think we should be willing to talk about what are we getting out of our partnership. When you sign a contract you are signing something that specifies what you get, what your lab gets, what your institution gets, in return for the work that you have done. If we sign a contract that limits what the manufacturer can do, that is counterproductive to what we are trying to do.

Mark Bromberg, Salt Lake City, Utah

Developing software in Windows format is important for research. Getting an EMG machine just because it has a specific software program is expensive. I am proposing that we simplify the package. PC computers are readily available. There are lab-computer interfaces that cost approximately a thousand dollars. There are amplifiers and stimulators that also cost several thousand dollars. With a relatively modest expense, a laboratory could have access to a variety of programs.

Jeremy Shefner, Syracuse, New York

I wonder if you could comment a little bit more, Wilson, on what it would take to show the validity of MUNE. I think statistical MUNE has been used in three multicenter trials, so I think to some extent the feasibility is partially answered.

Wilson Bryan, Rockville, Maryland

In that sense, the feasibility is being explored, but in some trials it was used at one or two centers in a small subset of the population. It you really want this to be an endpoint for a clinical trial, you have to be able to apply it to every patient who enters the study. If you have 100 patients entering the study and only 50 are willing to accept MUNE once a month, then that is a problem with feasibility. MUNE is now a secondary endpoint in trials, so you are in the process of exploring its use.

Richard Olney, San Francisco, California

How about validity? How much more needs to be done? I think there might be data that are available that can answer many of these questions once they get published and cross-correlated with other clinical measures. I think reproducibility has been shown to be good.

Wilson Bryan, Rockville, Maryland

That data may be available. Our policy at the FDA is that if you have a clinical trial and you want to use MUNE as an endpoint, you show us the data on reliability and the relationship of the surrogate endpoint to a clinically meaningful endpoint. If the data is convincing, then we will accept the surrogate. I will not pretend to know that data as well as this audience does, but we will want to see the reliability of that endpoint measure through the full range of the disease. That is, is MUNE reliable early in ALS, late in ALS, early in SMA, late in SMA, etc?

Kathryn Swoboda, Salt Lake City, Utah

What if you are talking about a population where the true endpoint is not feasible to measure? For instance, functional testing cannot be performed in SMA infants and young kids. You can look at time to death, but many of these patients are put on C-PAP and Bi-PAP and ventilated, so time of death is difficult to determine.

Wilson Bryan, Rockville, Maryland

This is one reason that we have had to use surrogate endpoints in some situations. If you are talking about a life-threatening disease where you cannot measure the true endpoint, it is possible to get accelerated approval of a drug based on a surrogate endpoint with the understanding that in the long term, you will try to look at the true clinical outcome. These diseases present particular challenges, and the FDA is open to discussing innovative ways to design trials. But you have to do what you can to learn about the endpoint measure in relationship to the disease process.

Clifton Gooch, New York, New York

Would you call strength a clinically relevant endpoint?

Wilson Bryan, Rockville, Maryland

Strength is clinically relevent. However, changes in strength may be too small to be clinically meaningful. For example, the clinical meaning of improving a manual muscle testing score from an average of 3.5 to an average of 4 is unclear. Function, such as ambulation, which is dependent on strength, is often more clearly clinically meaningful than a measure of strength. So I think that strength measurements often lack clinical meaning until you translate the strength measurements into patient function.

Clifton Gooch, New York, New York

You talk about MUNE not being a clinically relevant endpoint, but yet in some cases MUNE is actually a more accurate measure of what is happening at the actual disease level. MUNE tracks the disease process more closely than clinical endpoints; strength is being maintained yet the disease process is still ravaging on. MUNE sees the change yet the person can still walk. So if you relied on a clinical function test, you would be missing information that MUNE could provide you.

Wilson Bryan, Washington, DC

I agree. That is one reason that a trial needs more than one endpoint. A potential advantage of MUNE is that it may help you look at the pathophysiology of the disease. For instance, a hypothetical ALS clinical trial could produce strength measurement data suggesting that strength is maintained and MUNE data suggesting that motor neurons are steadily lost. One possible interpretation of such a trial would be that the intervention is acting to preserve strength through a mechanism (e.g., improved muscle contractility or more efficient reinnervation) other than preservation of motor neurons. I think there is a real value in looking at multiple endpoints to try to sort out what is happening in a clinical trial.

Jeremy Shefner, Syracuse, New York

I just wanted to point out that the distinction between a clinically relevant endpoint and an effective surrogate may not be as clear as you suggest. In terms of the distinction between strength and walking, you said that maybe an increase in strength from 3.5 to 4 may not translate into a direct clinical benefit. On the other hand, an increase in the ability to walk from three miles an hour to four miles an hour may also not translate to a direct clinical benefit even though that may be considered a relevant measure.

Wilson Bryan, Rockville, Maryland

There is some blurring in what is meaningful. What is meaningful to a patient is always going to be subjective. What is meaningful to one patient may not be meaningful to the next patient. When investigators submit a clinical trial to the FDA for review, we discuss the endpoint with the investigators, and we ask "Does this endpoint have clinical meaning?" We like to think we are reasonable and that we can work together with investigators to target an endpoint and design the trial to see an effect on an endpoint that most people would agree is clinically meaningful.

Mark Bromberg, Salt Lake City, Utah

Could you comment on what you think the FDA currently considers as the most clinically relevant endpoints for ALS; survival, FVC, ALSFRS?

Wilson Bryan, Rockville, Maryland

We want you to know that we are open to discussion of all endpoints. I think it is difficult to argue against survival as clinically meaningful. But there are problems with survival as an endpoint. So there is no endpoint that is right for every trial and every intervention.

Richard Olney, San Francisco, California

Survival has been repeatedly used as a primary endpoint in ALS trials. It would seem to me that if we can demonstrated in a multicenter setting that MUNE is predictive of survival in ALS patients, that would probably go a long way to fulfilling the criteria for making it linked to a valid clinical endpoint.

Wilson Bryan, Rockville, Maryland

Right, but I do not want you to overlook the fact that it may be just as easy to use survival as it is to use MUNE as an endpoint, and then the value of MUNE is as a supportive endpoint. MUNE is useful in phase 1 and phase 2 trials to look for an effect of the drug on the pathophysiology of the disease.

Richard Olney, San Francisco, California

Yes, but if we can demonstrated that it is highly predictive of survival, as several studies have already suggested, then as you said earlier in your talk, that would enable the design of a trial much shorter in duration that yields a more rapid answer.

Wilson Bryan, Rockville, Maryland

Potentially so. Again, that would depend on being able to show an effect of the intervention on MUNE prior to seeing the effect on survival. MUNE has potential as a surrogate marker in motor neuron diseases. Investigators must collect the data that demonstrates the value of MUNE as a surrogate for strength, survival, or some other clinically meaningful endpoint.

Kathryn Swoboda, Salt Lake City, Utah

I want to take the opportunity to ask one more pediatric question. Someone else from the FDA was at an SMA meeting told me that you are now requiring quality of life information for all FDA-approved trials?

Wilson Bryan, Washington, DC

At this time, the FDA does not require quality of life information for most trials.

Section XII

Consensus

Motor Unit Number Estimation (Supplements to Clinical Neurophysiology Vol. 55)
Editor: M.B. Bromberg

Chapter 40

Consensus

Mark B. Bromberg*

Department of Neurology, University of Utah, Salt Lake City, UT 84132, USA

Introduction

One of the goals of this symposium was to discuss issues related to standardizing the operational aspects of MUNE and to reach consensus on these issues. A number of issues were vigorously debated during the discussion sessions. Consensus was reached for some issues, but with others, consensus was tentative. What follows represents a review of the issues for which there was general agreement.

General MUNE methodology

There was consensus that investigators should be free to fully explore the field of MUNE, with no limitations on questions studied, methods used, and modes of data analysis. However, it was agreed that the methods sections of resultant publications should be detailed to provide readers with sufficient information for critical evaluation and reproduction of their work by others.

Nomenclature

A suggestion was made to simplify some of the nomenclature of the various recorded potentials (see table).

Recording electrodes

There was consensus that the stigmatic or active recording electrode should be placed over the motor point. Techniques to ensure this include the absence of an initial positive deflection in the CMAP, using a stimulating electrode to find the motor point, and moving the recording electrode to record the CMAP waveform with the highest amplitude and steepest rise time. Optimizing the placement of the recording electrode will minimize the effects of temporal dispersion on reconstructing CMAP caused by different latencies of SMUPs or macro potentials on.

Positive waveforms

It is recognized that while the maximal CMAP should have an initial negative deflection, some SMUPs or macro potentials may have an initial positive deflection. This is likely due to the fact that the recording electrode may be over the motor point for most of the motor units, but motor points for individual motor units are diffusely distributed over an area larger than covered by the recording electrode. Accordingly, SMUPs or macro waveforms that have an initial positive deflection followed by a major negative waveform should be acceptable.

The question of waveforms that are wholly or nearly wholly positive was debated. One stance was that these waveforms represented volume conduction of motor units from neighboring

**Correspondence to*: Department of Neurology, University of Utah, Salt Lake City, UT 84132, USA, e-mail: Mark.Bromberg@hsc.utah.edu

doi: 10.1016/S1567-424X(03)00041-2

SUGGESTED NOMENCLATURE

Recorded potential	Preferred term
Compound muscle action potential	CMAP
Single surface-recorded motor unit potential	SMUP or macro potential
Intramuscular potentials single motor unit potential	Micro potential

muscles, and therefore should not be considered part of the muscle or group of muscles under study. Another stance was that some volume conduction from neighboring muscles contributes to the CMAP, and therefore these SMUPs should be considered. Examples were given of positive single SMUP or macro waveforms that were associated with visible twitches in the primary muscle. Overall, the feeling was that waveforms that are wholly or primarily positive should be excluded, but if included they should be considered with caution and mentioned in the methods section.

Smallest single macro waveform

There were debates on whether very small SMUP or macro waveforms should be counted. A portion of the discussion was based on which MUNE technique was being used. With the statistical technique in particular, there was concern whether these small waveforms represented noise or true motor unit potentials. With other MUNE techniques, this question may be less problematic. A general consensus was reached that SMUP or macro waveforms whose negative peak amplitude was less than 10 μV or negative peak area was less than 25 μV ms should not be included. If very small macro waveforms are included, some measure of the magnitude and impact of their inclusion should be provided.

Number of single motor units sampled

An important variable in calculating MUNE values is the number of SMUPs collected and used to determine the average SMUP value. Several MUNE studies indicate that the variability of the MUNE calculation is reduced when 10–15 SMUPs are averaged. There was consensus that at least 10 units should be collected, although it was recognized that some subjects with severe degrees of denervation may not have 10 remaining motor units. Ideally, each MUNE project should include a determination of the effect on the number of SMUPs used for the average in the subject population and MUNE technique under study.

Primary metric for MUNE calculations

There were long discussions concerning which CMAP and SMUP metrics should be used in calculating the MUNE ratio. The major concern was the effects of phase cancellation as it relates to metrics that include biphasic components, such as peak-to-peak amplitude. The maximal CMAP includes phase cancellation between the different arrival times of the SMUPs that contribute to the waveform (temporal dispersion). In the incremental stimulation and statistical MUNE techniques both the CMAP and the SMUPs are evoked from the same stimulation site, and the effects of phase cancellation will be similar. There are concerns with the spike triggered averaging and multiple point stimulation MUNE techniques because the CMAP will be evoked at one site along the nerve while the SMUPs will be evoked at different sites. This will lead to different degrees of phase cancellation when calculating the average SMUP compared to the CMAP. Use of negative peak area or negative peak amplitude metrics will reduce the effects of phase cancellation. Ideally, for these later methods, individual SMUPs should be aligned based on their onsets, and an the average SMUP determined by a computer algorithm that calculates a negative peak average on a data point by data point bases. This process will best approximate the way the original CMAP was generated. It was recognized that these computer algorithms are not readily available, and there was consensus for using negative peak area or negative peak amplitude for the CMAP and SMUP or macro waveforms.

Choice of MUNE techniques

A large number of MUNE techniques and variations are described. Some may have methodologic and operational advantages. While there was no consensus to eliminate a MUNE technique, there was a general feeling that some techniques were more viable than others.

Favored MUNE techniques

- Incremental stimulation technique:
  Alternation a major problem.
  Can be used with any EMG machine.
  Temporal dispersion not a problem.
- Multiple point stimulation technique:
  Alternation not a problem.
  Temporal dispersion a problem.
- Adapted multiple point stimulation technique:
  Less influenced by alternation.
  More efficient compared to multiple point stimulation technique.
  Temporal dispersion a problem.
- Spike triggered averaging technique:
  Alternation not a problem.
  Includes intramuscular (micro) motor unit data.
  Can be used on proximal muscles.
  Temporal dispersion a problem.
- Decomposition enhanced spike triggered averaging technique:
  Similar to spike triggered averaging technique.
  Rapid data acquisition.
  Includes additional quantitative intramuscular (micro) motor unit.
- Statistical technique:
  Includes greater spectrum of motor units.
  Temporal dispersion not a problem.
  Calculation algorithms under continued development.

Less favored MUNE techniques

- Automated incremental stimulation technique:
  Dependent upon special software that is no longer available.
- F-wave technique:
  Challenging to identify single F-wave potentials.
  Facilitated by special software that is no longer available.
- Intraneural microelectrode stimulation technique:
  Time consuming; invasive.
  Alternation not a problem.
  Temporal dispersion not a problem.
- Integrated root mean square technique:
  Not fully developed.
- Motor unit index:
  Not fully developed.

Statistical expression of test–retest reliability

It was recognized that there are a variety of questions to answer with regards to MUNE reliability, and that no single statistical method for evaluating reliability will suffice. For example, trial-to-trial reproducibility of a MUNE technique may be assessed without removing and reapplying the electrodes, or reproducibility of MUNE in the same muscle may be assessed after removing and reapplying the electrodes. Reproducibility of the techniques with different operators and reproducibility over time can also be assessed. It was emphasized that the goals of the test and the methods of testing should be described in full in the methods sections.

For simple test–retest reproducibility, there was support for expressing the results as the absolute value of the difference between the first and second test value divided by the average of the two test values. However, this would lead to a standard deviation based on only two data points, which is appropriate for a within-subject standard deviation. Another way to present the data is the repeatability, which is 2.7 times the within-subject standard deviation ($2.77 = \text{square root of } 2 \times 1.96$ for 95% certainty). Accuracy can be improved by obtaining three or more observations.

Alternatively, reliability testing for a technique can be performed by the interclass correlation coefficient test. This results in a unitless R value. This statistic takes into account both within subject and between subject variability.

Ideally, the reproducibility of different MUNE techniques should not be directly compared by correlation coefficients. When available, the actual data sets produced by the different techniques should be analyzed using *t*-tests, comparing one set of coefficients of variation with another. If multiple tests are compared simultaneously, an ANOVA would be appropriate. This approach may not be practical for meta analysis of existing studies done by different investigators, but should be used when possible. If cross-study comparisons of reproducibility must be made using correlation coefficients, the limitations of this approach should be appreciated. Other measures of reproducibility may also be suitable, depending upon study design, but widely variant methods of analysis should be discouraged, to facilitate study-to-study comparisons.

Comparisons between MUNE techniques should include performance across a spectrum of large and small values and in healthy and subjects with disease, and sensitivity to change with change in disease. Other factors, such as the learning curve of the operator, ease of use, and the time necessary for testing should also be included.

Consensus on technical issues for statistical MUNE

The statistical MUNE technique is undergoing continued development. The technical issues presented below represent suggestions for the currently available software.

1. Record scan curve:
   a. Carefully set threshold and just maximal currents.
   b. Ensure that there are only a few responses at 0 and 100% CMAP amplitudes.
2. Determine if there are any true gaps $>10\%$ of total range (maximal CMAP amplitude $=100\%$):
   – if yes, each gap counts as 1 SMUP and% of gap is subtracted from 100% for number-weighted calculation (see 6).
3. Record SMUPs from four standard windows (except with gaps as described under 5c):
   a. If maximal CMAP >2.5 mV, set windows at 10–20%, 25–35%, 40–50%, 55–65%.
   b. If maximal CMAP <2.5 mV but >1.0 mV, use up to four windows of 250 μV each that are non-overlapping and as evenly spaced as possible to avoid gaps documented under 2 above.
   c. If maximal CMAP is <1.0 mV and more than one SMUP exists within any 250 μV range, record mean SMUP within this (these) window(s).
4. Within each recording window, vary stimulus intensity to verify that submaximal CMAPs are present in $>7\%$ of 10% range or in more than 175 μV of 250 μV range (that is, submaximal CMAPs fill more than two-thirds of the window):
   a. If yes, record 4–10 runs of 30; current set at one-quarter from bottom of window.
   b. If no, enlarge window to capture first SMUP beyond gap.
5. If true gaps found under 2:
   a. If one true gap was found (that is, a single SMUP had amplitude more than 10% [or more than 250 μV if maximal CMAP amplitude <2.5 mV], as described under 2 above), subtract this percentage of range from 100% for MUNE calculation and add 1 to MUNE.
   b. If 2 or more gaps, repeat this process as many times as large gaps found.
   c. In studies with one or more gaps, if any gaps occur within 5% of the recommended stimulus intensities (3 above), fewer than 4 mean SMUPs need be recorded:
      – If the first 1–3 recording encompass more than 40% of the CMAP range (or more than 1 mV of the CMAP range when CMAP <2.5 mV), or
      – If less than 40% of the CMAP range (or more than 1 mV of the CMAP range when CMAP <2.5 mV) is not interrupted by a $>10\%$ gap.
6. Calculate modified, number-weighted mean SMUP.

Conclusion

This consensus summary represents a work in progress. It is hoped that these issues will be discussed further, and reviewed at a future MUNE symposium.

Motor Unit Number Estimation (Supplements to Clinical Neurophysiology Vol. 55)
Editor: M.B. Bromberg

Chapter 41

Issues for the future

Mark B. Bromberg*

Department of Neurology, University of Utah, Salt Lake City, UT 84132, USA

Introduction

Motor unit number estimation (MUNE) has evolved over the 30 years from the description of the first technique in 1971 to include a dozen techniques and modifications. This symposium represents the first meeting devoted to MUNE. Many issues were discussed, and some consensus was reached. However, it is appropriate to look to the future and review issues that should be addressed before the next MUNE symposium.

MUNE reproducibility

Reproducibility remains a major concern to outside reviewers of the field. We have some consensus on the expression of trial-to-trial variability, and reliability values have improved to 10–15%. This is approaching the variability of the compound muscle action potential (CMAP) and quantitative muscle strength testing. Further efforts should be made to reduce variability and document variability in normal subjects and those with denervating illnesses.

MUNE in different diseases and disease states

MUNE is well suited to studying amyotrophic lateral sclerosis. Other suitable diseases include spinal muscular atrophy, old poliomyelitis, and Charcot Marie Tooth neuropathies, and MUNE is beginning to be used to study these disorders. MUNE may also provide information on the degree of motor involvement in polyneuropathies, such as diabetic neuropathies.

In addition to estimating the number of remaining motor units innervating a muscle, several MUNE techniques can provide additional insights into pathophysiologic changes associated with denervation and reinnervation. The spike triggered averaging technique in particular, with the decomposition algorithm, can provide information on the degree of collateral reinnervation, firing rates of the remaining motor units, and levels of motor activation.

Use as endpoint measure

The use of MUNE as an endpoint measure remains problematic from two points. The FDA requires that an endpoint measure be meaningful, and this has to be demonstrated in clinical trials. MUNE research is somewhat hampered in this

**Correspondence to*: Department of Neurology, University of Utah, Salt Lake City, UT 84132, USA. E-mail: Mark.Bromberg@hsc.utah.edu

doi: 10.1016/S1567-424X(03)00041-2

regard because there have been no successful clinical trial with which to compare MUNE to other endpoint measures. Reproducibility is a factor in multicenter trials, and several trials are using MUNE as a secondary endpoint measure and will generate MUNE data in this setting.

Availability of MUNE

There are a number of MUNE techniques and modifications described, but most have limited accessibility to the investigators. As different techniques are selected for their reproducibility and data yield, it will be important to make them readily available. There is a project underway to use Microsoft Windows® as a software base that would allow any MUNE program to run on a PC machine with the addition of an A/D interface and commercial amplifiers and stimulators.

Conclusions

MUNE has grown over the past 30 years in many directions. The goal of this symposium was to bring together clinical researchers, biomedical engineers and industry to discuss ideas and issues. It is hoped that various efforts can be focused to resolve issues and advance the field of MUNE.

Subject index